BETA-LACTAM ANTIBIOTICS

Edited by
SUSUMU MITSUHASHI

JAPAN SCIENTIFIC SOCIETIES PRESS, Tokyo
SPRINGER-VERLAG, Berlin Heidelberg New York

1981

ISBN 4-7622-0266-5

ISBN 3-540-10921-8 SPRINGER-VERLAG Berlin Heidelberg New York
ISBN 0-387-10921-8 SPRINGER-VERLAG New York Heidelberg Berlin

Sole distribution rights outside Japan granted to SPRINGER-VERLAG Berlin Heidelberg New York

Published jointly by
JAPAN SCIENTIFIC SOCIETIES PRESS Tokyo
                    and
SPRINGER-VERLAG Berlin Heidelberg New York

Printed in Japan

BETA-LACTAM
ANTIBIOTICS

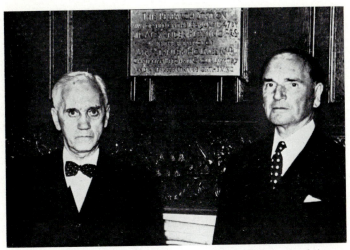

Sirs Alexander Fleming (left) and Stanley Holmes (right).

fish-breeding industries. The discovery of drug-resistance plasmids in Japan has clarified the reason for the rapid spread of multiply-resistant organisms all over the world, and in addition studies of drug-resistance plasmids have told us that wide gene exchanges occur among microorganisms through plasmids and among replicons through transposons.

Soon after returning from the Second World War, I was asked by Prof. S. Hosoya to begin studies on penicillium culture and penicillin purification during the period of Allied Occupation. We noticed that penicillin's activity was suddenly lost in some cases when culture filtrates of different bottles were combined together. I noticed accidentally that the destruction of penicillin was due to contamination of gram-negative bacteria from potatos used for the preculture of

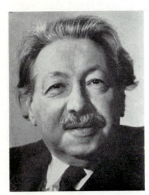

Professor Ernst B. Chain

penicillium. Owing to the advice of Prof. F. Egami, I purified the enzyme, penicillinase, without knowing of the published report on penicillinase by E.P. Abraham and E. Chain, because all literatures from foreign countries were only available in the U.S. Army Library in Japan. This was my first finding during the 35-year history of my life in research. Therefore, I have accepted with pleasure the task of editing this monograph on "Beta-Lactam Antibiotics" at the half century mark after the discovery of penicillin. The editor appreciates very much the support of all contributors, who are among the most eminent scholars in the world.

PREFACE

Paul Ehrlich opened the way for the study of experimental chemotherapy and introduced trypanred and salvarsan. His term "Chemotherapy" denotes the treatment of parasitic disease by direct chemical attack upon the invading organisms and the discovery of appropriate chemotherapeutic agents came about through human ingenuity. Therefore, advances in the field of chemotherapy were rather slow. Ehrlich's discoveries were followed by the advent of prontosil (G. Domagk, 1935) and of sulfonamide (G. Tréfouël, 1935), furazolidon (M. Dodd, 1947), p-aminobenzoic acid derivatives (PAS, isoniazid), furatrizine (K. Miura, 1961), nalidixic acid (G.Y. Lesher, 1962), etc.

The discovery of penicillin by Sir Alexander Fleming in 1929 was accidental but revolutionary. In 1938 Chain, Florey, and their associates purified the active principle from a culture filtrate of Penicillium notatum. The introduction of penicillin revolutionized the treatment of many infectious diseases and confirmed that many new chemotherapeutic agents may be found in organisms living in our surroundings, i.e., the soil, water, air, etc.

As practical example, Selman A. Waksman isolated streptomycin from Streptomyces griseus, a known soil organism, in 1943. In 1947, the antibiotic properties of chloramphenicol were first reported by J. Ehrlich, and Y. Koyama reported colistin in the same year. B.M. Duggar obtained chlortetracycline from Streptomyces aureofaciens in 1948. Thereafter, many antibiotics have been introduced in the treatment of infectious diseases, making our era the golden age of chemotherapy in the long history of medicine.

Half a century has passed since the discovery of penicillin and we are now faced with multiply-resistant microorganisms, which are resistant to chemotherapeutic agents formerly referred to as "magic bullets" in medicine and the livestock- and

I had asked Ernst B. Chain to write the foreword for our book. It was indeed unfortunate that he died suddenly last summer soon after he had accepted with pleasure.

April 1981

Susumu MITSUHASHI
Department of Microbiology
Laboratory of Bacterial Resistance
School of Medicine, Gunma University

FOREWORD

The body of scientific knowledge, like the murein sacculus, is a seamless web with many levels: each component is connected directly to a few others, and indirectly to all. The most spectacular connection of penicillin, is of course, to therapy, where its dramatic action has surely saved millions of lives. But this molecule is also remarkable for the variety of its other direct connections: *i.e.*, the principles, applications, and novel areas of study that it has generated. In industry penicillin initiated the systematic search for additional antibiotics, the isolation of mutants that increased the yield, and the development of aerobic "fermenters" with unprecedented capacities. Antibiotics have also made possible daring new kinds of major surgery, and they have advanced both virology and the study of cell biology by greatly simplifying animal cell culture. Organic chemists have found a wealth of challenging problems in the β-lactams, with their novel 4-membered ring; and the degradation products of these complex molecules have made possible model studies on the development of allergy to haptens.

In microbiology β-lactams continue to generate exciting new leads. Penicillin demonstrated earlier the remarkably selective toxicity of an inhibitor of a reaction unique to the parasite; it introduced the use of antibiotic resistance as a selective genetic marker; and its interference with a specific reaction in peptidoglycan synthesis was indispensable for the isolation of pieces small enough to analyze. More recently, refined studies have shown that β-lactams inhibit a number of different transpeptidases in the cell, and the regulation of these enzymes may well provide the key to the morphogenetic processes that divide a bacterial cell and determine its shape.

Perhaps the broadest contribution of antibiotics to biology has been the recognition that plasmids are ubiquitous, as originally shown in Japan. Moreover, they code not only for drug resistance but also for many other functions that are optional for the cell. Their use in molecular recombination of DNA *in vitro*, and in the study of special insertion sequences, is revolutionizing molecular genetics. Their role in gene transfer in evolution is increasingly recognized, and it may not be restricted to bacteria. Finally, studies with a variety of β-lactams are revealing a novel property of some enzymes, in which exposure to one ligand induces a relatively persistent conformational change that alters the subsequent reaction with another.

It is thus clear that work on β-lactams has led not only to immediate practical applications but also to many unexpected spinoffs. These provide strong support for two principles that need constant reiteration: basic and applied research are inextricably intertwined; and the most interesting and valuable discoveries are often unpredictable. This was true of Fleming's original observation; it was true of Chain's decision to purify a lytic agent that he assumed was an enzyme; and it will no doubt be true of many further discoveries involving the β-lactams.

Bernard D. DAVIS
Bacterial Physiology Unit
Harvard Medical School

CONTENTS

MODE OF ACTION

PHARMACOKINETICS

ALLERGY

1 HISTORY

A SHORT HISTORY OF THE β-LACTAM ANTIBIOTICS

E. P. ABRAHAM

*Sir William Dunn School of Pathology**

THE DISCOVERY OF PENICILLIN AND ITS CHEMOTHERAPEUTIC PROPERTIES

It is now more than half a century since Alexander Fleming observed the antibacterial action of penicillin on a plate seeded with staphylococci at St. Mary's Hospital, London, and nearly forty years since the work of Florey and Chain and their colleagues in Oxford demonstrated the remarkable therapeutic power of penicillin that led to its widespread use in medicine. These discoveries proved to be the forerunners of others which have led to the production of a large family of antibiotics, with established or potential clinical value, whose single common structural feature is the possession of a β-lactam ring. In this introductory chapter an attempt will be made to survey briefly how such developments came about.

Several aspects of the early work are worthy of comment, for numerous popular accounts of what happened have been notable mainly for the extent of their divergence from reality. Fleming's original observation of the production of penicillin after an accidental contamination of his plate on a laboratory bench by *Penicillium notatum* is not easily repeatable. Penicillin brings about the lysis of growing staphylococci, but not of resting organisms, and it appears that only unpredictable changes in the summer temperature made it possible for the fungus to grow and produce penicillin before the bacteria had completed their growth and become insensitive. However, Fleming cultured the fungus in broth and showed that the culture filtrates, which he called penicillin, were highly active against a variety of gram-positive bacteria. He also showed that the active broth was no more toxic than ordinary broth to animals and to leucocytes and used it in a few cases as a local antiseptic; but his interest in it for this purpose clearly waned, for he wrote in 1940: "the trouble of

* South Parks Road, Oxford OX1 3RE, U.K.

making it seemed not worth while." The idea that it might be introduced into the bloodstream and function as a systemic chemotherapeutic agent apparently never occurred to him.

Attempts to isolate penicillin in the decade following its discovery were soon abandoned, mainly because of difficulties arising from its instability. But, in 1938, the question was reopened when H. W. Florey and E. B. Chain decided to make a systematic investigation of antimicrobial substances produced by microorganisms in the Sir William Dunn School of Pathology, Oxford. This decision was a consequence of their interest in lysozyme. Penicillin was fortunately one of the first substances chosen for study, and the work of a small group of people led to its purification and to the demonstration by Florey and his colleagues of its remarkable therapeutic properties, first in mice and then in humans.

Despite the gratifying outcome of this work, which seemed at the time to be almost miraculous, the production of penicillin in war-time Britain in the quantities needed for its general medical use posed a virtually insoluble problem. Florey therefore went to the United States with N. G. Heatley, in 1941, to enlist American help. Subsequent work in the Northern Regional Research Laboratories in Peoria and in several American pharmaceutical companies was responsible for the addition of corn-steep liquor to the growth medium, the introduction of deep fermentation, and the isolation of higher-yielding strains of *Penicillium* which entirely changed the outlook for the large-scale production of penicillin. Thus, enough penicillin became available to treat all serious British and American casualties during the invasion of Europe in 1944.

During the war years the chemistry of penicillin became the subject of a massive and confidential Anglo-American investigation, involving many commercial and academic organisations, whose ultimate aim was to produce penicillin in quantity by chemical synthesis. The sodium salt of benzylpenicilin was crystallised at the Squibb Institute for Medical Research by Wintersterner and MacPhillamy in 1943 and soon afterwards a crystalline sodium salt was obtained from the purified 2-pentenylpenicillin of Abraham and Chain in Oxford. The β-lactam structure for penicillin (Fig. 1) was first proposed by Abraham and Chain in 1943. It was later strongly supported by R. B. Woodward, but was opposed by those committed to an alternative thiazolidine-oxazolone structure. However, the β-lactam structure was finally established beyond doubt in 1945 when an X-ray crystallographic analysis by Dorothy Hodgkin and Barbara Low came to a successful conclusion.

The outcome of the synthetic work during this time was disappointing, for no more than trace amounts of penicillin were ever obtained, and these in attempts to synthesise the thiazolidine-oxazolone structure.

By 1948 the outstanding value in medicine of benzylpenicillin had been firmly established. Many of its limitations, including a relatively low activity against gram-negative bacilli and the tubercle bacillus, were also known. In 1940 the first penicillinase had been discovered in *Escherichia coli* by Abraham and Chain, who suggested that the production of this enzyme was responsible, in some cases though not in

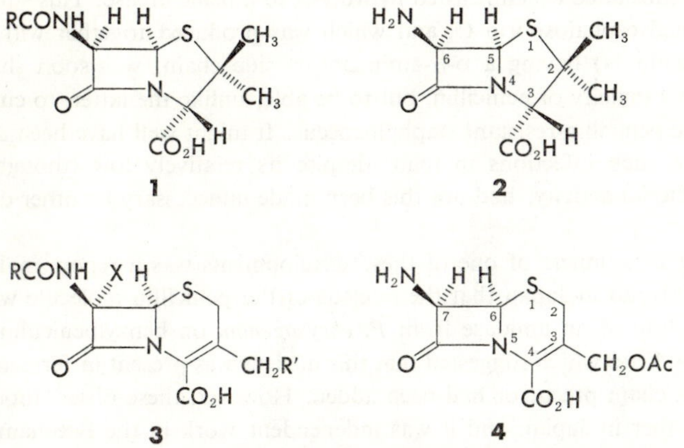

FIG. 1. Structures of: 1, penicillins; 2, 6-APA; 3, cephalosporins; and 4, 7-ACA. R is variable in the penicillins. In the cephalosporins R and R' are variable and X is H or OMe.

others, for bacterial resistance to penicillin. Within five years penicillinase had been found to be produced by a number of gram-negative and gram-positive pathogens, including some strains of *Staphylococcus aureus*, and in one case had been shown by Duthie to be an inducible enzyme. By this time it had also been shown that penicillins with different nonpolar side chains derived from mono-substituted acetic acids could be obtained by addition of appropriate side chain precursors to the fermentation of *Penicillium chrysogenum*; but none of the penicillins thus obtained had proved to be markedly superior to the benzylpenicillin then in use, although in 1954 the discovery of the relative acid-stability of phenoxymethylpenicillin (penicillin V) made the latter the first penicillin suitable for oral administration. Thus, towards the end of the 1940's the history of penicillin might have been regarded as that of a great medical discovery to which little more would be likely to be added. In the event, there were to be remarkable and unforeseeable further developments. These were to lead to the production of thousands of new β-lactam compounds, a number of which were to be responsible for significant advances in chemotherapy.

CEPHALOSPORIN C, 6-AMINOPENICILLANIC ACID, AND 7-AMINOCEPHALO-SPORANIC ACID

In the early 1950's a serious clinical problem arose from the emergence of penicillinase-producing staphylococci and the failure of the penicillins then available to cope with infections caused by these organisms. It was thus of some interest when Newton and Abraham, who were studying the production of antibiotics by a species of *Cephalosporium* that had been isolated by Brotzu in Sardinia, discovered in 1953 a penicillin-like substance which resisted hydrolysis to a penicillinase. This substance, which they named cephalosporin C, and which was produced together with a new penicillin (penicillin N) having a D-α-aminoadipyl side chain, was soon shown to have the very low toxicity of penicillin, but to be able, unlike the latter, to cure mice infected with the penicillin-resistant staphylococcus. It might well have been used for the treatment of such infections in man, despite its relatively low (though wide-ranging) antibacterial activity, had not this been made unnecessary by other developments.

The earliest forerunners of one of these developments was a report in 1950 by Sakaguchi and Murao in Japan that the nucleus of the penicillin molecule was produced by the action of an amidase from *P. chrysogenum* on benzylpenicillin and a report in 1953 by Kato which suggested that this nucleus was present in fermentations to which no side chain precursor had been added. However, these observations were not explored further in Japan, and it was independent work in the Beecham Laboratories by Rolinson and others which resulted, by 1959, in the isolation of the penicillin nucleus (6-aminopenicillanic acid, 6-APA, in Fig. 1) in quantity.

At about this time a definitive structure for cephalosporin C [Fig. 1, R=$^-$O$_2$CCH-(N$^+$H$_3$)(CH$_2$)$_3$, R'=OCOCH$_3$] was proposed by Abraham and Newton and confirmed, soon afterwards, by an X-ray crystallographic analysis by Hodgkin and Maslen. It was also found that the nucleus of cephalosporin C (7-aminocephalosporanic acid, 7-ACA, in Fig. 1) could be obtained, although in very small yield, by acid hydrolysis under controlled conditions and that acylation of 7-ACA with phenylacetyl chloride yielded a cephalosporin with very much higher activity than cephalosporin C itself against gram-positive bacteria. Furthermore, it was shown that the acetoxy group at C-3' in cephalosporin C could readily be replaced by a variety of nucleophiles to give compounds with higher activity. These compounds retained a resistance to hydrolysis by staphylococcal penicillinase, the resistance being due to the nature of the ring system.

SEMI-SYNTHETIC NEW PENICILLINS AND CEPHALOSPORINS

The finding that penicillin N, unlike benzylpenicillin, was as active against a number of gram-negative bacteria as it was against gram-positive organisms indicated that penicillins with other side chains, differing from those of the penicillins obtainable by fermentation of *P. chrysogenum*, might have interesting biological properties. Soon after the isolation of 6-APA, the Beecham Group began a fruitful study of new penicillins that could be prepared from it by chemical acylation. This led first to methicillin (R=2:6-dimethoxyphenyl in Fig. 1), which largely solved the clinical problem of the penicillin-resistant staphylococcus because of its stability in the presence of staphylococcal penicillinase. A major factor here was the very poor affinity of methicillin for the staphylococcal β-lactamase, which was associated with the presence of the two bulky methoxyl groups in its side chain close to the β-lactam ring. Methicillin was followed by oxacillin and cloxacillin which also resisted hydrolysis by the staphylococcal enzyme but which, unlike methicillin, were relatively stable to gastric acidity and were absorbed when given by mouth.

The first new penicillins showed very low activity against gram-negative bacteria. However, in 1961 ampicillin, with an amino group attached to the α-carbon atom of its side chain, was found to be considerably more active than benzylpenicillin against many gram-negative organisms. This α-aminobenzylpenicillin has been succeeded by the closely related amoxycillin. Both compounds are effective in the treatment of infections by a variety of gram-negative bacteria, but not infections by the penicillin-resistant staphylococcus, since they are readily hydrolysed by staphylococcal penicillinase.

While valuable new semi-synthetic penicillins were being produced by the Beecham Group the discovery in the Lilly Research Laboratories in 1962 of a chemical method for the removal of the α-aminoadipyl side chain of cephalosporin C in good yield and the production of 7-ACA in quantity opened the way to the extensive exploration by pharmaceutical companies of the potentialities of the cephalosporin ring system. A year later the Lilly group described a chemical route from the penicillin to the cephalosporin ring system which also proved to be of major importance.

Cephalothin, with a thienylacetyl side chain, was the first semi-synthetic cephalosporin to come into medical use. It was effective against a variety of gram-positive bacteria, including penicillinase-producing staphylococci, and also against a number of gram-negative bacilli. Cephalothin was followed by Glaxo's cephaloridine, in which the acetoxy group at C-3′ of cephalothin was replaced by a pyridinium group. The latter was not removed by acetyl esterases which converted cephalothin to the less active deacetylcephalothin *in vivo*. Later cefazolin was produced by Fujisawa in Japan and was the first of a number of cephalosporins in which the acetoxy group was replaced by a heterocycle carrying a thiol group.

The early cephalosporins were not absorbed from the gastrointestinal tract, despite their relative stability to acid. However, cephalosporins with a D-phenylglycyl side chain (that of ampicillin) were readily absorbed when given by mouth. The first of these compounds, introduced by Eli Lilly, was cephalexin, which also contained a methyl group in place of an acetoxymethyl group at C-3′. A related compound, cephradine, containing a cyclohexadienylglycyl side chain, was then produced by Squibb.

The availability and use of β-lactam antibiotics able to cope with infections by gram-positive bacteria, together with changing patterns of infection, focused attention on a growing problem of resistance in gram-negative bacteria. In some cases and particularly with *Pseudomonas aeruginosa*, resistance was partly due to the poor ability of β-lactam antibiotics to penetrate the cell wall and reach their sites of action on the cytoplasmic membrane. But another important factor was the ability of many of the resistant organisms to produce a cell-bound β-lactamase. It became evident that there were many β-lactamases with different substrate profiles and that while some of them were chromosomal others were mediated by plasmids which could be transferred from one organism to another.

In 1967 the Beecham Group introduced carbenicillin, a penicillin with a carboxyl group in place of the amino group of ampicillin. This compound showed a wide range of activity and, unlike earlier β-lactam antibiotics, was effective against some strains of *P. aeruginosa*. More recently ticacillin, the ureidopenicillin azlocillin, and piperacillin have been rivals reported to be superior to carbenicillin as broad-spectrum penicillins. Among other derivatives of 6-APA, mecillinam, with an amidino side chain which endows it with a higher activity against gram-negative than against gram-positive bacteria, has found limited clinical use.

NEW CEPHALOSPORINS

The first "cephalosporinase" was found in culture filtrates of *Bacillus cereus* by Newton and Abraham in 1956. The 1970's have seen the appearance of a second generation of semi-synthetic cephalosporins with a higher resistance than their predecessors to hydrolysis by a considerable number of β-lactamases. Cephamandole, produced by Eli Lilly, has a side chain derived from mandelic acid. Cefuroxime, from Glaxo, has a methoximino group at the α-carbon of its side chain and was produced after the potential value of an oximino group in this position had been found during a chemical study in which it was used to generate an amino group. A third compound, cefoxitin, was an outcome of findings in the Lilly and Merck laboratories that 7α-methoxycephalosporins with a D-α-aminoadipyl side chain are produced by certain species of *Streptomyces*. Cefoxitin, a semi synthetic 7α-methoxycephalosporin from Merck, Sharp & Dohme, is a 7α-methoxycephalosporin with a thienylacetyl side chain and a carbamoyloxy group at C′-3. It is notable for its stability in the presence of a variety of β-lactamases. Cefmetazole, also a 7α-methoxycephalosporin, has been produced by Sankyo.

Following these compounds, there is now a third generation of cephalosporins which is likely to extend the range of infections that can be treated successfully with members of this family. They include cefotiam from Japan; cefsulodin from Takeda and Ciba Geigy, which has a sulphonic acid group at the α-position of its side chain and is active specifically against *P. aeruginosa*; cefoperazone from Toyama and Pfizer; cefotaxime, with a methoximino group and an aminothiazole ring in the side chain, from Hoechst-Roussel Uclaf, which shows an exceptionally wide spectrum of activity; and a broad spectrum 1-oxa cephalosporin from Shionogi and Lilly which contains oxygen in place of sulphur in its six-membered ring and also a 7α-methoxy group.

NEW β-LACTAMS FROM *STREPTOMYCES* SPP.

Further screening of *Streptomyces* spp. has revealed new and potentially useful β-lactams which are neither penicillins nor cephalosporins. Thienamycin, discovered in the Merck laboratories in 1976, has a fused β-lactam-pyrroline ring system. It has a broad spectrum of activity and a high resistance to many β-lactamases. Screening by the Beecham group for β-lactamase inhibitors rather than for antibacterial activity revealed clavulanic acid, with a fused β-lactam-oxazolidine ring system, and the olivanic acids, related to thienamycin. These substances are inactivators of certain β-lactamases. The use of a test organism supersensitive to β-lactam antibiotics led to the discovery of a family of monocyclic β-lactams (the nocardicins) by Fujisawa.

TOTAL CHEMICAL SYNTHESIS AND BIOSYNTHESIS

With the exception of benzylpenicillin and phenoxymethylpenicillin, most of the β-lactam antibiotics that have found a place in medicine are semi-synthetic compounds derived from natural products isolated from fermentations of *Penicillium, Cephalosporium*, or *Streptomyces* spp. Total chemical synthesis has been unable to compete in efficiency with the biosynthetic processes of microorganisms. Nevertheless, it has turned out to be an area in which organic chemists have made outstanding advances. Following the disappointing outcome of the Anglo-American effort to synthesise penicillin in the 1940's rational total synthesis of phenoxymethylpenicillin and of 6-APA was accomplished by Sheehan and his colleagues at the Massachusetts Institute of Technology in 1958–1959; and in 1966 R. B. Woodward and others reported a total synthesis of cephalosporin C. The synthesis of cephalosporin C was succeeded in the 1970's by others accomplished by the Woodward, Merck, and Smith, Kline, and French groups. Nuclear analogues of the penicillin or cephalosporin ring system were made, in which sulphur was replaced by oxygen or moved to a different position in the ring. A penem, in which a β-lactam was fused with a thiazoline ring, was also synthesised. These compounds showed significant antibacterial activity. Work on the synthesis of compounds related to other β-lactams such as clavulanic acid and thienamycin, may well throw further light on structure-activity relationships.

In parallel with these extensive chemical studies there have been others on biosynthesis, dating from the discovery in the 1940's by Behrens and others that a variety of penicillins with nonpolar side chains could be produced from *P. chrysogenum* by feeding appropriate side chain precursors (which were nonpolar monosubstituted acetic acids) to the fermentation medium. The work of Arnstein and others in the 1950's established that L-cysteine and L-valine were the precursors of the penicillin ring system. Experiments in the 1960's in Oxford showed that the biosynthesis of penicillin N and cephalosporin C by the *Cephalosporium* sp. resembled that of the penicillins by *P. chrysogenum*, but differed from it in some respects. For example, L-cysteine and L-valine were precursors of the ring systems, but the D-α-aminoadipyl side chain of the compounds produced by the *Cephalosporium* could not be varied by the addition of precursors. Further progress came from work with cell-free systems in Oxford and at the Massachusetts Institute of Technology and from the use of mutants, isolated in Ciba Geigy, in the Lilly Research Laboratories, and in Japan, which were blocked at certain stages in the biosynthetic pathways. It now seems that the tripeptide δ(L-α-aminoadipyl)-L-cysteinyl-D-valine is a precursor of isopenicillin N (which has an L-α-aminoadipyl side chain) and that the latter is a common intermediate in the biosynthesis both of other penicillins and of cephalosporins. The methoxyl group of the 7α-methoxycephalosporins from *Streptomyces* spp. appears to be introduced after the cephalosporin ring system has been formed.

PENICILLIN-BINDING PROTEINS AND β-LACTAMASES

In 1940 A. D. Gardner observed that bacteria grown in the presence of subinhibitory concentrations of penicillin became swollen or filamentous. In 1942 Gladys Hobby and others showed that penicillin was bactericidal only to growing organisms and in 1946 Abraham and Duthie reported that killing preceded lysis. Lederberg found in 1957 that cells of *E. coli* were converted to protoplasts when grown in the presence of penicillin in a hypertonic medium and proposed that penicillin inhibited cell wall synthesis.

The discovery by Park in 1952 that certain uridine nucleotides accumulated in staphylococci damaged by penicillin was the prelude to an extensive series of studies by Strominger and his colleagues and by Ghuysen, Spratt, Tomasz, and others. These studies have thrown light on the sequence of reactions involved in wall synthesis, on the points at which inhibition by β-lactam antibiotics occurs, on its mechanism, and on the various penicillin- and cephalosporin-binding proteins in bacterial cell membranes which are transpeptidases or carboxypeptidases. It appears that β-lactam antibiotics inactivate such enzymes by acylating a serine residue in their amino acid sequences.

In 1956 Pollock, Kogut, and Tridgell obtained β-lactamase I from *B. cereus* in crystalline form. This was followed by the purification of a variety of different β-lactamases by Richmond, Kuwabara, Davies, and Abraham, and others. During the present decade the amino acid sequences of four different β-lactamases have been found by Ambler to show considerable homology and it may be that there is significant homology between the sequences of the β-lactamases and the cell-membrane DD-carboxypeptidases.

Although the first β-lactamase was discovered nearly 40 years ago it is only recently that definitive progress has been made towards the elucidation of the active sites of these enzymes. The ability of cephalosporin C to act as a competitive inhibitor of a β-lactamase was observed in Oxford in 1956; and the inactivation of β-lactamases during hydrolysis of certain substrates was reported in 1962 and studied further by Dyke in 1967. Work by several groups with new substrates that act as inactivators has now shown that such compounds form an acyl-enzyme intermediate which undergoes a further change that interrupts the normal catalytic process. Studies by Waley and his colleagues have indicated that the intermediate is formed by the acylation of a serine residue. Thus the mechanisms of action of certain β-lactamases and DD-carboxypeptidases have features in common.

β-Lactamase inhibitors and inactivators have been shown to act as synergistic agents with other β-lactam antibiotics. But whether they will find extensive clinical use for this reason is still uncertain.

REFERENCES

1. Abraham, E. P. 1977. β-Lactam Antibiotics and Related Substances XXX, Suppl 1–26.
2. Abraham E. P. 1979. *Rev. Infect. Dis.*, **1**, 99–105.
3. A Discussion on Penicillin 50 years after Fleming. Organised by J. Baddiley and E. P. Abraham 1980. *Phil. Trans. Roy. Soc. Lond. B*, **289**, 165–378.
4. Hans T. Clarke, John R. Johnson, and Sir Robert Robinson (Editorial Board) 1949. "The Chemistry of Penicillin," Princeton Univ. Press, Princeton, New Jersey.
5. Florey, H.W., Chain, E., Heatley, N. G., Jennings, M. A., Sanders, A. G., Abraham, E. P., and Florey, M. E. 1949. "Antibiotics," Vol. II, Oxford Univ. Press, London and New York.
6. Mitsuhashi, S. (ed.). 1977. "R Factor-Drug Resistance Plasmid," Japan Sci. Soc. Press, Tokyo.
7. Hare, R. 1970. "The Birth of Penicillin," George Allen and Unwin Ltd.

2 EPIDEMIOLOGY AND GENETICS OF RESISTANCE

EPIDEMIOLOGY AND GENETICS OF RESISTANCE TO β-LACTAM ANTIBIOTICS

Susumu Mitsuhashi and Matsuhisa Inoue

*Department of Microbiology, Laboratory of Bacterial Resistance, School of Medicine, Gunma University**

The first paper on penicillin was published in 1929 by Alexander Fleming (see p. 3) but we had to wait about 20 years to put the drug into practical use because this was the first experience of producing an antibiotic in medical history. The introduction of sulfanilamide (SA) and penicillin G (PCG) opened a dramatic age in chemotherapy and we celebrated the 50th anniversary of penicillins discovery in 1979. Following the introduction of a number of chemotherapeutic agents, many observations on bacterial drug resistance have been reported, for example, reports of resistance to SA by Maclean *et al.* (*16*), to PCG by Abraham *et al.* (*1*), and to streptomycin (SM) by Murray *et al.* (*29*). The author discovered by chance in Japan that the activity of penicillin in collected broth from many cultured bottles was sometimes suddenly decreased in the purification process due to mixing of contaminated bacteria, *i.e.*, penicillinase (PCase) in culture filtrate (*11*). Now we are aware of the rapid spread of multiple resistance in bacteria isolated from clinical materials, livestock, and cultured fish (*23, 26, 27*).

PENICILLIN G(PCG) RESISTANCE

PCG is effective against *Staphylococcus aureus*, *S. epidermidis*, *Streptococcus pyogenes*, *S. pneumoniae*, *S. viridans*, *Neisseria meningitidis*, and *N. gonorrhoeae*. The fact that most strains of streptococci and the *Nesseria* group are still sensitive to PCG should be noted from the evolutionary process of the plasmid spread mediating the production of PCase. However, nonconjugative(r) plasmids governing PCase production have recently been found in *N. gonorrhoeae*, *Haemophilus influenzae* (*30, 32*), and *S. pyogenes*, which may cause the rapid spread of penicillin resistance in the organisms.

Nonconjugative(r) plasmids were first demonstrated in *S. aureus* strains (*17, 20,*

---

* Showa-machi 3-39-22, Maebashi 371, Japan.

TABLE I.   Isolation Frequency of Drug-resistant Strains of *S. aureus*

Drug	Resistant strains (%) isolated in											
	1961	1962	1963	1964	1965	1966	1967	1968	1969	1970	1974	1976
SA	98	95	99	95	95	94	96	98	98	98	96	98
SM	41	34	31	20	25	28	34	26	23	31	23	35
TC	29	37	36	35	37	36	41	33	40	38	22	30
PC	50	54	63	55	43	70	78	78	77	69	70	74

The results are based on surveys of 6,930 strains isolated between 1961 and 1976.

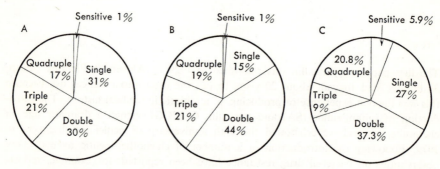

FIG. 1.   Patterns of resistance in *S. aureus* to TC, SM, SA, and PC.
Quadruple resistance, TC.SA.SM.PC; triple resistance, TC.PC.SA, SM.SA.TC, SM.SA.PC, and TC.PC.SM; double resistance, TC.SA, PC.SM, SA.PC, and SM.SA. A: summary of results from 2,099 strains isolated between 1961 and 1965.   B: summary of results from 4,293 strains isolated between 1966 and 1972.   C: summary of results from 538 strains isolated between 1974 and 1976.

22) (Fig. 5B). Most staphylococci are lysogenic and the staphylococcal r plasmids are transmitted from cell to cell by lysogenic phage lysates, suggesting the spread of r plasmids by phages (*18, 20, 22*). Among the gram-positive bacteria, the isolation frequency of PCG-resistant strains is extremely high in *S. aureus* strains, reaching a maximum of about 70% of PCG-resistant strains (Table I). Resistance to tetracycline TC, SM, PCG, and SA is predominant in *S. aureus* strains (Fig. 1). The isolation frequencies of strains resistant to macrolide antibiotics (Mac), chloramphenicol (CM), kanamycin (KM), methicillin (DMP), and noboviocin (NB) are much higher from triply-and quadruply resistant strains to TC, SM, PCG, and SA. These results indicate that multiply-resistant staphylococci become easily resistant when new drugs are introduced in practical use (Table II) (*20, 21*).

Streptococcus pyogenes strains isolated in Europe are still singly TC-resistant. The strains of *S. pyogenes* isolated 10 years before in Japan were also singly-TC-

TABLE II. Isolation Frequency of Strains Resistant to Mac, CM, KM, DMP, and NB among Strains Resistant to TC, SA, SM, and PC

Patterns of resistance to TC, SA, SM, and PC		Isolation frequency (%) of strains resistant to				
		Mac	CM	KM	DMP	NB
Single						
1961–1965	(31)[a]	9. 6	11. 8	8. 3	11. 8	37. 0
1966–1969	(15)	9. 9	11. 0	14. 1	16. 7	11. 0
1970	(17)	4. 0	12. 0	8. 0	12. 0	12. 0
1972	(18)	6. 0	8. 0	10. 0	10. 0	0
1974	(27)	4. 8	0	0	0	0
1975	(31)	6. 5	5. 3	7. 9	20	25
1976	(35)	11. 0	8. 8	2. 4	0	0
Double						
1961–1965	(30)	21. 2	27. 4	24. 9	31. 0	22. 3
1966–1969	(42)	21. 4	27. 6	36. 1	27. 8	27. 8
1970	(50)	18. 0	36. 0	39. 0	44. 0	52. 0
1972	(44)	18. 0	19. 0	18. 0	33. 0	9. 0
1974	(46)	19. 0	8. 3	6. 7	0	0
1975	(45)	31. 0	3. 0	9. 5	20	20
1976	(28)	20. 0	14. 7	12. 0	0	33
Triple and quadruple						
1961–1965	(38)	69. 2	60. 8	66. 8	57. 2	40. 7
1966–1969	(43)	68. 7	61. 4	49. 8	55. 5	61. 2
1970	(33)	78. 0	52. 0	53. 0	44. 0	38. 0
1972	(25)	76. 0	71. 0	74. 0	57. 0	91. 0
1974	(27)	76. 2	91. 7	93. 3	0	100
1975	(24)	62. 5	91. 7	82. 6	60	55
1976	(37)	69. 0	76. 5	85. 6	100	67

The isolation frequency indicates the distribution of strains resistant to each drug among strains carrying single, double, triple, and quadruple resistance to TC, SA, SM, and PC during the survey period.
[a] Figures in brackets indicate total isolation frequency (%) for each resistance pattern during the survey period.

resistant (Fig. 2). However, the number of triply-and doubly-resistant strains to Mac, CM, and TC has increased in Japan (*12, 19, 21, 30–32*). It should be noted that most *S. pyogenes* strains are still sensitive to PCG except for a very few cases of PCG-resistant *S. pyogenes* strains reported in South Africa (Fig. 3).

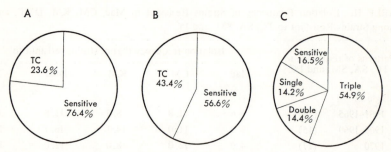

FIG. 2.   Resistance patterns of *S. pyogenes* strains isolated in Japan and Europe. A: 258 strains isolated in Europe between 1976 and 1977.   B: 780 strains isolated in Japan between 1963 and 1964.   C: 1,021 strains isolated in Japan between 1974 and 1975.   Triple, Mac.TC.CM.   Double, Mac.TC, TC.CM, and Mac.CM.

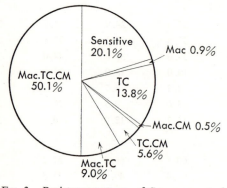

FIG. 3.   Resistance patterns of *S. pyogenes* strains.

Among *S. pneumoniae* strains, strains resistant to TC, CM, and Mac have been isolated from clinical materials but PCG-resistant strains have not been isolated thus far (Table III) (*31*). Similarly, PCG has been effective thus far toward *N. gonorrhoeae*. However, *N. gonorrhoeae* carrying PCG-resistant r plasmids was isolated and these organisms are increasing in number all over the world (*12*).

AMPICILLIN (APC) RESISTANCE

PCG is only effective against gram-positive bacteria, but the introduction of APC has broadened the antibacterial spectrum toward gram-negative bacteria. After the use of a large amount of APC in practical medicine, APC-resistant strains of bacteria have appeared in clinical isolates. However, the isolation frequency of APC-resistant strains is different in each bacterial species similar to that of PCG-resistant strains in gram-positive bacterial species. The isolation frequencies of APC-resistant strains are rather low in *Shigella, Salmonella*, the indole-negative *Proteus* group, and *Escherichia coli*. By contrast, APC-resistant strains are frequently isolated in the indole-positive *Proteus* group, *Klebsiella pneumoniae, K. oxytoca, Serratia marcescens*,

TABLE III.   Drug Resistance of *S. pneumoniae*

Drug-resistance pattern	Isolation frequency (%)
TC. CM. Mac	2.0
TC. CM	53.0
TC	12.0
CM	3.0
Sensitive strains	30.0

Results are based on surveys of 470 strains isolated between 1975 and 1977.

TABLE IV.   Bacterial Patterns of Resistance to TC, CM, SM, and SA

Resistance pattern	Organism				
	Shigella	*E. coli*	*K. pneumoniae*	*Proteus*	*S. marcescens*
Quadruple	74.9	45.0	52.0	23.9	72.8
Triple	5.3	12.1	22.6	13.5	16.8
Double	3.1	20.1	13.4	14.0	10.4
Single	16.7	22.8	12.0	47.9	0

Patterns of resistance to TC, CM, SM, and SA found in enterobacteria isolated from clinical sources.   Results are from a survey of 12,800 strains.

TABLE V.   Isolation Frequency of APC-resistant Strains and Demonstration Frequency of R Factors Carrying APC Resistance

Organism	Isolation frequency of strains resistant to APC (%)	Isolation frequency of R factors carrying APC resistance
		From APC-resistant strains
Shigella	2.9	77.5[a]
E. coli	19.2	81.3
Salmonella	2.9	48.7
K. pneumoniae	91.2	40.4
P. aeruginosa[b]	8.1	22.7

Summary of results from 12,242 strains of *Shigella*, 338 strains of *E. coli*, 2,920 strains of *Salmonella*, 335 strains of *K. pneumoniae*, and 204 strains of *P. aeruginosa*.
[a] The number of R[+] strains/total number of APC-resistant strains.   [b] Highly resistant to carbenicillin (CPC).   Most of *P. aeruginosa* strains are resistant to CPC (87.0%).

Enterobacter cloacae, Citrobacter freundii, etc. APC is not effective toward *Pseudomonas aeruginosa*, and carbenicillin (CPC) and sulbenicillin (SPC) have been used for the treatment of *P. aeruginosa* infections. However, CPC- and SPC-resistant strains of *P. aeruginosa* are now frequently isolated from clinical materials (Table III).

In gram-negative bacteria, strains resistant to TC, CM, SM, and SA are often isolated from clinical sources, and especially strains with quadruple resistance to these four drugs are frequently seen, followed by those with single, triple, and double resistance in that order (Table IV). APC-resistant strains are often seen in quadruply- and triply-resistant strains to the four drugs, indicating that APC-resistant strains are usually multiply resistant (Table V).

DRUG RESISTANCE PLASMIDS

The conjugative(R) and nonconjugative(r) resistance plasmids are widly distributed in bacteria isolated from clinical materials, livestock, and cultured fish (*23, 26, 27*). The R plasmids are often seen in gram-negative bacteria and demonstrated from multiply resistant strains of bacteria to TC, CM, SM, SA, aminoglycoside antibiotics, and to β-lactam antibiotics (Fig. 5A). As shown in Table VI, R plasmids are frequently seen from quadruply- and triply-resistant strains to TC, CM, SM, and SA. APC resistance is also mostly due to the presence of R or r plasmids (Table VII).

In relation to resistance to TC, CM, SM, and SA, R plasmids carrying (TC.CM. SM.SA), (TC.SM.SA), or (CM.SM.SA) resistance are seen at high frequencies (more than 95%) and those carrying resistance to other combinations of the four drugs are rarely seen in clinical isolates. R plasmids carrying double resistance to TC, CM, SM, and SA are shown in Table VIII. R plasmids with (SM.SA) resistance are most frequently seen in bacterial isolates. R plasmids with single TC resistance are isolated most frequently, followed by those carrying resistance to mercury (Hg), and by APC resistance, in that order (Table IX).

The resistance patterns of R plasmids specifying APC-resistance are shown in Table X, indicating that the APC plasmids with multiple resistance are often seen in clinical isolates.

In relation to resistance to TC, CM, SM, and SA, the R plasmids carrying single CM or double (TC.CM; CM.SM; CM.SA) resistance are rarely isolated. The CM-mediating R plasmids with triple resistance (TC.CM.SA; TC.CM.SM) are rarely seen, although R(CM.SM.SA) plasmids are often seen in clinical isolates. However, R plasmids carrying (CM.APC), (CM.SA.APC), (CM.SM.APC), (TC.CM.APC), and (TC.CM.SA.APC) resistance are isolated, eventhough rare in number, from clinical isolates. These results suggest that R(APC) plasmids pick up the resistance determinants, *i.e.*, (TC.CM.SA), (TC.SM), (CM.SM), (CM.SA), and (CM) which are extremely rarely found, resulting in the formation of R(TC.CM.SA.APC), R(TC. CM.APC), R(CM.SM.APC), R(CM.SA.APC), and R(CM.APC) plasmids (Table XI).

TABLE VI. Isolation Frequency of R Plasmids from Strains Resistant to TC, CM, SM, and SA

Resistance pattern	Isolation frequency of R plasmids from strains resistant to							
	E. coli	Shigella	Salmonella	Proteus Ind. (+)	Proteus Ind. (−)	Klebsiella	E. cloacae	S. marcescens
Quadruple	59.7	79.7	84.3	61.8	50.0	63.2	60.0	84.7
Triple	55.6	82.4	75.6	45.2	36.4	43.0	62.5	41.3
Double	19.7	41.3	36.5	14.7	19.0	27.7	19.4	23.0
Single	9.2	10.8	6.1	1.2	0	7.1	0	0

[a] Resistance pattern to TC, CM, SM, and SA.

TABLE VII. Isolation Frequency of R Plasmids Specifying APC or KM Resistance from Resistant Strains

Drug	No. of R⁺ strains								
	E. coli	Shigella	Salmonella	Proteus Ind. (−)	Proteus Ind. (+)	K. pneumoniae	S. marcescens	E. cloacae	P. aeruginosa
APC	74.4	73.3	77.0	36.1	11.1	40.3	68.0	60.0	45.3[a]
KM	69.8	75.9	73.0	62.1	50.0	55.1	66.3	58.3	56.5

[a] R plasmids from highly resistant strains to CPC or KM.

TABLE VIII.   R plasmids Encoding Double Resistance to TC, CM, SM, and SA

Organism	No. of plasmids	R plasmids encoding double resistance to				
		SM SA	TC SM	CM SA	CM TC	TC SA
Shigella	747	79	1	8	0	0
E. coli	247	15	3	1	0	0
Salmonella	330	27	11	0	0	0
K. pneumoniae	360	22	6	1	0	0
Proteus	303	63	3	1	1	0
S. marcescens	304	181	0	0	0	0
Total	2,291	315	24	11	1	0

TABLE IX.   R plasmids Encoding Single Resistance

Organism	No. of plasmids examined	R plasmids encoding single resistance to							
		TC	CM	SM	SA	KM	APC	GM	Hg
Shigella	747	49	0	0	0	4	11	0	0
E. coli	247	20	0	0	1	4	9	0	0
Salmonella	330	61	0	1	1	0	5	0	0
K. pneumoniae	360	14	0	0	0	3	7	0	0
Proteus	303	0	0	0	5	0	13	0	0
P. aeruginosa	318	0	0	4	4	0	0	0	95
S. marcescens	304	0	0	0	0	10	1	0	0
Total	2,609	144	0	5	11	21	46	0	59

TABLE X.   Resistance Patterns of R Plasmids Carrying APC Resistance

R plasmid carrying	No. of R plasmids (%)	
APC resistance		
TC. CM. SM. SA. KM. APC	87	(11.9)
Quintuple resistance	252	(34.6)
Quadruple resistance	219	(30.0)
Triple resistance	75	(10.3)
Double resistance	50	(6.9)
Single APC resistance	46	(6.3)
Total	729	

The R plasmids were isolated from 15,884 strains of gram-negative bacteria including *E. coli*, *Shigella*, *Salmonella*, *K. pneumoniae*, *Proteus*, and *S. marcescens*.

TABLE XI. Resistance Patterns of R Plasmids Carrying CM Resistance

Resistance patterns	No. of R plasmids		(%)
TC.CM.SM.SA	1,980		
TC.CM.SM.SA.APC	390	2,421	(56.9)
TC.CM.SM.SA.KM	19		
TC.CM.SM.SA.KM.APC	32		
CM.SM.SA	1,659		
CM.SM.SA.APC	58	1,779	
CM.SM.SA.KM	38		
CM.SM.SA.KM.APC	24		
TC.CM.SM	0		
TC.CM.SM.APC	0	0	1,783 (41.9)
TC.CM.SM.KM	0		
TC.CM.SA	0		
TC.CM.SA.APC	4	4	
TC.CM.SA.KM	0		
TC.CM	0		
TC.CM.APC	19	19	
TC.CM.KM	0		
CM.SM	0		
CM.SM.APC	20	20	40 (0.9)
CM.SM.KM	0		
CM.SA	0		
CM.SA.APC	1	1	
CM.SA.KM	0		
CM	3		
CM.APC	7	10	10 (0.2)
CM.KM	0		
Total	4,254		

NONCONJUGATIVE RESISTANCE(r) PLASMIDS

Nonconjugative(r) plasmids were first demonstrated in *S. aureus* strains (*12, 17, 20, 22*). The r plasmids are smaller in size than R plasmids and lack the determinants governing conjugal transferability. They usually confer single resistance on their host and exist in multiple copies in a cell. Isolation frequencies of r plasmids from gram-positive and gram-negative bacteria are shown in Table XII, indicating a high dem-

TABLE XII.   Isolation Frequency of Nonconjugative r Plasmids from Resistant Strains

Organism	Isolation frequency of r plasmids (%)
S. aureus	85. 0
S. pyogenes	95. 0
H. influenzae	60. 0
E. coli	96. 0
Shigella	98. 0
Salmonella	95. 0
P. mirabilis	67. 0
S. marcescens	63. 0

Resistant strains without R plasmids were used for the demonstration of r plasmids.

1. r

2. $r_1 + r_2 + r_3 \cdots \cdots$

3. R

4. $R_1 + R_2$

5. R+r

FIG. 4.   Type of the plasmid-mediated resistance in bacteria.

onstration frequency of r plasmids. Then the plasmid-mediated resistance patterns of bacteria are summarized as shown in Fig. 4. Resistance patterns of *S. aureus* strains are of type 2 and those of gram-negative bacteria are mostly of type 3 or of type 5.

The appearance of penicillin-resistant strains of *N. gonorrhoeae* and *H. influenzae* (*32*) is thought to be due to the presence of r plasmids mediating the production of PCase. PCG resistance in *S. aureus* is mostly due to the presence of r plasmids governing the formation of PCase. From these results, it can be concluded that penicillin resistance in gram-positive and gram-negative bacteria is mostly due to the production of PCase, which is mediated by conjugative(R) or nonconjugative(r) plasmids. Electron micrographs of plasmids are shown in Fig. 5.

By contrast, cephalosporin resistance in gram-negative bacteria is due mostly to the production of cephalosporinase (CSase) which is mediated by the chromosome. Therefore, β-lactam resistance in gram-negative bacteria is often biphasic, *i.e.*, due to the production of CSase and of PCase mediated by plasmids.

β-Lactam resistance in bacteria is partly due to a decrease in the permeability of the drugs into bacterial cells. But epidemiological studies are not complete and biochemical mechanisms of this type of resistance have not been fully elucidated.

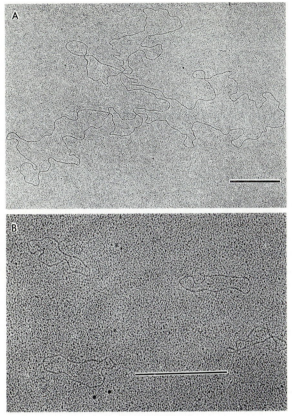

Fig. 5.   Electron micrograph of plasmids.
Bar represents 1 μm.   A: R(TC.CM.SM.SA) plasmid.   B: r(APC) plasmid.

TRANSPOSON SPECIFYING APC RESISTANCE (TnA)

In the transduction of R_{ms10} (TC.CM.SM.SA) with bacteriophage ε, the TC resistance determinant (*tet*) on the R plasmid was integrated into the bacterial chromosome between *pro* and *lac*. When TC-resistant transductant was infected with an F plasmid, we obtained a recombinant F-*tet*. When *E. coli*/F-*tet* was infected with the R plasmid, R-*tet* was obtained (*4, 5, 19, 24–26*).

In the transduction of the R_{ms14} plasmid with bacteriophage P1, we obtained an active phage P1-*cml* capable of conferring CM resistance. The CM resistance determinant (*cml*) on P1-*cml* was easily translocated to the F or R plasmid, resulting in the formation of F-*cml* or R-*cml* (*13, 14, 19, 24–26*). These findings are the first reports of the translocable resistance determinants on the R plasmid, *i.e.*, "transposons."

Plasmid-mediated resistance to penicillins and cephalosporins is almost universally associated with the elaboration of a β-lactamase. Four general classes of drug resistance factor mediated penicillin β-lactamase are now recognized (26), and the properties of the four penicillin β-lactamases (PCases) can be summarized as follows. Type I PCase may be identical to TEM-PCase which is mediated by R6K (3, 6). Type II PCase (so called oxacillin hydrolyzing enzyme) mediated by the R factor is able to hydrolyze the semi-synthetic penicillins, i.e., DMP, oxacillin, and its derivatives. Type III PCase has an isoelectric point of 8.3, is highly active against phenethicillin, oxacillin, and PCG, and is inhibited by NaCl but not by ferrous ions. Type IV PCase is able to hydrolyze CPC at a high rate. Type I PCase is the most common R-factor mediated β-lactamase and is found in a wide variety of naturally occurring plasmids (6). The other type of R-factor mediated β-lactamase is not so common as type I PCase, but type II and type IV β-lactamases mediated by R plasmids were isolated from our stock cultures of gram-negative bacteria.

The most striking feature of Datta's study (2) was the finding of determinants for a type I like β-lactamase on plasmids with a wide variety of compatibility properties from a broad taxonomic range of bacteria which were isolated from four continents. They tested 29 APC resistance plasmids, and type I PCase was very uniform with respect to substrate specificity but heterogeneous in a absolute levels of β-lactamase activity. Type I β-lactamase was determined by R-factors of compatibility groups FII, Iα, Iε, N, C, A, T, W, P, L, and X, and by prophage ϕAmp. However, type II was less common and was determined by R-factors of compatibility groups FI, Iα, N, C, and O (6), and these data were supported by Heffron et al. (9). They uggested that type I and type II PCases would be translocated from one replicon to another.

Evidence has been accumulated that type I β-lactamase gene is sometimes situated on a sequence of deoxyribonucleic acid that is capable of being translocated from one replicon to another

Datta et al. (2) have shown the translocation of type I β-lactamase from RP4 to the I compatibility plasmid R64. Richmond and Sykes (33) later showed the translocation of type I β-lactamase from RP1 to the E. coli chromosome. Soon after, Hedges and Jacob (7) isolated a series of plasmid derivatives which received type I APC resistance from RP4. These plasmids showed an increased molecular weight accompanying the change to APC resistance and, in turn, were able to translocate type I APC-resistance to other plasmids. This finding has been of considerable importance from the epidemiological view point of certain infectious diseases. The translocable sequence, i.e., the DNA translocable from RP4 to the derivative plasmids and including the structural information for the type I β-lactamase formation, was termed transposon A(TnA). TnA is capable of transposition from the replicon independently of the normal rec functions of the host cell.

Heffron et al. (8, 9) demonstrated that a sequence of DNA 2.7×10^6 to 3×10^6 daltons in size is common to naturally occurring plasmids of a variety of compatibility groups that specify type I-mediated APC resistance. APC resistance residues in a 3×10^6-dalton DNA segment, TnA, which is bounded by inverted complementary sequences of about 140 bp. Like IS sequences, insertions of TnA are mutagenic and occur, without circular permutation, in two different orientations. Insertions in one orientation are strongly polar on distal gene expression, whereas insertion in the other orientation is less polar and may have a promoter effect (8).

Furthermore, TnA insertion occurs independently of the *E. coli recA* function (15). For example, Tn4 (isolated from R1*drd*) is able to insert into 19 distinct sites on the genome of one of the nonconjugative plasmids, RSF1010. Insertion is non-random, suggesting that Tn4 may recognize a specific, but fairly common, nucleotide sequence at or near the site of insertion into the recipient genome. These results were supported by other transposons TnA suggesting that transposons TnA are able to insert into several sites on the DNA replicon. Several transposons TnA have been reported in many papers (10). Recently Yamamoto *et al.* (34) reported that Tn2601 and Tn2062, which are carried by Rms212 and Rms325, respectively, are about 4,700 base pair long APC transposons encoding so called type I PCase and share a high degree of DNA sequence homology with each other. Electron microscopic examination of denatured DNAs containing Tn2601 or Tn2602 reveals that both transposons TnA have inverted repeat sequences at the ends of them which are similar to other known transposons. Both the transposons are very similar to the known APC transposon, Tn3, in size, endonuclease cleavage sites, and possesion of a short inverted repeat sequence at both ends. Differences in the cleavage pattern among the three transposons were observed in the region around the BamHI site which is assumed to be a part of the repressor gene for a transposon.

Epidemiological studies show that transposition of antibiotic resistance in nature has played a key role in the evolution of R plasmids. Indeed, we isolated several plasmids which encoded type II and type IV β-lactamases isolated from our stock cultures. Then we tested the APC-resistance genes on R plasmids (Katsu *et al.*, in preparation; Nakazawa *et al.*, in preparation). APC-resistance mediated by type II PCase plasmid was transposed to pACYC184 and isolated different mutants which carried either the CM- or TC-resistance gene together with APC resistance. Sometimes, APC resistance was translocated on *E. coli* host chromosome. Katsu *et al.* have collected type IV PCase mediated by R plasmids and tested the compatibility groups of those plasmids. Type IV PCases were determined by R plasmids of compatibility groups P, V, and W. These data suggested that even type IV PCase would be translocated from one replicon to other. They found that type IV PCases were translocated to plasmids, such as pACYC184, pCR1, and pSC101. However, both type II and type IV PCase transposons were always accompanied by SM and SA resistance, that is, Tn*Ap.Sm.Su*. The molecular weight of these transposons is about 11×10^6 daltons.

NEWLY INTRODUCED β-LACTAM ANTIBIOTICS

It is well known that β-lactam antibiotics have been used for bacterial infections

TABLE XIII.   Chemical Structures of Newly Introduced Penicillins

Penicillins		R_1	R_2
Apalcillin (PC-904)	(APL)		-COONa
Piperacillin (T-1220)	(PIP)		-COONa
Talampicillin	(TAP)[a]		

[a] Oral administration.

and have shown excellent effectiveness in clinical medicine. However, the incidence of infections caused by bacteria resistant to known β-lactam antibiotics has increased recently, and therefore, it has been necessary to develop new β-lactam antibiotics which have potent antibacterial activity, a broader antibacterial spectrum, and effectiveness against resistant bacteria. Recently, many β-lactam antibiotics have been introduced and we have investigated their antibacterial activities and biochemical properties. Newly introduced β-lactam antibiotics have broadened their antibacterial spectra and have become effective even against *P. aeruginosa* and *S. marcescens*. Apalcillin (APL) and piperacillin (PIP) are APC derivatives (Table XIII) and are highly active against *P. aeruginosa* (Fig. 6). The chemical structures of newly introduced cephalosporins are shown in Table XIV and their activities against *P. aeruginosa* indicate the chemotherapeutic effectiveness due to broad spectra and high antibacterial activities (Fig. 7). Cephamycin derivatives (Table XV) are known to be resistant to β-lactamases but are less active against *P. aeurginosa* than other β-lactam antibiotics.

Moxalactam (MXA, 6059-S) is characteristic in its chemical structure and is stable to β-lactamases due to the presence of a 7-methoxy group (Table XVI). MXA is highly active and has a broad spectrum except against *P. aeruginosa* (Fig. 8). It should be noted that thienamycin (THM, MK-0787) is quite stable to β-lactamases and highly active against gram-positive and gram-negative bacteria. A comparison of the antibacterial activities of newly introduced drugs are shown in Figs. 6–9.

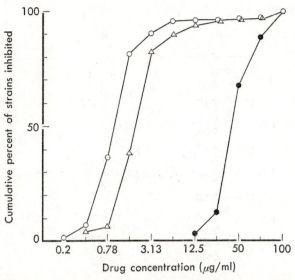

FIG. 6.   Antibacterial activities of penicillins against *P. aeruginosa* strains. Clinical isolates of 580 *P. aeruginosa* strains were used.   ○ APL; △ PIP; ● CPC.

TABLE XIV.   Chemical Structures of Newly Introduced Cephalosporins

Cephalosporins	R_1	R_2	R_3
Cefamandole (CMD)	⟨phenyl⟩–CHCO– | OH	–CH₂S–⟨tetrazole N—N/N-N, CH₃⟩	–COONa
Cefsulodin (CFS) (SCE-129)	⟨phenyl⟩–CHCO– | SO₃Na	–CH₂–N⁺⟨pyridine⟩–CONH₂	–COO⁻
Cefotiam (CTM) (SCE-963)	⟨aminothiazole H₂N⟩–CH₂CO–	–CH₂S–⟨tetrazole⟩ ·2HCl, CH₂CH₂N(CH₃)₂	–COOH
Cefuroxime (CXM)	⟨furan O⟩–C-CO– | N | OCH₃	–CH₂OCONH₂	–COONa
Cefotaxime (CTX) (HR-756)	⟨aminothiazole H₂N⟩–C-CO– | N | OCH₃	–CH₂OCOCH₃	–COONa

TABLE XIV. (continued)

Cephalosporins	R_1	R_2	R_3
Ceftizoxime (CZX) (FK-749)	(aminothiazole-methoxyimino group, HN= form) N—C-CO-, N-OCH$_3$	-H	-COONa
Cefmenoxime (CMT) (SCE-1365)	H$_2$N—thiazole—C-CO-, N-OCH$_3$	-CH$_2$S-(1-methyltetrazol-5-yl) ·1/2HCl	-COOH
Ro 13-9904	H$_2$N—thiazole—C-CO-, N-OCH$_3$	-CH$_2$S-(2-methyl-5-oxo-6-oxo-triazinyl)-ONa ·3.5H$_2$O	-COONa
GR-20263	H$_2$N—thiazole—C-CO-, N-O-C(CH$_3$)$_2$-COONa	-CH$_2$-N$^+$(pyridinium)	-COO$^-$
Cefoperazone (CFP) (T-1551)	H$_5$C$_2$-N(2,3-dioxopiperazine)N-CONHCHCO- (p-hydroxyphenyl, OH)	-CH$_2$S-(1-methyltetrazol-5-yl)	-COONa
SM-1652	(4-hydroxy-2-methylpyridine-5-carbonyl) OH, H$_3$C-pyridine-CONHCHCO- (p-hydroxyphenyl, OH)	-CH$_2$S-(1-methyltetrazol-5-yl)	-COONa
E-0702	(6,7-dihydroxy-4-oxo-chromone-3-)CONHCHCO- (p-hydroxyphenyl, OH), HO, HO	-CH$_2$S-(1-carboxymethyltetrazol-5-yl) CH$_2$COONa	-COONa
AC-1370	NaOOC-(imidazole,NH)-CONHCHCO-(phenyl)	-CH$_2$-N$^+$(pyridinium)-CH$_2$CH$_2$SO$_3^-$	-COONa
Cefroxadine (CXD)[a] (CGP-9000)	(phenyl)-CHCO-, NH$_2$	-OCH$_3$·2H$_2$O	-COOH
Cefaclor (CCL)[a]	(phenyl)-CHCO-, NH$_2$	-Cl	-COOH

[a] Oral administration.

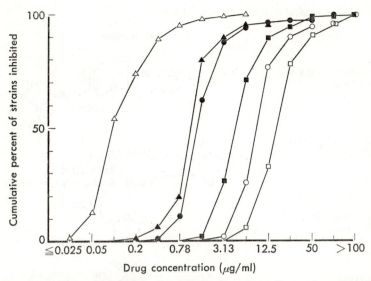

Fig. 7.   Antibacterial activities of cephalosporins against *P. aeruginosa* strains. Clinical isolates of 1,260 *P. aeruginosa* strains were used.   △ E-0702;   ▲ CFS; ● SM-1652; ▆ CFP; ○ CMT; □ CTX.

TABLE XV.   Chemical Structures of Cephamycins

Cephamycin	R_1	R_2	R_3
Cefoxitin (CFX)	$\boxed{}_S\!-CH_2CO-$	$-CH_2OCONH_2$	$-COONa$
Cefmetazole (CMZ)	$N\equiv C-CH_2-S-CH_2CO-$	$-CH_2S-\!\!\begin{smallmatrix}N-N\\N-N\\CH_3\end{smallmatrix}$	$-COONa$
YM-09330	$\begin{smallmatrix}NaOOC\\H_2NOC\end{smallmatrix}\!C\!=\!C\!\begin{smallmatrix}S\\S\end{smallmatrix}\!CHCO-$	$-CH_2S-\!\!\begin{smallmatrix}N-N\\N-N\\CH_3\end{smallmatrix}$	$-COONa$

As shown in Table XVII, CEZ is only effective against 50% of *E. coli* and *K. pneumoniae* strains, and CPC is active toward *E. coli* and *Proteus* strains. The ID_{50} value of CPC against recent isolates of *P. aeruginosa* strains was about 50 $\mu g/ml$.

TABLE XVI. Chemical Structure of New β-Lactams

Drug	Chemical structure
Moxalactam (MXA) (6059-S)	
Thienamycin (THM) (MK-0787)	R : NH$_2$, THM R : NHCH=NH , MK-0787
Clavulanic acid (CVA)	
CP-45899	
Carpetimycin (CPM)	R : H ,CPM-A R : SO$_3$H , CPM-B
PS-5	

Other newly introduced drugs, *i.e.*, CZX, CMT, CTX, MKA, and YM-09330, were effective against most genera of gram-negative bacteria except *P. aeruginosa* strains. It should be noted that newly introduced β-lactam antibiotics effective toward gram-negative organisms are less active against gram-positive bacteria than CEZ, PCG, and APC. From the effectiveness of β-lactam antibiotics, therefore, three groups of bacteria, *i.e.*, gram-negative bacteria including *P. aeruginosa*, gram-negative organisms except *P. aeruginosa*, and gram-positive bacteria, exist in clinical isolates, whose bacterial cell wall structures cause the difference in the effectiveness of β-lactam antibiotics.

As shown in Table XVIII, the MIC_{90} values of CFP, THM, APL, and PIP indicate that effectiveness of these drugs toward *P. aeruginosa* strains. However, the MIC_{90} values of APL and PIP tell us of the presence of organisms resistant to these drugs due to their lability to PCases. By contrast, the MIC_{90} values of CZX, CMT,

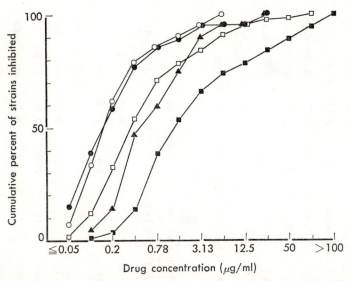

FIG. 8.   Antibacterial activities of new β-lactam antibiotics against *S. marcescens* strains.
Clinical isolates of 540 *S. marcescens* strains were used.   ● CZX; ○ CMT; □ CTX;
▲ MXA; ■ YM-09330.

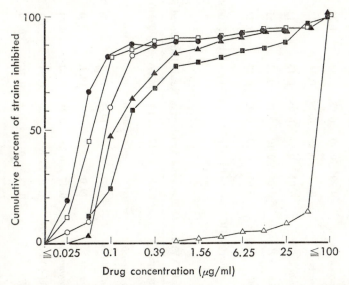

FIG. 9.   Antibacterial activities of new β-lactam antibiotics against *E. cloacae.*
Clinical isolates of 520 *E. cloacae* strains were used.   ● CZX; □ CTX; ▲ MXA;
○ CMT; ■ CFP; △ CEZ.

TABLE XVII.   Antibacterial Activities of Newly Introduced β-Lactam Antibiotics against Clinical Isolates of Bacteria

Organism	CZX	CMT	CTX	MXA	YM-09330	CFP	MK-0787	GR-20263	AC-1370	E-0702	APL	PIP
P. aeruginosa	24.3	8.70	14.3	25.7	100	3.60	0.8	2.05	6.0	0.09	1.39	2.95
S. marcescens	0.29	0.30	0.88	0.84	1.27	4.40	0.2	0.25	3.6	0.10	89.0	5.15
E. cloacae	0.32	0.16	0.29	0.16	3.13	0.16	0.15	0.42	2.6	0.27	5.20	4.10
K. pneumoniae	0.03	0.09	0.05	0.13	0.13	0.21	0.1	0.18	2.5	0.02	6.0	8.10
Indole(+) Proteus	0.05	0.10	0.11	0.13	0.51	1.80	0.5	0.08	0.6	0.10	0.94	0.81
E. coli	0.05	0.10	0.07	0.13	0.28	0.19	0.05	0.32	2.3	0.01	1.47	1.70

Data indicate MIC_{50} values (μg/ml) of each drug.   About 500 strains were used as test organisms in each species of bacteria.

TABLE XVIII.   Antibacterial Activities of Newly Introduced β-Lactam Antibiotics against Clinical Isolates of Bacteria

Organism	CZX	CMT	CTX	MXA	YM-09330	CFP	MK-0787	GR-20263	AC-1370	E-0702	APL	PIP
P. aeruginosa	>100	48.5	48.0	50	>100	12.7	1.56	8.3	20.0	0.45	5.0	7.5
S. marcescens	5.80	3.9	14.2	16.7	55.0	96.0	0.8	0.5	100	56.0	>100	>100
E. cloacae	79.0	25.0	47.0	19.1	75.0	30.3	0.2	20.0	50.0	2.2	>100	>100
K. pneumoniae	0.17	0.28	0.28	0.40	0.24	5.32	0.1	0.79	47.5	0.20	>100	>100
Indole(+) Proteus	1.25	1.5	1.5	0.34	5.3	7.57	1.56	3.10	30.0	1.0	3.0	27.0
E. coli	0.18	0.2	0.2	0.36	0.54	3.43	0.07	1.47	23.8	0.10	>100	>100

Data indicate MIC_{90} values (μg/ml) of each drug that are required to inhibit the growth of 90% of isolates.   About 500 strains were used as test organisms in each species of bacteria.

TABLE XIX. Antibacterial Spectrum of β-Lactam Antibiotics

Organism	Cephalosporin	Penicillin	New β-lactam
Gram-negative bacteria including *P. aeruginosa*	CFP, SM-1652 GR-20263, AC-1370 E-0702	APL, PIP	THM
Gram-negative bacteria except for *P. aeruginosa*	CMD, CTM, CMT CXM, CTX, CZX Cephamycins RO 13-9904	TIC	MXA, CPM
P. aeruginosa	CFS		

CTX, MXA, YM-09330, CFP, and THM indicate the effectiveness of these drugs toward *K. pneumoniae, Proteus,* and *E. coli* strains due to their resistance to β-lactamases. It should be noted that CZX, CMT, CTX, MXA, and THM are effective against 90% of *S. marcescens* strains.

The antibacterial spectra of new β-lactams can be classified into three groups (28): (1) gram-negative bacteria including *P. aeruginosa*, (2) gram-negative bacteria except for *P. aeruginosa*, and (3) active only against *P. aeruginosa*. THM, PIP, APL, SM-1652, E-0702, AC-1370, and cefoperazone belong to group I, with broader antibacterial spectra and potent antipseudomonal activity. Other compounds (group 2) have broader spectra than known β-lactam antibiotics but are less active against *P. aeruginosa*. It should be noted that cefsulodine (SCE-129) is active only against *P. aeruginosa* strains. These results indicate that *P. aeruginosa* has a specific cell wall structure which prevents the penetrability of drugs (Table XIX).

β-Lactam antibiotics have been used extensively owing to their low toxicity resulting from the biochemical mechanism of their antibacterial activity. Accordingly, bacterial strains resistant to β-lactams have appeared and spread all over the world. β-Lactam resistance was found to be due mainly to two biochemical mechanisms: (1) a decrease in penetrability of the drug into bacterial cells; and (2) the formation of β-lactamase (see p. 41). PCase production was mediated by conjugative(R) or nonconjugative(r) resistance plasmids or by transposons. The findings of drug resistance plasmids and APC transposons have disclosed the rapid spread of strains resistant to β-lactams. CSase production in gram-negative bacilli is chromosomally mediated (see p. 44). Therefore, highly β-lactam-resistant strains of gram-negative bacteria are known to be due to the presence of two types of β-lactamase, *i.e.*, chromosomally mediated CSase and plasmid-mediated PCase.

The newly introduced β-lactams have been shown to have broader antibacterial spectra and potent activities against various species of bacteria which are often seen in clinical specimens. However, the 50-year history of antibiotics tells us the appearance of bacteria resistant to new β-lactams occurs in parallel with the use of these antibiotics.

REFERENCES

1. Abraham, E. P., Chain, E., Fletcher, C. M., Florey, H. W., Gardner, A. D., Heatley, N. G., and Jennings, M. A. 1941. *Lancet*, ii, 177–181.
2. Datta, N., Hedges, R. W., Show, E. J., Sykes, R., and Richmond M. H. 1971. *J. Bacteriol.*, **108**, 1244–1249.
3. Egawa, R., Sawai, T., and Mitsuhashi, S. 1967. *Japan. J. Microbiol.*, **11**, 173–178.
4. Harada, K., Kameda, M., Suzuki, M., and Mitsuhashi, S. 1963. *J. Bacteriol.*, **86**, 1332–1338.
5. Harada, K., Kameda, M., Suzuki, M., and Mitsuhashi, S. 1965. *J. Bacteriol.*, **88**, 1257–1265.
6. Hedges, R. W., Datta, N., Kontomichalou, P., and Smith, J. T. 1974. *J. Bacteriol.*, **117**, 56–62.
7. Hedges, R. W. and Jacob, A. 1974. *Mol. Gen. Genet.*, **132**, 31–41.
8. Heffron, F. Rubens, C., and Falkow, S. 1975. *Proc. Natl. Acad. Sci. U.S.A.*, **72**, 72, 3623–3627.
9. Heffron, F., Sublett, R., Hedges, R. W., Jacob, A., and Falkow, S. 1975. *J. Bacteriol.*, **122**, 250–256.
10. Heffron, F., Rubens, C., and Falkow, S. 1977. *In* "DNA Insertion Elements, Plasmids, and Episomes," ed. by A. I. Bukhari, J. A. Shapiro, and S. L. Adhya, Cold Spring Harbor Lab., New York, p. 161.
11. Hosoya, S., Mitsuhashi, S., Nomura, T., and Soeda, M. 1947. *Penicillin*, **1**, 1–5.
12. Inoue, M. and Mitsuhashi, S. 1980. *In* "Bacterial Drug Resistance—R Plasmids," ed. by S. Mitsuhashi, Kodansha, Tokyo, pp. 19–29.
13. Kondo, E. and Mitsuhashi, S. 1964. *J. Bacteriol.*, **88**, 1266–1276.
14. Kondo, E. and Mitsuhashi, S. 1966. *J. Bacteriol.*, **91**, 1787–1794.
15. Kopecko, D. J. and Choen, S. 1975. *Proc. Natl. Acad. Sci. U.S.A.*, **72**, 1373.
16. Maclean, I. H., Rogers, K. B., and Fleming, A. 1939. *Lancet*, i, 562–568.
17. Mitsuhashi, S., Morimura, M., Kono, M., and Oshima, H. 1963. *J. Bacteriol.*, **86**, 162–164.
18. Mitsuhashi, S., Oshima, H., Kawarada, U., and Hashimoto, H. 1965. *J. Bacteriol.*, **89**, 967–976.
19. Mitsuhashi, S. 1971. *In* "The Problems of Drug-resistant Pathogenic Bacteria," ed. by E. L. Dulaney and A. I. Laskin, New York Acad. Sci., New York, pp. 141–152.
20. Mitsuhashi, S., Inoue, M., Kawabe, H., Oshima, H., and Okubo, T. 1973. *In* "Contributions to Microbiology and Immunology, Staphylococci and Staphylococcal Infections," ed. by J. Jeljaszewicz, Karger, Basel, Vol. 1 pp. 144–165.
21. Mitsuhashi, S., Inoue, M., Fuse, A., Kaneko, Y., and Oba, T. 1974. *Japan. J. Microbiol.*, **18**, 98–99.
22. Mitsuhashi, S., Inoue, M., Oshima, H., Okubo, T., and Saito, T. 1976. *In*

"Staphylococci and Staphylococcal Diseases," ed. by J. Jeljaszewicz, Gustav Fisher Verlag, Stuttgart and New York, pp. 267–278.

23. Mitsuhashi, S. 1977. *In* "R Factor—Drug Resistance Plasmid," ed. by S. Mitsuhashi, Japan Sci. Soc. Press, Tokyo/Univ. Park Press, Baltimore, pp. 3–48.

24. Mitsuhashi, S. 1977. *In* "R Factor—Drug Resistance Plasmid," ed. by S. Mitsuhashi, Japan Sci. Soc. Press, Tokyo/Univ. Park Press, Baltimore, pp. 73–88.

25. Mitsuhashi, S., Hashimoto, H., Iyobe, S., and Inoue, M. 1977. *In* "DNA Insertion Elements, Plasmids, and Episomes," ed. by A. I. Bukhari, J. A. Shapiro, and S. L. Adhya, Cold Spring Harbor Lab., New York, pp. 139–146.

26. Mitsuhashi, S. 1979. *Mol. Cell Biochem.*, **26**, 135–180.

27. Mitsuhashi, S. 1980. *In* "Bacterial Drug Resistance—R Plasmid," ed. by S. Mitsuhashi, Kodansha, Tokyo, pp. 6–15.

28. Mitsuhashi, S. and Inoue M. 1981. "New β-Lactam Antibiotics: Antibacterial Activities and Inducibility," Academic Press, New York, in press.

29. Murray, R., Kilham, L., Wilcox, C., and Finland, M. 1964. *Proc. Soc. Exp. Biol. Med.*, **63**, 470–474.

30. Nakae, M., Murai, T., Kaneko, Y., and Mitsuhashi, S. 1977. *Antimicrob. Agents Chemother.*, **12**, 427–428.

31. Nakae, M., Inoue, M., and Mitsuhashi, S. 1980. *In* "Bacterial Drug Resistance—R Plasmid," ed. by S. Mitsuhashi, Kodansha, Tokyo, pp. 43–46.

32. Nake, M., Matsumoto, K., Saito, K., and Mitsuhashi, S. 1981. *Microbiol. Immunol.*, in press.

33. Richmond, M. H. and Sykes, R. B. 1972. *Genet. Res.*, **20**, 885.

34. Yamamoto, T., Katoh, R., Shimazu, A., and Yamagishi, S. 1980. *Microbiol. Immunol.*, **24**, 479.

3 BIOCHEMICAL MECHANISMS OF RESISTANCE

MECHANISMS OF RESISTANCE TO β-LACTAM ANTIBIOTICS

Susumu Mɪᴛsᴜʜᴀsʜɪ and Matsuhisa Iɴᴏᴜᴇ

Department of Microbiology, Laboratory of Bacterial Resistance
*School of Medicine, Gunma University**

The introduction of chemotherapeutic agents into practical medicine, livestock farming, and the fish culturing industry has brought about emergence of resistant bacteria, which are of prime importance in medicine and pharmaceutical science. Epidemiological studies have disclosed that resistance to β-lactam antibiotics is mainly due to the production of β-lactamases by resistant organisms (*1*, *2*), and to a decrease in the permeability of the drugs into bacterial cells.

β-LACTAMASE

β-Lactamases are classified into three groups according to their substrate profiles, *i.e.*, penicillin β-lactamase (PCase), cephalosporine β-lactamase (CSase), and cefuroxime (CXM) β-lactamase (CXase) (*3*) (Table I).

Recently, new β-lactam antibiotics have been synthesized and we have had a chance to study their antibacterial spectra, antibacterial activities, and resistance to inactivation by β-lactamases (*3*). Accordingly, these newly introduced drugs have enabled us to study the enzymological properties of β-lactamases in more detail.

1. Penicillinases (PCase)

Genetic and epidemiological studies have disclosed that the genes (*bla*) governing the formation of PCases are mostly located on plasmids or are mediated by transposons. According to their substrate profiles, they are classified into five types, *i.e.*, types, I, II, III, IV, and V (Table II). Most of the PCases mediated by plasmids are of type I.

The formation of PCases is mostly constitutive except for *Staphylococcus aureus* PCase. The substrate profiles of PCases are shown in Fig. 1. Type I PCase (TEM type, 5) hydrolyzes penicillin G (PCG), ampicillin (APC), 6-aminopenicillanic acid

---

* Showa-machi 3-39-22, Maebashi 371, Japan.

TABLE I. Classification of β-Lactamases

Group	Type	Localization of bla gene	Organism	Inducibility of β-lactamase formation	Classification by M.H. Richmond (4)
PCase	PCase I	R plasmid	Gram-negative bacteria	c	Class IIIa (TEM type)
		r plasmid	Neisseria gonorrhoeae	c	
			Haemophilus influenzae	c	
	PCase II	R plasmid	Gram-negative bacteria	c	Class Va/b
	PCase III	R plasmid	Gram-negative bacteria	c	
	PCase IV	R plasmid	Gram-negative bacteria	c	Class Vc
	PCase V	r plasmid	S. aureus	i(c)	Class Ia
CSase		Host chromosome	Gram-negative bacteria	i(c)	Class Ib, Ic, and Id
					Class II
CXase		Host chromosome	B. fragilis	c	
			P. vulgaris	i	
			P. cepacia	i	

i, inducible; c, constitutive.

TABLE II. Substrate Profiles of PCases

β-Lactamase produced by	Type of PCase	Relative rate of hydrolysis (V_{max})							
		PCG	APC	CPC	CLX	PPC	PIP	APL	CER
E. coli W3630/Rms212	Type I	100	115	11	2	32	89	64	130
E. coli W3630/Rms213	Type II	100	454	40	292	155	118	133	263
E. coli W3630/Rte16	Type III	100	131	54	310	413	90	85	23
P. aeruginosa M1/Rms 139	Type IV	100	105	110	2	84	5	47	20
S. aureus MS258/rMS258	Type V	100	194	50	1	90	430	180	10

Hydrolysis of each substrate is expressed as the relative rate of hydrolysis, taking the absolute rate of PCG as 100. R, conjugative resistance plasmid; r, nonconjugative resistance plasmid.

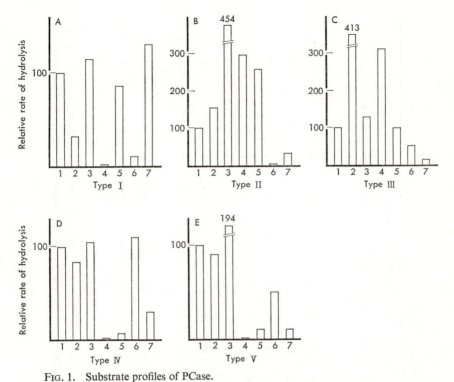

FIG. 1.   Substrate profiles of PCase.
Hydrolysis of each substrate is expressed as the relative rate of hydrolysis, taking the absolute rate of PCG. A: *E. coli* W3630/Rms212. B: *E. coli* W3630/Rms213. C: *E. coli* W3630/Rte 16. D: *P. aeruginosa* M1/Rms139. E: *S. aureus*/rMS258. R, conjugative resistance plasmid; r, nonconjugative resistance plasmid. Substrates. 1, PCG; 2, pheneticillin; 3, APC; 4, cloxacillin; 5, 6-APA; 6, CPC; 7, cephaloridine.

(6-APA), and cephaloridine (CER) at a high rate. Type II and type III PCases are characteristic in hydrolyzing cloxacillin (CLX) at a high rate, and are called cloxacillin-hydrolyzing enzymes. Type IV PCase is a carbenicillin(CPC)-hydrolyzing enzyme. Each type of PCase is immunologically specific (see below).

2.   Cephalosporinase (CSase)

Gram-negative bacteria without plasmids produce chromosome-mediated β-lactamases. The substrate profiles are almost the same in each organism belonging to the same species. Representative results are shown in Fig. 2. One organism was selected from each species of bacteria and the enzyme was purified by column chromatography. All purified enzymes have a single protein band upon polyacrylamide gel electrophoretic analysis. The substrate profiles are shown in Talbe III. The enzymes produced by *Escherichia coli, Enterobacter cloacea, Citrobacter freundii, Serratia marcescens,*

TABLE III.   Substrate Profiles of Chromosome-mediated β-Lactamases

β-Lactamases produced by	Relative rate of hydrolysis (V_{max})[a]															
	CER	CET	CEZ	CEX	CMD	CTM	CFS	CFP	SM-1652	CXM	CTX	CZX	CMT	CFX	PCG	APC
CSase																
E. coli GN5482	100	269	311	29	5	88	<1	4	<1	<1	<1	<1	<1	<1	63	<1
E. cloacae GN7471	100	189	100	14	<1	29	<1	1	<1	<1	<1	<1	<1	<1	12	<1
C. freundii GN7391	100	125	116	80	<1	8	<1	1	<1	<1	<1	<1	<1	<1	3	<1
S. marcescens GN10857	100	88	198	6	<1	16	<1	2	9	<1	<1	<1	<1	<1	3	<1
P. retigeri GN4430	100	85	99	8	<1	4	<1	<1	<1	<1	<1	<1	<1	<1	3	<1
P. morganii GN5407	100	46	20	4	<1	8	<1	<1	<1	<1	<1	<1	<1	<1	16	<1
P. aeruginosa GN10362	100	139	222	64	<1	12	<1	5	<1	<1	<1	<1	<1	<1	29	<1
CXase																
P. vulgaris GN7919	100	173	387	274	278	222	9	15	12	1,140	84	<1	39	<1	20	12
P. cepacia GN11164	100	323	156	58	452	161	161	10	15	239	174	29	97	<1	161	323
B. fragilis GN11478	100	81	60	<1	6	8	3	7	5	50	7	2	3	<1	3	<1

a Hydrolysis rate of substrates is expressed in percent hydrolysis of CER. V_{max}, maximum rate of hydrolysis. Maximum rate of hydrolysis (relative V_{max}) is expressed in μmol of substrate hydrolyzed per min per mg of enzyme and was determined from Lineweaver-Burke plots.

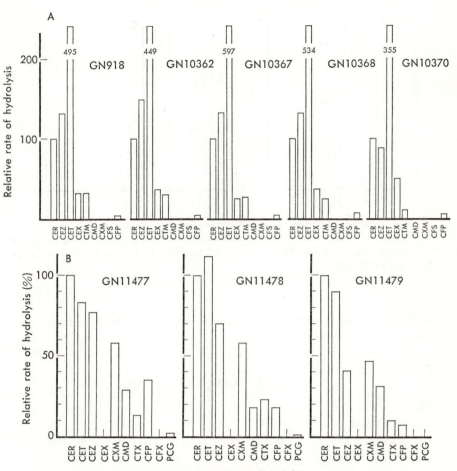

FIG. 2.   Substrate profiles of chromosome-mediated β-lactamases.
Hydrolysis of each substrate is expressed as the relative rate of hydrolysis, taking the
absolute rate of CER as 100. A: *P. aeruginosa* strains. B: *B. fragilis* strains.

Proteus rettgeri, P. morganii, and *Pseudomonas aeruginosa* easily hydrolyzed CER, cephalothin (CET), cefazolin (CEZ), cephalexin (CEX), cefotiam (CTM), and PCG. On the contrary, the newly introduced drugs such as CXM, cefamandole (CMD), cefsulodine (CFS), cefotaxime (CTX), cefoperazone (CFP), SM-1652, and cefoxitine (CFX) were stable to inactivation by these enzymes. Penicillins such as APC, CPC, and CLX were quite stable to these enzymes, indicating that these enzymes are of the CSase type.

The enzymes produced by *Proteus vulgaris, Pseudomonas cepacia,* and *Bacteroides fragilis* had a unique substrate profile and hydrolyzed the new cephalosphorins in-

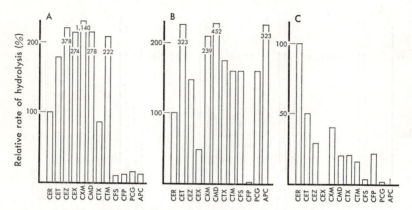

FIG. 3. Substrate profiles of chromosome-mediated cefuroximases. Hydrolysis of each substrate is expressed as the relative rate of hydrolysis, taking the absolute rate of CER as 100. A: *P. vulgaris* GN7919. B: *P. cepacia* GN11164. C: *B. fragilis* GN11477.

TABLE IV. Inhibitor Constants for the Hydrolysis of Cephalothin by β-Lactamases in the Presence of Various β-Lactam Antibiotics

β-Lactamases produced by	K_i (μM)					
	CXM	CTX	CZX	APC	CPC	CLX
CSase						
E. coli GN5482	0.04	0.13	0.73	2.60	0.35	0.01
E. cloacae GN7471	0.18	0.05	1.15	15.00	0.48	0.02
C. freundii GN7391	0.001	N.T.	0.035	0.044	0.005	0.0006
S. marcescens GN10857	0.49	3.36	7.70	0.02	0.13	0.001
P. rettgeri GN4430	10.00	2.07	1.02	0.2	1.39	0.30
P. morganii GN5407	0.05	0.07	0.24	1.00	0.01	0.0015
P. aeruginosa GN10362	0.003	0.27	2.00	10.00	1.50	0.006
CXase						
P. vulgaris GN7919	—	—	—	1.20	0.85	0.20
P. cepacia GN11164	—	—	—	—	—	3.40
B. fragilis GN11477	—	—	—	0.60	0.60	0.40

Dissociation constants for enzyme-inhibitor complexes were determined from both Lineweaver-Burke and Dixon plots with CER as a substrate.

TABLE V. Kinetic Constants for the Hydrolysis of Cephaloridine or Cephalothin by β-Lactamases in the Presence of Inhibitors

Enzyme source		K_m (μM)	K_i (μM)[b]						
			CVA	CP-45899	CFX	CMZ	YM-09330	MXA	MK-0787
CSase									
E. coli GN5482		63	—	—	0.11	0.57	0.22	0.86	0.84
E. cloacae GN7471		105	—	—	0.50	0.64	0.22	0.81	0.95
C. freundii GN7391		16	—	—	0.33	0.19	0.09	0.07	0.78
S. marcescens GN10857		44	—	—	0.15	0.39	0.44	13.0	0.39
P. aeruginosa GN10362		71	—	—	0.23	0.10	0.15	0.39	3.13
P. rettgeri GN4430		125	—	—	0.34	4.31	3.64	102	0.68
P. morganii GN5407		33	—	—	0.22	0.40	0.11	0.16	0.95
CXase									
P. vulgaris GN7919		61	1.07	0.91	12.40	5.22	13.30	107	0.40
P. cepacia GN11164		70	1.72	1.82	—	—	—	—	2.55
B. fragilis GN11477		100	0.20	0.30	0.50	0.20	0.20	0.10	0.02
PCase									
E. coli W3630/Rms212	(type I)	400[a]	0.47	0.47	—	—	—	—	1.42
E. coli W3630/Rms213	(type II)	333[a]	18.30	154	245	116	8.53	16.70	1.02
E. coli W3630/Rte16	(type III)	83[a]	21.70	3.57	16.70	2.74	1.02	27.80	0.03
P. aeruginosa M1/Rms139	(type IV)	111[a]	2.50	0.73	—	—	—	—	—

Enzyme activity was photometrically determined and CET was used as a substrate. —, not inhibited. [a] CER was used as a substrate. [b] The reaction was run without preincubation with inhibitor.

cluding CXM, CTX, ceftizoxime (CZX), and cefumenoxime (CMX). The enzymes produced by these three organisms are called cefuroxime-hydrolyzing β-lactamase (CXase). In addition to known cephalosporins, CMD, CFS, CFP, and SM-1652 were easily hydrolyzed by these enzymes, indicating their broad substrate profiles (Fig. 3). It should be noted that these enzymes are inhibited by clavulanic acid (CVA) and CP-45899, which are known to be PCase inhibitors (see below).

New cephalosporins, *i.e.*, CXM, CTX, CZX, *etc.* had low K_i values against the CET-hydrolyzing activities of CSases produced by various gram-negative rods. However, CXM, CTX, and CZX were easily hydrolyzed by CXases and could not inhibit the CET-hydrolyzing activities of CXases. Ampicillin, CPC, and CLX has low K_i values against the CET-hydrolyzing activities of both CSases and CXases (Table IV).

β-Lactamase inhibitors, *i.e.*, CVA and CP-45899 could not inhibit CSase activities. But they could inhibit CXase and PCase (types I and IV) activities (Table V).

As shown in Table V, the cephamycin group β-lactams could inhibit CSase activities except for *P. rettgeri* CSase and they inhibited *B. fragilis* CXase. It should

TABLE VI.   Physicochemical Properties of β-Lactamases

β-Lactamases produced by	M.W.	Opt. temperature (°C)	Opt. pH	pI
CSase				
E. coli	39,000	40	8.0	8.7
E. cloacae	44,000	40	8.5	8.4
C. freundii	37,000	45	8.0	8.6
S. marcescens	38,000	40	8.0	8.9
P. aeruginosa	37,000	40	8.0	8.7
P. rettgeri	42,000	50	8.0	8.7
P. morganii	42,000	40	8.5	8.7
CXase				
P. vulgaris	30,000	45	7.0	8.8
P. cepacia	24,000	45	8.0	9.3
B. fragilis	32,000	37	7.2	4.9
PCase				
PCase type I[a]	20,600	45	7.0	5.4
PCase type II[a]	23,300	35	7.6	8.3
PCase type III[a]	46,000	40	7.5	8.3
PCase type IV[b]	21,000	45	7.5	5.7
PCase type V[c]	29,600	N.T.	5.9	8.7

[a] Host, *E. coli* W3630.   [b] Host, *P. aeruginosa* M1.   [c] Host, *S. aureus* MS258.

be noted that MK-0787 is rather stable to all types of β-lactamase including CSase, CXase, and PCase and has a high inhibitory activity against the hydrolysis of CER or CET by CSases, CXases, and PCases.

The physicochemical properties of β-lactamases are summarized in Table VI. The molecular weights of CSases are between 37,000 and 44,000. Those of CXases and PCases are between 20,000 and 32,000, except for type III PCase. The pI values of *B. fragilis* CXase, types I and IV PCases are acidic. Those of the other β-lactamases are alkaline.

The K_m values of CSases and CXases are shown in Table VII. CSases have high K_m values toward CER, CEZ, and CET, but low K_m values toward CMD and CXM. By contrast, CXases have high K_m values against various β-lactams including CMD, CTM, and CXM.

TABLE VII. K_m values of Chromosome-mediated β-Lactamases

β-Lactamases produced by	K_m (μM)								
	CER	CET	CEZ	CEX	CMD	CTM	CFP	CXM	PCG
CSase									
E. coli GN5482	105	63	400	10	22	154	80	—	7
E. cloacae GN7471	570	105	800	61	6	100	250	—	10
C. freundii GN7391	58	3	450	6	—	—	—	—	—
S. marcescens GN10857	167	46	200	50	—	26	14	—	18
P. rettgeri GN4430	500	125	150	22	24	48	—	—	21
P. morganii GN5407	500.	37	83	6	33	19	167	—	26
P. aeruginosa GN10362	167	71	667	42	15	83	23	—	34
CXase									
P. vulgaris GN7919	61	56	54	357	278	222	28	769	N.T.
P. cepacia GN11164	70	71	40	30	183	133	—	105	47
B. fragilis GN11478	83	91	125	91	10	28	56	143	7

K_m values were expressed in μmol of substrate hydrolyzed per min per mg of enzyme protein and were determined from Lineweaver-Burke plots. N.T., not tested.

3. Immunological Properties of Purified β-Lactamases

Anti-β-lactamase rabbit sera were prepared by immunizing rabbits with purified β-lactamases and the effects of antibodies on the purified enzymes were studied by a neutralization curve using constant antigen titration. One of the representative results is shown in Fig. 4. The standard curve was obtained when increasing quantities of the antibody were added to a fixed quantity of the purified enzyme. The maximum

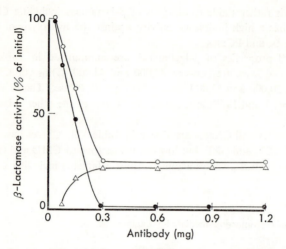

FIG. 4.   Neutralization curve obtained for titration of β-lactamase from C. freundii GN7391 with anti-GN7391 antibody (constant antigen titration). Purified enzyme (4 units) was incubated with various amounts of antibody at 37°C for 20 min and then left at 5°C for 18 hr. Portions of each reaction mixture were assayed for β-lactamase activity (○). The remaining reaction mixture was centrifuged at 6,000×g for 30 min to separate immunoprecipitates and supernatants. The precipitates were washed once with saline, and then the β-lactamase activities of the supernatant fractions (●) and suspended precipitates (△) were assayed.

degree of neutralization of the purified enzyme was approximately 80%, even when an excess of the antibody was used. The reaction mixture was centrifuged to separate the supernatants from the immunoprecipitates. The supernatants had no β-lactamase activity with an excess of antibody. The remaining enzyme activity (some 20% of the initial activity) was not due to the presence of a different kind of β-lactamase which was unreactive with the antibody, but rather due to precipitation of the antigen-antibody complex possessing some enzyme activity.

Plasmid-mediated PCases were purified and their immunological properties were examined. As shown in Table VIII, R-mediated PCases are immunologically specific and did not show any cross reaction with chromosome-mediated CSases or with CXases. However, the anti-type I (TEM) PCase antibody neutralized PCases from *Klebsiella pneumoniae* strains (50–75%), which are known to be PCase producers but not CSase producers. From these results, the possibility of the origin of the type I PCase gene on R plasmids was presented to be from *K. pneumoniae*.

Anti-CSase sera neutralized the CSase activity of the same species of bacteria (95–100%) but did not affect CSases from other species of bacteria at all (Table IX). There were no reactions with R plasmid-mediated PCases. Anti-*Bacteroides* enzyme sera neutralized the enzyme activities from *B. fragilis* and *B. thetaiotaomicron* strains

TABLE VIII. Immunological Properties of PCase

β-Lactamases produced by	Anti-serum against			
	PCase type I (Rms212)	PCase type II (Rms213)	PCase type III (Rte 16)	PCase type IV (Rms139)
E. coli W3630/Rms212 PCase type I	100	0	0	0
E. coli W3630/Rms213 PCase type II	0	98	0	0
E.coli W3630/Rte16 PCase type III	0	0	100	0
P. aeruginosa M1/Rms139 PCase type IV	0	0	0	82

Rabbits were immunized with purified β-lactamase.

TABLE IX. Inhibition of CPase Activity by Anti-CSase Serum

Enzyme source	Inhibition rate (%)	Enzyme source	Inhibition rate (%)
C. freundii GN7391[a]	100	P. cepacia GN11164[a]	100
GN299	97	GN11127	100
GN324	99	GN11152	94
GN346	96	GN11155	92
GN7093	100	P. aeruginosa GN10362[a]	100
GN7099	98	GN918	100
S. marcescens GN10857[a]	97	GN10367	100
GN7647	98	B. thetaiotaomicron GN11478[a]	100
GN10788	97	GN11484	91
GN10815	96	GN11483	77
P. vulgaris GN7919[a]	100	B. fragilis GN11477	85
GN76	96	GN11480	71
GN4413	98	GN11482	81
E. cloacae GN7471[a]	100	GN11479	67
GN7476	92	B. fragilis other GN11499	28
GN5797	100		

[a] Anti-CSase sera were produced by injecting rabbits with purified CSases prepared from each of the indicated strains.

(70–100%). These results indicate that the active sites of plasmid-mediated PCases and chromosome-mediated β-lactamases are immunologically specific and do not show any cross-reaction with each other, although β-lactamases are widely distributed among all species of bacteria.

TABLE X.   Neutralization of β-Lactamase Activities with Anti-β-lactamase Sera

β-Lactamases produced by	Neutralization of β-lactamase activities with anti-sera against (%)[a]			
	P. vulgaris GN7919 β-lactamase	C. freundii GN346 β-lactamase	E. cloacae GN7471 β-lactamase	E. coli GN5482 β-lactamase
P. vulgaris GN7919	100	0	0	0
GN76	96	0	0	0
GN4413	98	0	0	0
P. cepacia GN11164	87	0	0	0
GN11127	89	0	0	0
GN11152	90	0	0	0
GN11155	86	0	0	0
E. cloacae GN7471	0	92	100	6
GN7467	0	96	92	8
GN5797	0	92	100	0
E. coli GN5482	0	0	62	96
GN11754	0	0	65	100
C. freundii GN346	0	100	0	0
GN7391	0	100	0	0

[a] Neutralization of β-lactamase activity was expressed by the following equation: $a-b/b(\%)$. a, enzyme activity without antiserum; b, enzyme activity with antiserum.

It should be noted, however, that anti-sera against P. vulgaris, C. freundii, E. cloacae, and E. coli β-lactamases showed crossreactions, respectively, with β-lactamases from P. cepacia and E. cloacae strains (Table X). It is interesting to note that these cross reactions are only one-way and cannot reverse.

4.   Inducer Activity of β-Lactamase by β-Lactams

Penicillinase formation in S. aureus is inducible, but plasmid-mediated PCase formation is mostly constitutive. It is well known, however, that many gram-negative bacteria produce inducible and species-specific β-lactamase, i.e., CSase and CXase (Table I). The inducer activities of β-lactam antibiotics were investigated using E. cloacae GN5797 which produces a large amount of inducible CSase. The kinetics of CSase formation in E. cloacae GN5797 after the addition of an inducer were investigated. An overnight culture in broth was diluted 20-fold with fresh broth and incubated with shaking at 37°C. After 2 hr of incubation, an inducer (CFX) was added to a final concentration of 10 μg/ml. The induced cells were harvested by centrifugation at the indicated times after the addition of CFX, and the β-lactamase activities were determined (Fig. 5). Without the addition of an inducer, CSase

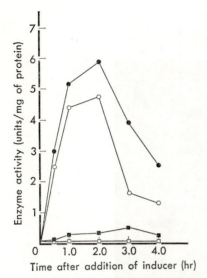

FIG. 5.   The kinetics of β-lactamase formation after addition of cefoxitin as an inducer.
○ at the start of incubation (lag phase);   ● 2 hr after incubation (mid-log phase);
■ 4 hr after incubation (stationary phase);   □ without inducer.

activity was almost undetectable during all phases of growth. The maximum specific activity was obtained 2 hr after the addition of an inducer to cells in the mid-log phase. Addition of the drug in the lag phase gave somewhat lower activity, and in the stationary phase, induction was at a very low degree.

To determine inducibility with β-lactam antibiotics, various concentrations of drugs were added to the culture at the mid log phase (about 10^9 cells/ml), and the cultures were incubated with shaking at 37°C for a further 2 hr before the organisms were harvested. Under these conditions most of the drugs showed little or no effect on the growth of E. cloacae GN5797 when their concentrations were less than 100 μg/ml. Many drugs repressed the growth of the culture or lysed the cells at 1,000 μg/ml, but methicillin (MTC), cloxacillin (CLX), PCG, CER, CEZ, CET, CEX, and CTM did not show any effect on the culture growth even at 1,000 μg/ml, probably due to the low penetrability of MTC and CLX and to the rapid enzyme hydrolysis of CER, CEZ, CET, CEX, CTM, and PCG.

The inducibility of CSase by β-lactam antibiotics in E. cloacae GN5797 is shown in Fig. 6. Based on their inducibility, the β-lactam antibiotics can be classified into three groups, i.e., with high (A), intermediate (B), or low (C) inducer activity. Ampicillin and cephamycin derivatives such as CFX, cefmetazole, YM09330, and moxalactam (MXA) showed high inducer activity, at lower concentrations than for CER, CEZ, CET, CEX, CTM, and PCG which are in the same group and easily hydrolyzed

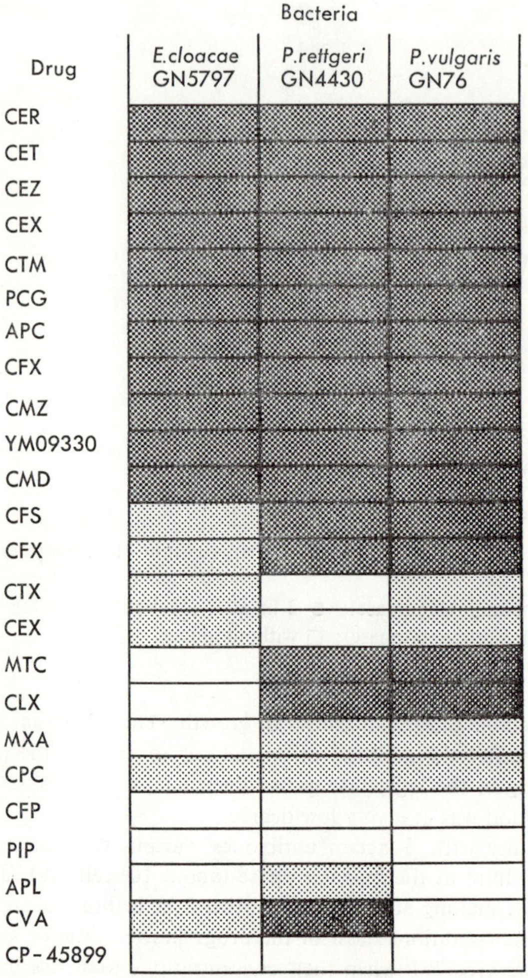

FIG. 6.   Inducer activities of β-lactam antibiotics for β-lactamase formation. *E. cloacae* GN5797, *P. rettgeri* GN4430, and *P. vulgaris* GN76 were used. Various concentrations of each drug were used as inducers and the largest amount of CSase formation was scored. ▓ high inducibility; ▒ intermediate inducibility; ☐ low (or no) inducibility.

by the enzyme. Cefuroxime-type cephalosporins and CPC belong to group B. Piperacillin (PIP), CFP, apalcillin (APL), and CFS, which are newly-introduced drugs, showed a low inducibility (group C). Methicillin and CLX showed the lowest inducibility among the drugs tested, possibly due to low penetrability of these drugs into bacterial cells.

In other gram-negative bacteria, *i.e.*, *P. rettgeri* and *P. vulgaris*, it was also recognized that PIP and CFP showed low inducer activity (Fig. 6).

The high antibacterial activity of PIP and CFP against *E. cloacae, P. rettgeri,* and *P. vulgaris* would be due to not only their stability to CSase but also their low inducer activity for CSase production. Furthermore, it seems likely that the low inducer activity of PIP and CFP contributes to their broad antibacterial spectrum against gram-negative bacteria.

DECREASE IN β-LACTAM PERMEABILITY

Bacteria resist the action of antibiotics by various mechanisms including enzymatic inactivation of the antibiotic, barriers to its entry into the bacterial cell, and alterations in the site of action of the antibiotic. Each of these mechanisms may show different levels of resistance to antibiotics. Multiple mechanisms may also be present in some bacterial cells. The usefulness of an antibiotic is probably limited by the number of resistance mechanisms and by the prevalence of resistant bacteria.

A gram-negative bacteria which is resistant to penicillin or cephalosporin antibiotics usually contains different types of β-lactamase. However, the resistance levels of bacteria to different β-lactam antibiotics do not correlate with the rates at which these antibiotics are hydrolyzed by the β-lactamase released from the bacteria. Thus, one of the resistance mechanisms to some β-lactam antibiotics is attributed to the impermeability of drugs into bacterial cells. Methicillin resistance in *Staphylococcus aureus* was found to be due to its inability to hydrolyze the drug. The *S. aureus mec* (methicillin resistance) strain conferred methicillin resistance due to its impermeability into host cells. Biochemical studies of this type of resistance have explained the following facts: (a) it does not hydrolyze β-lactam antibiotics; and (b) there is a decrease in the level of drug resistance after treatment with EDTA. However, the biochemical mechanism of this resistance still remains unknown.

Investigations have shown that methicillin resistance is usually associated with morphological changes in the bacterial cell envelope, and it has been concluded that these alterations in some way interfere with the drug's reaching its sensitive target (5) and with the synthesis of cell wall peptidoglycan. Unfortunately there is no direct evidence for the relationship between cell wall changes and resistance. Accordingly, it has been suggested that methicillin resistant strains may also have other special properties (6). Studies of the penicillin binding proteins have opened an exciting area of bacterial membrane biology (7), but no one yet knows how β-lactam antibiotics get into cells and exactly which one of their target sites is decisive in their mode of action.

REFERENCES

1. Mitsuhashi, S., Yamagishi, S., Sawai, T., and Kawabe, H. 1977. *In* "R Factor—

Drug Resistance Plasmid," ed. by S. Mitsuhashi, Japan Sci. Soc. Press, Tokyo/ Univ. Park Press, Baltimore, pp. 195–254.
2. Mitsuhashi, S. 1979. *Mol. Cell Biochem.*, **26**, 135–180.
3. Mitsuhashi, S. and Inoue, M. 1981. Beta-lactam Antibiotics, Academic Press, New York, in press.
4. Richmond, M.H. and Sykes, R.S. 1972. *Genet. Res.*, **20**, 885.
5. Sabath, L.D. 1977. *J. Antimicrob. Chemother.*, **3**, 47–51.
6. Sabath, L.D. and Wallace, S.J. 1971. *Ann. N.Y. Acad. Sci.*, **182**, 256–266.
7. Spratt, B.G. 1977. *Eur. J. Biochem.*, **72**, 341–342.

4 STRUCTURE AND FUNCTION RELATIONSHIPS

STRUCTURE-ACTIVITY RELATIONSHIP

Hiroshi Noguchi and Susumu Mitsuhashi

Department of Microbiology, School of Medicine, Gunma University*

Since the discovery of penicillin by Alexander Fleming in 1929, many β-lactam antibiotivs have been developed and several of them are being used in clinical medicine. Compared to other antibiotics, β-lactam antibiotics can be more easily and extensively modified by chemical synthesis. The introduction of specific side chains to the "nucleus" of β-lactam-thiazolidine and β-lactam-dihydrothiazine has resulted in a variety of changes in biological properties: expansion of the antibacterial spectrum, an increase in stability against β-lactamase and improved pharmacokinetic properties. Chemical modification of the "nucleus" itself has recently led to a new series of compounds with characteristic biological activities. Due to endless efforts in research and development of new derivatives, β-lactam antibiotics still remain the most important chemotherapeutic agents among antibacterial drugs because of a high intrinsic antibacterial activity, wide spectrum, and high selective toxicity.

In the history of β-lactam antibiotic development up to 1970, penicillin G, cloxacillin, ampicillin, cephaloridine, cefazolin, and cephalexin were milestones. Penicillin G is the first penicillin possessing an excellent chemotherapeutic potency against gram-positive coccal infections. Isoxazoyl penicillins such as cloxacillin are effective toward penicillin G-resistant gram-positive cocci because of their resistance to hydrolysis by β-lactamase. Ampicillin, developed in 1961 as both an oral and parenteral β-lactam, expanded its antibacterial spectrum to gram-negative organisms in addition to gram-positive organisms. After 1962, cephalosporin derivatives (cephalothin, cephaloridine) with a 6-membered dihydrothiazine ring in place of the 5-membered thiazolidine ring of the penicillin molecule were semi-synthesized and introduced into treatment of infectious diseases. They are active against gram-negative organisms and also against penicillin-resistant gram-positive cocci, and show improved *in vivo* chemotherapeutic effects. Furthermore, cefazolin, developed in

* Showa-machi 3-39-22, Maebashi 371, Japan.

1967, has improved pharmacokinetic antibiotic properties and show high activity against infections caused by gram-negative rods. Cephalexin, developed in 1967, possesses high oral absorbability and is used against mild infections caused by gram-positive and gram-negative organisms.

There are many reviews and articles concerning the history and antibacterial and pharmacokinetic properties of the old-type penicillins and cephalosporins briefly mentioned above. This article is mainly concerned with the structure-activity relationships of β-lactam antibiotics developed in the past decade. We will present an overview of their structure and characteristic properties, and in addition will describe the critical points for evaluating a new derivative at the preclinical stage.

We can classify many β-lactam antibiotics into four classes according to the clinical usefulness and pharmacokinetic properties of the drugs: (I) parenteral penicillins (Fig. 1), (II) parenteral cephalosporins (Fig. 2), (III) oral penicillins and cephalosporins (Fig. 3), and (IV) nonclassical β-lactam antibiotics including β-lactamase inhibitors (Fig. 4). Furthermore, we have tentatively divided them into 19 subclasses as showin in Figs. 1–4, according to the structure and antibacterial spectrum of the derivative. The structure of the antibiotics is depicted in Tables I–VIII.

In the 1970's, gram-negative rods were isolated with increasing frequency in parallel with the decrease in the isolation frequency of pathogenic gram-positive cocci. Among the gram-negative rods isolated in Japan from 1973 to 1974, *Escheri-*

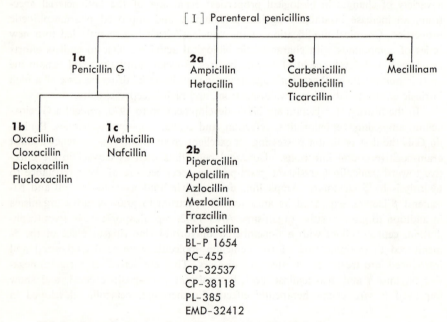

FIG. 1. Recently developed parenteral penicillins in clinical use.

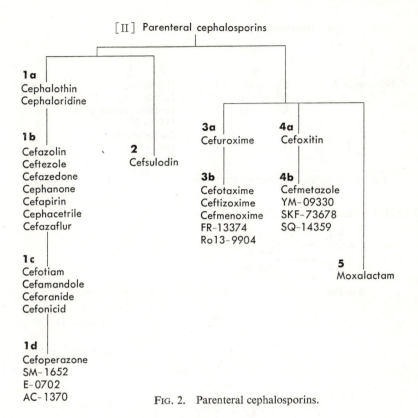

FIG. 2.   Parenteral cephalosporins.

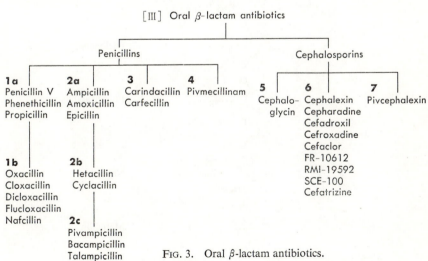

FIG. 3.   Oral β-lactam antibiotics.

[Ⅳ] Nonclassical β-lactam antibiotics

1	2	3
Nocardicin A	Clavulanic acid CP-45899 CP-47904	Thienamycin Epithienamycin A N-acetylthienamycin MK-0787 Carpetimycin MM-4550 PS-4-7

FIG. 4.   Nonclassical β-lactam antibiotics.

TABLE I.   The Structure of [I]-1a-c

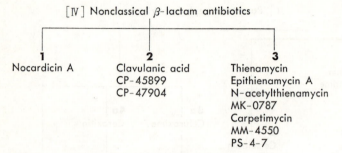

Subclass	R	Name
1a	—CH₂—	Penicillin G
1b		Oxacillin
		Cloxacillin
		Dicloxacillin
1c		Flucloxacillin
		Nafcillin
		Meticillin

TABLE II.   The Structure of [I]-2a, b

Subclass	R_1	R_2	Name
2a	H	H	Ampicillin
2b		H	Piperacillin (T-1220)
		H	Apalcillin (PC-904)
		H	Azlocillin (Bay e6905)
		H	Mezlocillin (Bay f1353)
		OH	Frazcillin (Bay k4999)
		H	Pirbenicillin
	$NH_2-\underset{\underset{NH}{\parallel}}{C}-NH-CO-$	H	BL-P 1654
		OH	PC-455
		H	CP-32537
	$NH_2-\underset{\underset{NH}{\parallel}}{C}-NH-CO-NH-CH_2-CO-$	OH	CP-38118

TABLE II. (continued)

Subclass	R_1	R_2	Name
2b	(structure: CHO-N-piperazine-pyrimido-pyridinone with CO- group)	OH	PL-385
	(structure: OH-substituted naphthyridine with NH-CO- group)	OH	EMD-32412
2a	(structure: phenyl-CH-C(=O) with HN, CH₃ CH₃ ring, penicillin nucleus S, CH₃ CH₃, N, COOH)		Hetacillin

TABLE III. The Structure of [I]-3 and 4

Subclass	R	Name
3	(structure: phenyl-CH(COOH)-C(=O)-NH- penicillin nucleus S, CH₃ CH₃, N, COOH)	Carbenicillin
	(structure: phenyl-CH(SO₃H)-C(=O)-NH- penicillin nucleus)	Sulbenicillin
	(structure: thienyl-CH(COOH)-C(=O)-NH- penicillin nucleus)	Ticarcillin (BRL-2288)
4	(structure: azepane ring-N-CH=N- penicillin nucleus S, CH₃ CH₃, N, COOH)	Mecillinam (FL-1060)

chia coli was most frequently isolated (28%), followed by genus *Klebsiella* (24%), genus *Pseudomonas* (18%), and genus *Proteus* (13%). Broad-spectrum β-lactam antibiotics developed in the 1960's, such as ampicillin, cefazolin, and cephalexin, were commonly and frequently used in treatment against gram-negative infections. As a result, one-third of *E. coli* isolates acquired resistance to the old-type penicillins, and strains resistant to the old-type cephalosporins have emerged. In addition, the isolation frequency of *P. aeruginosa*, indole-positive *Proteus*, *Serratia*, and *Entero-bacter* not susceptible to commonly used β-lactam antibiotics rose.

TABLE IV. The Structure of [II]-1 and 2

Subclass	R_1	R_2	Name
1a		$-OCOCH_3$	Cephalothin
			Cephaloridine
1b			Cefazolin
			Ceftezole
			Cefazedone (EMD-30087)
			Cephanone
		$-OCOCH_3$	Cephapirin
	$NCCH_2-$	$-OCOCH_3$	Cephacetrile
	CF_3SCH_2-		Cefazaflur
1c		$\cdot 2HCl$	Cefotiam (SCE-963, CGP-14221/E)
			Cefamandole (Lilly 106223)
			Ceforanide (BL-S 786)

TABLE IV.   (continued)

Subclass	R_1	R_2	Name
			Cefonicid (SKF-75073)
1d			Cefoperazone (T-1551)
			SM-1652
			E-0702
			AC-1370
2			Cefsulodin (SCE-129, CGP-7174)

As a result of the change in the refractory organisms and on the isolation frequency of pathogens, much effort was directed toward developing β-lactams possessing (a) a higher intrinsic activity and wider spectrum than those of ampicillin and cefazolin, especially against *P. aeruginosa* and genus *Serratia*; (b) stability to hydrolysis of β-lactamase produced, especially by gram-negative organisms; and (c) a higher oral absorbability than that of ampicillin and cephalexin.

Eventually, these efforts achieved success in the development of (a) new anti-pseudomonal penicillins and cephalosporins, (b) new types of β-lactamase-resistant cephalosporins, oxime-type cephalosporins and cephamycins, (c) nonclassical β-lactam

TABLE V.   The Structure of [II]-3–5

Subclass	R_1	R_2	R_3	Name
3a		$-CH_2OCONH_2$	$-H$	Cefuroxime (640/359)
3b		$-CH_2OCOCH_3$	$-H$	Cefotaxime (RH-756)
		$-H$	$-H$	Ceftizoxime (FK-749)
			$-H$	Cefmenoxime (SCE-1365)
		$-H$	$-CH_3$	FR-13374
			$-H$	Ro-13-9904

antibiotics possessing β-lactamase inhibitory action, and (d) improved oral absorbability and semi-synthetic conversion to an orally available form.

ANTIPSEUDOMONAL PENICILLINS AND CEPHALOSPORINS

Carbenicillin, developed in 1967, is the first parenteral penicillin active against *P. aeruginosa*. Because the average MIC of this drug is relatively high, ranging from 50 to 100 μg/ml, large amounts of carbenicillin (10 to 30 g/day) are administered by drip infusion to attain sufficient therapeutic results. This massive amount of therapy sometimes induces undesirable side effects such as imbalance of electrolytes in body fluid, haemolysis, and hepatic and renal toxicity.

Following carbenicillin, sulbenicillin, which possesses a sulfonic group in the α position, was developed in 1968. Although this compound is superior to carbenicillin in its stability in powder from neutral pH, it has almost the same antibacterial activity and pharmacokinetic properties as those of carbenicillin. In addition, ticarcillin possessing the 3-thienyl ring in lieu of the phenyl ring in the 6-side chain of carbenicillin was developed in 1974. Although this modification gave an approxi-

TABLE V. (continued)

Subclass	R_1	R_2	X	Name
4a	(thiophene)$-CH_2-$	$-CH_2OCONH_2$	S	Cefoxitin
4b	$NC-CH_2-S-CH_2-$	$-CH_2S-$(tetrazole, CH_3)	S	Cefmetazole (CS-1170)
	$HOOC$, H_2NOC $C=C$ (dithiole) $CH-$	$-CH_2-S-$(tetrazole, CH_3)	S	YM-09330
	(thiophene)$-CH-$ NH CO NH_2	$-CH_2-S-$(tetrazole, CH_3)	S	SQ-14359
	CF_3SCH_2-	$-CH_2-S-$(tetrazole, CH_3)	S	SKF-73678
5	$HO-$(phenyl)$-CH-$ $COOH$	$-CH_2-S-$(tetrazole, CH_3)	O	Moxalactam (6059-S, LY-127935)

mately 2-fold increase in *in vitro* activity, large doses were still required to achieve effective therapy.

An acidic functional group was introduced to the 7-position of the cephalosporin molecule, in expectation of the increased antipseudomonal activity seen in penicillin. Cefsulodin, α-sulfophenylacetamido cephem having the 4-carbamoylpyridinium group at the 3-methylene position, was developed in 1976 and showed suprisingly potent antipseudomonal activity (average MIC: 0.78 to 1.56 μg/ml), although its spectrum was narrow and showed only moderate activity against *E. coli* and genus *Klebsiella*. The high antipseudomonal activity of cefsulodin is likely to be caused not only by the α-sulfonic group but also by the positively charged nitrogen at the 4-carbamoyl-pyridinium group. A dose of 0.5 to 2 g/day is reported to be effective against pseudomonal infections.

On the other hand, in the 1970's many researchers focused their efforts on modification at the α-amino group of ampicillin and amoxicillin, because acylation with

TABLE VI. The Structure of [III]-1–4

Subclass	R	Name
1a	⟨benzene⟩–CH₂–	Penicillin G
	⟨benzene⟩–O–CH₂–	Penicillin V
	⟨benzene⟩–O–CH– CH₃	Phenethicillin
	⟨benzene⟩–O–CH– CH₂CH₃	Propicillin
1b	See Table I	

Subclass	R	Name
2a	⟨phenyl⟩–	Ampicillin
	HO–⟨phenyl⟩–	Amoxicillin
	⟨cyclohexadienyl⟩–	Epicillin (SQ-11302)
2b		Hetacillin
		Cyclacillin

TABLE VI. (continued)

Subclass	R	Name
2c	$-CH_2OCOC(CH_3)_3$	Pivampicillin
	CH_3 $-CHOCOOC_2H_5$	Bacampicillin
		Talampicillin

Subclass	R	Name
3		Carindacillin
		Carfecillin
4		Pivmecillinam (FL-1039)

aliphatic, aromatic, and heteroaromatic carboxylic acids gave an expanded spectrum with especially increased activity against *P. aeruginosa*. The representative compounds obtained were piperacillin, apalcillin, and azlocillin, which were semi-synthesized by acylating the α-amino group of ampicillin with piperazine carboxylic acid, naphthyridine carboxylic acid, and imidazolidine carboxylic acid, respectively. They show very low MICs, ranging from 0.78 to 6.25 μg/ml against *P. aeruginosa* clinical isolates. This modification also endows higher antibacterial activity against genus *Serratia*, genus *Klebsiella*, indole-positive *Proteus*, and genus *Enterobacter*. Acylation of α-amino group at the 7-position of the cephalosporin molecule as well as at the 6-position of the penicillin molecule led to increased antipseudomonal activity, the

TABLE VII. The Structure of [III]-5–7

Subclass	R_1	R_2	Name
5	$-CH-$ NH_2	$-CH_2OCOCH_3$	Cephaloglycin
6	$-CH-$ NH_2	$-CH_3$	Cephalexin
	$-CH-$ NH_2	$-CH_3$	Cephradine
	HO $-CH-$ NH_2	$-CH_3$	Cefadroxil (BLS-578)
	$-CH-$ NH_2	$-OCH_3$	Cefroxadine (CGP-9000)
	$-CH-$ NH_2	$-Cl$	Cefaclor (Lilly 99638)
	$-CH$ NH_2 CH_3SO_2NH	$-CH_3$	FR-10612
	$-CH-$ NH_2	$-CH_3$	RMI-19592
	$-CH-$ NH_2	$-CH_3$	SCE-100
	HO $-CH-$ NH_2	$-CH_2-S$	Cefatrizine (BL-S640)
7	$-CHCONH-$ NH_2		Pivcephalexin (ST-21)

TABLE VIII. The Structure of [IV]-1–3

Subclass	R	Name
1		Nocardicin A
2		Clavulanic acid (MM 14151)
		CP-45899
		CP-47904
3		Thienamycin
		Epithienamycin A
		N-acetyl thienamycin
		N-formimidoyl thienamycin (MK-0787)

representative compounds being cefoperazone and SM-1652. However, the MICs and minimal bactericidal concentrations (MBCs) of these acylamino penam and acylamino chephem derivatives usually become larger with increasing inoculum size.

The mode of action (including antipseudomonal mechanism) of 6-acylamino penam and 7-acylamino cephem derivatives is likely to be much different from those of α-acidic group-substituted β-lactams such as carbenicillin and cefsulodin. The former compounds are moderately active against carbenicillin-type β-lactam-resistant

TABLE VIII.   (continued)

Subclass	R	Name
		MM-4550
		PS-5
		Carpetimycin A
		Carpetimycin B

clinical isolates. Almost all the carbenicillin-resistant clinical isolates of *P. aeruginosa* produce so-called carbenicillinase, mediated by R plasmids, which preferentially degrades carbenicillin-type β-lactams at an extremely high rate, in contrast to acylamino β-lactams which are relatively stable. In Enterobacteriaceae such as *E. coli* and *Klebsiella*, one third of isolates show extremely high resistance to carbenicillin, their resistance being considered to be caused not by carbenicillinase but by the interaction with chromosomally mediated β-lactamase. Carbenicillin-type compounds have too high an affinity for chromosomally-mediated β-lactamase to exert inhibitory activity against these enzymes, which trap β-lactam molecules preventing their action on target proteins. In contrast, acylamino β-lactams have low affinity for β-lactamase and do not have β-lactamase inhibitory activity. In addition, acylamino β-lactams have higher affinities for penicillin target proteins, penicillin-binding proteins (PBPs), than the latter, suggesting the high intrinsic activities of the former compounds. Almost all the acylamino derivatives possess extremely high affinity for PBP-3 in *P. aeruginosa*, which is likely to be involved in septum formation of cells, causing morphological change into long filaments.

Bacteriostatic and bactericidal activities of carbenicillin-type β-lactams are less influenced by inoculum size than are acylamino β-lactams. This advantage over acylamino derivatives leads to higher *in vivo* chemotherapeutic activity than expected from *in vitro* activity. Although the reason is now open to question, we should consider the following as the causes: β-lactamase inhibitory activity, the effect on β-lactamase induction, direct damage to the cell wall, and interaction with lytic enzymes, *etc.*

Several new compounds, structurally classified into two types, have already been approved for clinical use and marketing. In the near future we will learn the reason for the fundamental difference between the two in mode of action and how it affects clinical usefulness and effectiveness.

β-LACTAMASE-RESISTANT CEPHALOSPORINS AND CEPHAMYCINS

The history of antibiotic development is also that of our fight against resistant organisms. With the increase in the isolation frequency of gram-negative pathogens resistant to the old-type β-lactams in the 1970's, we succeeded in chemically developing two types of cephalosporins effective against resistant strains.

One is a series of compounds possessing a *syn*-configurated methoxyimino group at the 7β-position of cephalosporin, that is, an oxime-type cephalosporin. The first compound developed was cefuroxime (in 1975). This compound showed resistance to hydrolysis by β-lactamase although its antibacterial activity was comparable to the established cephalosporins. The anti-configuration of this compound does not give resistance to hydrolysis by β-lactamase. It is thought that the *syn*-configurated methoxyimino group prevents access of the β-lactamase molecule to the β-lactam ring. Thus, hydrolysis of the β-lactam ring cannot occur. Further, introduction of the aminothiazole group as a substitute for the furyl moiety of cefuroxime has resulted in a wider spectrum and greatly heightened activity, with examples of this type of compound being cefotaxime, ceftizoxime, and cefmenoxime. These compounds are active against penicillin-resistant gram-negative organisms and are also moderately active against *P. aeruginosa*.

Another is a cephamycin group, *i.e.*, 7α-methoxycephalosporin. Since Strominger's hypothesis on penicillin action in 1965 and the discovery of naturally occurring cephamycin C by Najarajan *et al.* in 1971, intensive research has focused on the modification of natural products and on the chemical methoxylation of the "nucleus" of β-lactams. Chemical modification by any substitute, except for the methoxy group such as the methyl, ethyl, methylthio, acetoxy, and carboxy groups, in place of the 7α-hydrogen of cephalosporin did not lead to any improvement in antibacterial activity. The first cephamycin derivative available in clinics was cefoxitin (in 1972), followed by cefmetazole, and YM-09330. The latter two compounds have the advantage of a wider spectrum and higher activity than cefoxitin. These 7α-methoxy analogs are more active against *Serratia marcescens*, indole-positive *Proteus*, β-lactam-resistant strains of gram-negative rods, and anaerobes such as *Bacteroides* than their 7-hydrogen congener, although in general these cephamycins have lower activity against gram-positive organisms than the corresponding cephalosporins. The 7α-methoxy substitute conferred resistance against β-lactam hydrolysis by cephalosporinase.

In 1978, moxalactam (6059-S), an oxacephem derivative possessing oxygen in lieu of sulfur atom of the cephalosporin nucleus and a 7α-methoxy substituent has chemically been transformed from penicillin and developed for clinical use. This compound has an expanded antibacterial spectrum and even has a moderate level of antipseudomonal activity.

Compared to oxime-type cephalosporins, 7α-cephalosporins possess higher resistance to hydrolysis by cephalosporinase and also inhibitory activity against these enzymes, their MICs being less influenced by inoculum size.

NONCLASSICAL β-LACATAMS AND β-LACTAMASE INHIBITORS

We now refer to old-type β-lactam antibiotics possessing a penam and cephem nucleus as "classical β-lactams" and to those with an unusual nucleus as "nonclassical β-lactams." According to this criterion, although we should mention oxacephems such as moxalactam in this section, we included them in the cephamycins because moxalactam has the same biological properties as other cephamycins.

In 1976, nocardicins were reported as a single-β-lactam antibiotic, possessing moderate activity against gram-negative organisms including *P. aeruginosa*. Attractively, nocardicin A exerted a higher *in vivo* activity than expected from *in vitro* antibacterial activity and showed resistance against both plasmid- and chromosome-mediated β-lactamases. The MICs were much influenced by the component of media used and its bactericidal activity was potentiated by the addition of serum and leukocytes.

Screening for a substance possessing β-lactamase inhibitory action in fermentation broth led to the discovery of clavulanic acid in 1976. Clavulanic acid strongly inhibits penicillinase and exerts a synergistic effect on antibacterial activity when it is combined with β-lactamase-susceptible penicillins such as ampicillin, amoxicillin, and ticarcillin. Against cephalosporinase, however, its inhibitory activity is very weak. Clinical trials of augmentin which consists of amoxicillin and clavulanic acid (2:1) are now in progress. The antibacterial activity of clavulanic acid is moderately weak against *S. aureus* and gram-negative organisms except for *Neisseria gonorrohoeae*, against which clavulanic acid shows an extremely low MIC.

CP-45899 and its prodrug CP-47904 have been developed, their advantage over clavulanic acid being prolonged stability in buffer and body fluids.

In 1976, Merck researchers reported they were successful in extracting and purifying a new type of β-lactam possessing a wide antibacterial spectrum and high β-lactamase inhibitory activity, thienamycin. This compound is highly active against almost all microorganisms including *P. aeruginosa* and anaerobe *Bacteroides*. It is worth mentioning that this compound is also active against β-lactam resistant strains because it is not only resistant to hydrolysis by β-lactamase but also inactivates the destructive enzymes. However, this compound is extremely unstable in buffer and body fluids. Further chemical modification toward a more stable compound is in progress.

Like thienamycin, many substances have been extracted from fermentation broth and purified, such as olivanic acid, PS-5, and carpetimycin.

IMPROVEMENT OF PHARMACOKINETIC PROPERTIES

Investigations have been focused on the improvement of oral absorbability. Estification of carboxic acid at the 3-position of ampicillin has resulted in a 2- to 3-fold increase in serum level and a higher urinary recovery after oral administration compared to ampicillin. The clinical candidates are pivaloyloxymethylester (pivampicillin), phthalidylester (talampicillin), and 1'-ethoxycarbonyloxyethylester (bacampicillin) of ampicillin. These "prodrugs" are *in vivo* rapidly hydrolyzed to the parent compounds. However, these estified compounds of ampicillin induce side effects such as gastrointestinal tract disturbances at a moderately high incidence.

On the other hand, introduction of the hydroxy group at the *para*-position of the benzene ring of ampicillin, amoxicillin, conferred a 2-fold higher serum level and urinary recovery, and higher bactericidal activity than ampicillin without changing the antibacterial spectrum. Amoxicillin is absorbed, excreted, and exerts its activity without being metabolized.

As had been seen in pivampicillin, estification of mecillinam has resulted in an orally available form, pivmecillinam. Pivmecillinam as well as mecillinam has an unique antibacterial spectrum, is especially active against Enterobacteriaceae and is resistant to β-lactamase hydrolysis.

As previously mentioned, compounds with antipseudomonal activity have been developed, but not all of them can be administered orally. As a result, some workers have tried to convert carbenicillin, the first antipseudomonal β-lactam, to its orally available form by estifying the α-carboxy group to protect its labile group. Among the many esters of carbenicillin, compounds which are acid stable and rapidly hydrolyzed to carbenicillin by esterase have been selected. Clinical candidates are phenyl (carfecillin) and 5-indanylester (carindacillin) of carbenicillin.

In contrast to estified ampicillin, these esters of carbenicillin possess a different antibacterial spectrum from the parent compound. That is, carindacillin and carfecillin show activity inferior to carbenicillin against gram-negative rods although they show activity superior to the latter against gram-positive cocci. When orally administered, the parent compound was absorbed *via* the gastrointestinal tract, and produced by ester hydrolysis. The chemotherapeutic effects of these esters depend upon the rate of hydrolysis. Effective treatment with these compounds would be restricted to urinary infections because their serum levels are too low to attain *in vivo* activity.

In contrast, efforts to improve the oral absorbability of cephalosporins, focusing on modification of the benzene ring in the 7β-aminophenylglycyl moiety and the 3-methyl moiety of cephalexin, have encountered difficulty. Cefradine and cefadroxil have almost the same pharmacokinetic and antibacterial properties as those of cephalexin. Cefroxadine and cefaclor show improved *in vivo* activity by their higher bactericidal activities although they are absorbed and distributed into tissues at a level similar to cephalexin.

In addition to the improvement in oral absorbability, some compounds have acquired a prolonged serum level by chemical modification. Cefazolin has a longer half-life (about 2 hr after parenteral administration in humans) than cephalothin and cephaloridine. Ceforanide and cefonicid possessing a carboxyl- or sulfo-methyl tetrazolethiomethyl side chain at the 3-position show 1.5- to 2-fold longer half-lives than cefazolin after being administered parenterally. Furthermore, YM-09330 and SM-1652 also show longer serum level half-lives than cefazolin. It is interesting that most of the compounds with prolonged serum levels have relatively high rates of serum protein binding. Although it was believed that high protein binding diminished *in vivo* activity, some recently developed β-lactams show prolonged serum levels, high penetrability into inflammatory tissues, and high *in vivo* activity, even though they are bound to serum protein at a high rate.

In addition, some of the recently developed compounds, such as apalcillin, cefoperazone, and SM-1652, show high recovery into the bile-tract, ranging from 30 to 60% of the administered drugs. Although ampicillin and cefazolin are known to be excreted into the bile at a relatively high rate until now, their levels in bile were insufficient to achieve clinical effectiveness against biliary infections.

PRECLINICAL POINTS FOR DEVELOPING A NEW DERIVATIVE OF β-LACTAM

Once one desires to develop a new drug for clinical use, one should critically and extensively evaluate its many properties before subjecting it to clinical trials. The critical points for the evaluation of a new derivative of β-lactam antibiotics at the preclinical stage are listed in Table IX.

One of the most important goals is to obtain highly purified products with high reproducibility, as contamination with by-products such as polymers could cause allergic reaction. β-Lactams are relatively unstable in the solid state. For commercial use it is required that the derivative of the product be stable for at least 1.5 years in a refrigerator, and if possible at room temperature. In solution it is also required to be stable at a physiological pH. A derivative that is stable in acidic solution at pH 2 would be a candidate for oral use.

Almost all the binding rates of β-lactams to serum protein are low. Before the development of cefazolin it was believed that a high rate of protein binding diminished antibacterial activity. Even if cefazolin binds to serum protein at a rate of over 90%, this drug exerts high *in vivo* antibacterial activity. In addition it was recently reported that drugs which bound to serum protein at a high rate but reversibly have a prolonged half-life in serum and a higher penetrability into inflammatory tissues than do drugs with low binding rates. The reversibility of binding is likely to be very important.

The first screening for newly synthesized derivatives and fermented products is in many cases *in vitro* antibacterial assay. Many methods and many organisms are used in this assay. We usually use a dilution method with agar or broth, and the disc method. In the latter method, a disc containing an appropriate concentration

TABLE IX.   Critical Points in Preclinical Evaluation of β-Lactam Antibiotics

Physicochemical properties	Purity
	Solubility
	Stability (solid, solution; acidic and neutral pH)
	Serum protein binding (rate, reversibility)
In vitro activity	Antibacterial spectrum
	MIC (agar, broth) against clinical isolates
	Inoculum-size effect
	Factors (the kind of medium, pH, *etc.*) which affect MIC and MBC
	MBC against clinical isolates
	Cross-resistance
	Activity in combination with other drugs
	Activation by natural and immunological defense systems
Mode of action	Stability to β-lactamase (V_{max}, K_m, K_i)
	Permeability through outer membrane
	Morphological changes induced by drug
	Affinity to target proteins, including PBPs
	Inhibition of peptidoglycan-synthesizing enzymes
	Interaction with lytic enzymes and their inhibitors
	Selective toxicity on the synthesis of biomacromolecules
In vivo activity	Systemic infection in animals
	Urinary infection
	Respiratory infection
	Biliary infection
Pharmacokinetic properties	Blood and body fluid level (C_{max}, half-life, distribution volume)
	Tissue distribution (kidney, liver, lung, *etc.*)
	Excretion to urine and bile
	Drug penetration to inflammatory tissue
	Metabolism
	Oral absorption (absorption in intestines)
Pharmacological and toxicological properties	General pharmacology
	Acute toxicity (LD_{50})
	Subacute toxicity
	Chronic toxicity
	Reproduction test
	Local safety test
	Haemolysis (direct and immunological)
	Allergy (antigenecity, cross-reaction)
	Effect on normal flora
	Mutagenicity test

of the drug is overlayered onto an agar plate seeded with the test organism and antibacterial activity is determined by measuring the diameter of the inhibitory zone around the disc. Different kinds of test organisms should be used as the isolation frequency of pathogens changes from year to year. Recently, *P. aeruginosa, Proteus,* β-lactam-resistant and supersensitive strains have been used as test organisms in preliminary screening in lieu of *B. subtilis, S. aureus, Micrococcus luteus,* and *E. coli.* Antibacterially active derivatives selected in the first preliminary screening are usually subjected to evaluation of their antibacterial spectrum and activity against clinical isolates. The clinical isolates used should be freshly isolated and derived from at least several hospitals in different areas because the nature of these isolates will be different from year to year and from area to area.

Evaluation of antibacterial activity against strains resistant to the already established β-lactams is also important. Resistance to β-lactam antibiotics is mainly caused by hydrolyzing enzymes, that is, β-lactamases (see p. 41). β-Lactamases are classified on the basis of substrate profile, isoelectric point, molecular weight, *etc.* Among β-lactamases coded by plasmids, R_{TEM} (classified by Richmond *et al.*) or type I (classified by Mitsuhashi *et al.*) is mainly responsible for resistance in Enterobacteriaceae. In *P. aeruginosa,* carbenicillinase is frequently detected, which degrades carbenicillin at a particularly high rate. Chromosomally mediated β-lactamases are species specific and exert a high level of resistance to cephaloridine and cephalothin.

Generally, antibacterial activity is expressed in terms of the MIC, the minimal concentration required to visually inhibit the growth of cells. Bactericidal activity is expressed in terms of the MBC, the minimal concentration required to completely (more than 99.99%) kill bacteria. Although the old-type penicillins such as penicillin G are known to act bactericidally against gram-positive organisms, most of the recently developed β-lactam derivatives active against pathogens such as *P. aeruginosa* act bacteriostatically and their MBCs are frequently higher than their MICs. Bactericidal activity as well as bacteriostatic activity especially dropped when test organisms were inoculated at a high concentration. Therefore it is necessary to evaluate the effect of inoculum size on MICs and MBCs.

In addition to the above mentioned evaluation, we should investigate: (1) synergy in the combination of a derivative with β-lactamase inhibitors and drugs other than β-lactam antibiotics; and (2) its immunopotentiating activity.

Studies on the mode of action of drugs and the mechanisms of drug resistance would contribute to the "drug design" of new derivatives and rational chemotherapy in clinics. Through studies on their mode of action, the microbiologically characteristic properties of drugs can be better understood. β-Lactams irreversibly bind to target enzymes and inhibit specific enzymes which are involved in biosynthesis of the bacterial cell wall. An easy and reproducible method ofr measuring the binding affinity of a derivative to target proteins, PBPs, was developed by Spratt and Pardee (see p. 204). They showed that the structure of a derivative determins its binding affinity for target proteins, and thus causes different morphological changes in the cell. This method is useful for understanding structure-activity relationships and in the design of new derivatives

In gram-positive cocci, penicillin is known to activate an autolytic enzyme (autolysin) by triggering the inhibitor of its complex. On the other hand, an interaction of β-lactams with endogenous lytic enzymes is still open to question in gram-negative organisms. To exert its antibacterial activity, a drug must be able to penetrate through the outer membrane to the inner membrane where target proteins are located, without being degraded by β-lactamase. The penetrability of a drug through the outer membrane is also one of the important points for evaluating and improving its antibacterial activity, as well as resistance to β-lactamase and affinity for target proteins. The following methods for measuring the penetrability of drugs have been developed: (1) incorporation of a radiolabeled drug into intact cells; (2) competition of an unlabeled drug with the incorporation and the binding to PBPs of [^{14}C]-labeled penicillin G using intact cells; (3) comparison of the β-lactamase degrading rate or the binding affinity to PBPs of a drug in a system of intact cells with that in a system of disrupted cells which do not have a permeability barrier; (4) comparison of the MIC against a mutant defective in the permeability barrier with the MIC against the parent strain; and (5) comparison of the penetrability of a drug into liposome. However, these methods for measuring the permeability of drugs are not always easy, convenient, or reproducible.

In most cases, β-lactam antibiotics are first selected by *in vitro* testing, followed by *in vivo* testing. Drugs are administered parenterally or orally to rodents systemically infected with virulent pathogens and activity is determined by the mortality of the infected rodents. Although this system provides a simple method of examining *in vivo* activity, it should be remembered that systemic infections in rodents are very different from those in humans. Urinary, respiratory, and biliary infection systems in mice, rats, guinea pigs, rabbits, and dogs are useful and are more appropriate for predicting the chemotherapeutic potency against infections in humans. In these systems the antibacterial activity of a drug is determined not only by mortality but also by the number of viable cells in infected organs. Sometimes, there exists a great discrepancy between *in vitro* and *in vivo* activities. This gap can mostly be explained by examining the pharmacokinetic properties of the drug. If a drug shows poorer *in vivo* antibacterial activity than expected from its *in vitro* activity, in most cases the drug would be poorly absorbed into body fluid and tissues, inactivated by highly irreversible binding to serum and tissue components, rapidly excreted, or rapidly metabolized to an inactive form. Structural modification of the drug could improve its pharmacokinetic properties. An example of the activity-structure relationship on pharmacokinetic properties can be seen in the following pages. The serum or plasma level, half-life in blood, and urinary recovery of a drug administered are good indicators of the other pharmacokinetic properties. Generally all penicillins and cephalosporins are rapidly excreted and have short half-lives in blood after administration. Therefore three or four administrations per day are required to achieve an effective therapy. The long half-life-type drugs give prolonged activities *in vivo*, high chemotherapeutic effects and are convenient for doctors to administer to patients because of the low frequency of administration. In process of developing a new derivative into clinically available drug, investigations of toxicological and pharmacological properties are very important. Although β-lactam antibiotics have a high toxicity against bacterial parasites, they commonly have low toxicities and little effect on the respiratory and central nervous systems. Nevertheless, much attention must be paid to toxicological and pharmacological evaluations because chemical modification could cause unpredictable toxicity in humans.

AMPICILLIN

G. N. ROLINSON

*Beecham Pharmaceuticals Research Division**

Ampicillin (APC) is a semi-synthetic penicillin prepared from 6-aminopenicillanic acid. Compared with benzylpenicillin (PCG) APC shows a broad spectrum of activity against gram-positive and gram-negative bacteria. Unlike PCG, APC is highly acid stable and is well absorbed when given by mouth. For oral administration APC is available in the form of the free acid. For parenteral administration the sodium salt is available.

APC was introduced into clinical practice in 1961 with reports on the microbiological (*4*) and the pharmacokinetic (*3*) properties. Data on the antibacterial activity of APC *in vitro* and *in vivo* are shown in Table I.

Against the pyogenic cocci APC shows a level of activity very similar to that of PCG, streptococci and non-β-lactamase-producing staphylococci being inhibited at a concentration of 0.02–0.05 μg/ml or less. APC is not stable to staphylococcal β-lactamase and therefore is not active against the penicillin-resistant strains of *Staphylococcus aureus*. Against *Streptococcus faecalis* APC is 2–4 times more active than PCG. Among the gram-positive bacteria APC is also active against *Corynebacterium diphtheriae*, *Listeria monocytogenes*, and *Clostridium* species, with the level of activity being similar to that of PCG. APC is highly active against the meningococcus and comparable with PCG. APC is also active against non-β-lactamase-producing strains of *Neisseria gonorrhoeae* and *Haemophilus influenzae*.

Among the Enterobacteriaceae, APC is active against *Escherichia coli*, *Proteus mirabilis*, *Salmonella* species, and *Shigella* species. β-Lactamase-producing strains however are resistant. APC is not active against the indole-positive *Proteus* species, *Klebsiella*, *Enterobacter*, *Serratia*, and *Pseudomonas aeruginosa*.

APC is bactericidal and following repeated subculture resistant variants arise in a slow stepwise fashion. The antibacterial activity of APC is not markedly affected

* Brockham Park, Betchworth, Surrey, RH3 7AJ, U.K.

TABLE I. Structure-activity Relationship of Antibacterial Activity

Compound		*In vitro* antibacterial activity[b]			
Code No. (Name)	Structure	% of key compound			
	R	*S. aureus*[a]	*E. coli*[a]	*P. mira-bilis*	*P. aeru-ginosa*
Key compound APC	CH·CO– NH₂ (phenyl-CH(NH$_2$)CO–)	100 (0.05)	100 (5.0)	100 (1.25)	100 (>250) μg/ml
Reference compound PCG	CH₂·CO– (phenyl-CH$_2$CO–)	250 (0.02)	10 (50.0)	25 (5.0)	100 (>250) μg/ml

[a] Non-β-lactamase producing. [b] MIC values determined by serial dilution in agar. Ino-Antibiotic administered as single dose immediately after infection.

TABLE II. Structure-activity Relationship of Pharmacokinetic Properties

Compound	Relative activity (%)			Relative toxicity (%)[c] compared to a key compound
Code No. (Name)	Serum level[a] at peak	Urinary[b] recovery	Biliary[b] recovery	
Key compound APC	100 (4.6 μg/ml)	100 (31.3%)	100 (9.6%)	100 (>5,000 mg/kg)
Reference compound PCG	44 (2.01 μg/ml)	80 (25.0%)	156 (15.0%)	—

[a] Intramuscular administration of 5 mg/kg in dogs (2). [b] Intramuscular administration of 100 mg/kg in rats (1). [c] LD$_{50}$ (mg/kg) subcutaneous dosage in mice (2).

by the presence of serum and in human serum only 18% is bound to plasma proteins.

Against intraperitoneal infections with staphylococci and streptococci in mice the activity of APC is comparable with that of PCG (2). Against infections with members of the Enterobacteriaceae APC is more active than PCG. Unlike PCG,

(Ref. *4*)		*In vivo* antibacterial activity (Ref. *2*) CD_{50} (mg/kg) [c]			
ID_{50} (μg/ml)		% of key compound			
		S. aureus		S. typhimurium	
S. aureus[a]	E. coli[a]	Oral	Subcut.	Oral	Subcut.
0.05	5.0	100 (0.3)	100 (0.3)	100 (18)	100 (12.8) mg/kg
0.02	50.0	5 (5.8)	100 (0.3)	<5 (>400)	16 (82) mg/kg

culum: one drop undiluted overnight broth culture. [c] Intraperitoneal infection in mice.

TABLE III. Structure-activity Relationship of Physicochemical Properties

Compound	Molecular weight	Partition[a] coefficient	Serum protein binding rate[b]	Acid[c] stability
Code No. (Name)				
Key compound APC	349.4	−2.68	18%	(+)
Reference compound PCG	334.4	−1.82	59%	(−)

[a] log P, *n*-octanol/water, pH 7.2 (*6*).   [b] % bound in human serum determined by ultrafiltration (*5*).   [c] (+) indicates half-life at pH 2 at 37°C >2 hr.

APC is effective against experimental infections when administered by mouth. Data on the pharmacokinetic properties of APC are shown in Table II. In humans approximately 30–50% of the dose is absorbed following oral administration. Certain esters of APC (pivampicillin, talampicillin, and bacampicillin) are more completely absorbed and give rise to higher levels of APC in the body than are obtained when APC itself is administered. APC is excreted largely in the urine and also in the bile. In rats approximately 10% of the dose can be recovered in the bile following intramuscular administration.

The toxicity of APC in experimental animals and in humans is low.

REFERENCES

1. Acred, P. and Brown, D. M. 1967. *In* "Proceedings of the Vth International Congress of Chemotherapy," ed. by K. H. Spitzy and H. Haschek, Wiener Medizinischen Akademie, Vienna, Vol. V, pp. 273–277.
2. Acred, P., Brown, D. M., Turner, D. H., and Wilson, M. J. 1962. *Br. J. Pharmacol. Chemother.*, **18**, 356–369.
3. Knudsen, E. T., Rolinson, G. N., and Stevens, S. 1961. *Br. Med. J.*, **2**, 198–200.
4. Rolinson, G. N. and Stevens, S. 1961. *Br. Med. J.*, **2**, 191–196.
5. Rolinson, G. N. and Sutherland, R. 1965. *Br. J. Pharmacol.*, **25**, 638–650.
6. Sobotka, P. and Safanda, J. 1976. *J. Mol. Med.*, **1**, 151–159.

APALCILLIN (PC-904) AND ITS RELATED COMPOUNDS

Toshiaki KOMATSU, Hiroshi NOGUCHI, Hisao TOBIKI, and Takenari NAKA-GOME

Research Department, Pharmaceuticals Division, Sumitomo Chemical Co., Ltd.*

In 1977, Price described the future objectives of penicillins as follows (*12*): "Screening emphasis is being directed toward identifying new compounds that may be effective against a particularly troublesome group of organisms; *e.g.*, carbenicillin against *P. aeruginosa.*"

Carbenicillin or sulbenicillin that had been marketed was moderate in anti-pseudomonal activity and required a high dose to achieve successful therapeutic results against severe infections. The authors had therefore started to search for more active compounds than carbenicillin against gram-negative bacilli (GNB), especially *Pseudomonas aeruginosa*, since 1969.

At an early stage, it was found in our research laboratories that a monochloro-acetamido-derivative of the α-amino group of ampicillin synthesized as an inter-mediate of ampicillin derivatives exhibited weak antipseudomonal activity. Some N-acyl derivatives of ampicillin had been reported, but their antibacterial activities were very weak (*2, 3*).

Various N-acylated ampicillin derivatives have been, therefore, synthesized in our research laboratories with the expectation of obtaining a much more potent anti-pseudomonal penicillin with a broad spectrum of activity. Of these compounds, apalcillin (PC-904) was selected as a candidate for a further clinical evaluation (*9*). Fundamental and clinical evaluations were carried out by the Japan Society of Chemotherapy (*5*). This article is concerned with the structure-activity relationships of apalcillin and its related ampicillin derivatives.

ANTIBACTERIAL ACTIVITIES

The structure-activity relationships of antibacterial activities are demonstrated in Table I.

* Takatsukasa 4-2-1, Takarazuka, 665, Japan.

TABLE I.   Structure-activity Relationship of Antibacterial Activity

R_1-CONHCHCONH ... CH_3 CH_3 COOX (S, N, O, R_2)

No. (Name)	Structure			In vitro antibacterial activity							In vivo antibacterial activity		Ref.
	R₁	R₂	X	% of key compound				ID₅₀ (μg/ml)			% of key compound		
				S. aureus	E. coli	K. pneumoniae	P. aeruginosa	S. aureus	E. coli	P. aeruginosa	E. coli	P. aeruginosa	
1 Apalcillin	OH-quinoline	phenyl-methyl	Na	100 (0.39)	100 (0.78)	100 (3.13)	100 (0.78 μg/ml)[a]	0.5	1.4	1.4	100 (18–160)	100 (4–60) mg/kg[b]	9, 14
2	pyridine-methyl	phenyl-methyl	K	50	0.8	0.4	3	—	—	—	—	—	14
3	Cl-pyridine	phenyl-methyl	H	100	0.8	6	3	—	—	—	—	—	13
4	OH-pyridine	phenyl-methyl	Na	100	6	13	25	—	6.0	3.4	<30	19–38	14

No.	Structure (heterocycle)	Aryl	Salt										
5	5-methyl-2-hydroxypyridine (HO, N)	phenyl (toluene)	K	25	1.6	<1.6	1.6	—	—	—	—	8	*13*
6	3-methyl-2-OH-pyridine (OH, N)	phenyl	K	100	6	13	13	—	—	—	—	—	*14*
7	(OH, CH₃–CH, OH, CH₃, N)	phenyl	K	50	3	25	13	—	6.0	9.0	24-32	17	*13*
8	(N, OH)	phenyl	K	100	3	13	6	—	—	—	—	—	*14*
9	(OH, N=N)	phenyl	Na	200	25	50	25	0.8	8.3	6.2	43	12-38	*14*
10	(OH, N=N)	phenyl	K	100	1.6	1.6	3	—	—	—	—	—	*13*
11	(OH, N)	phenyl	K	100	3	3	25	—	—	—	—	—	*14*
12	(O, N–C₂H₅, CH₃ quinolone)	phenyl	K	100	3	1.6	6	—	—	—	—	—	*14*

TABLE I. (continued)

No.	Structure	M										Ref.
13	OCH_3 quinoline (CH₃)	H	200	3	1.6	6	—	—	—	—	—	*14*
14	OH quinoline (CH₃)	K	200	13	6	13	—	1.5	6.0	24–32	15	*14*
15	OH (CH₃)	K	50	6	50	13	—	—	—	—	13	*14*
16	OH (CH₃), CH_3	K	100	25	200	25	—	—	54	—	—	*14*
1	OH (CH₃)	Na	100	100	100	100	0.5	1.4	1.4	100	100	*9, 14*
17	OH (CH₃), H_3C–N(H_3C)	K	50	200	400	25	—	1.0	4.6	—	10	*14*
18	OH (CH₃), H_3CS	K	50	100	400	25	—	1.2	9.2	—	5	*13*

No.	Structure	Substituent	Metal											Ref.
19	OH / CH₃ core, H₃CO-substituted naphthyridinol	(phenyl, CH₃)	K	50	50	100	25	—	—	2.0	8.3	—	<5	*13*
20	OH / CH₃ naphthyridinol	(cyclohexadienyl, CH₃)	Na	100	50	100	50	—	—	—	—	—	38–153	*13*
21	OH / CH₃ naphthyridinol	(cyclohexenyl, CH₃)	Na	50	50	50	25	—	—	—	—	—	38	*13*
22	OH / CH₃ naphthyridinol	(cyclohexyl, CH₃)	Na	25	25	13	13	—	—	—	—	—	33	*13*
23	OH / CH₃ naphthyridinol	$-CH_2$ (phenyl)	Na	25	3	3	6	—	—	—	—	—	—	*13*
24 (DL-threo)	OH / CH₃ naphthyridinol	$-CH$, OH (phenyl)	Na	13	3	<1.6	3	—	—	—	—	—	—	*13*
25 (DL)	OH / CH₃ naphthyridinol	$-CH_2-CH$, CH_3, CH_3	Na	13	13	13	13	—	—	—	—	—	—	*13*
26 (DL)	OH / CH₃ naphthyridinol	$-CH-CH_3$, C_2H_5	Na	50	6	6	13	—	—	—	—	—	32–50	*13*

TABLE I. (continued)

No.	Structure	Salt										Ref.
27 (DL)	OH, -(CH₂)₃CH₃	Na	25	6	13	6	—	—	—	—	15	13
28 (DL)	OH, -CH(CH₃)CH₃	Na	13	3	3	3	—	—	—	—	—	13
29	OH, phenyl, CH₃S	K	100	13	50	6	—	—	—	—	—	14
30	OH, phenyl	K	100	25	50	13	—	—	—	—	26	13
31	phenyl	K	100	6	13	13	—	—	—	—	18	13
32	OH, phenyl	K	25	3	1.6	6	—	—	—	—	10	13
Carbenicillin			50 (0.78)	13 (6.25)	1.6 (200)	3 (25 µg/ml)	1.6	6.0	49	100 (15–180)	10–25 (50–60 mg/kg)	9, 14

[a] MIC (µg/ml): inoculum size, 10^6/ml. [b] ED$_{50}$ (mg/kg): challenge, i.p.; treatment, 1 and 4 hr after challenge, s.c.

Antibacterial activities against *Staphylococcus aureus*, the gram-positive cocci of these derivatives, were not significantly influenced by the substitution of the N-acyl group of ampicillin, and so the structure-activity relationships on GNB including *P. aeruginosa* will be mainly discussed.

1. Monocyclic Heteroaromatic Derivatives

At first, the influence of antibacterial activities due to the change of R_1 in the general formulae in Table I will be discussed.

When the α-amino group of ampicillin was acylated with pyridinecarboxylic acid (2), its activities on GNB such as *Escherichia coli, Klebsiella pneumoniae*, and *P. aeruginosa* were very low as compared with the key compound, apalcillin (1).

Introduction of Cl into the pyridine nucleus (3) did not influence the activities, but the introduction of OH into the pyridine nucleus heightened the antibacterial activities on GNB as seen in compounds 4 and 6. This OH introducing effect was limited to the *ortho*-position of the carbon atom of the pyridine ring having amido-linkage, and was very weak in the *para*-position (5). This effect was also confirmed in the case of the pyridazine and pyrimidine nuclei (9 and 11).

Maximum activities were achieved in compound 9, but its potency was still one fourth to one-half that of apalcillin (1).

2. Bicyclic Heteroaromatic Derivatives

Bicyclic heteroaromatic compounds such as quinolinecarboxamido or naphthyridine-carboxamido derivatives of ampicillin were synthesized in an attempt to obtain more active derivatives.

4-Hydroxy-3-quinolinecarboxamido derivative (14) exhibited fairly potent activities, while N-alkylation of the quinoline nucleus (12) or OCH_3 displacement of OH (13) weakened the activities. 4-Hydroxy-1,6-naphthyridine (15) and 4-hydroxy-1,8-naphthyridine group (16) reduced the activities against *E. coli* and *P. aeruginosa*, but did not against *S. aureus* and *K. pneumoniae* as compared with the key compound.

Various 1,5-naphthyridine derivatives (1 and 17–28) were investigated. When R_1 was 4-hydroxy-1,5-naphthyridine and the R_2 phenyl group (1, apalcillin), pronounced potent effects against *E. coli, K. pneumoniae*, and particularly against *P. aeruginosa* were achieved. It exhibited the most potent activity on *P. aeruginosa* among the derivatives tested.

Substitution of the 6-position of 1,5-naphthyridine with the methylmercapto (17), dimethylamino (18), or methoxy (19) group resulted in the reduction of activity against *P. aeruginosa* but in a rise in activity against *K. pneumoniae*.

When the phenyl group at R_2 was displaced with the cyclohexadienyl (20), cyclohexenyl (21), or cyclohexanyl (22) group, their antibacterial activities were reduced in that order. When R_2 was on aliphatic (C_3-C_4) or benzyl group, their *in vitro* activities fell markedly as seen in compounds 23–28. Therefore, when R_2 was phenyl, the strongest activity among the derivatives tested was observed.

Some hydroxy-N-containing bicyclic heteroaromatic derivatives other than 1,5-

TABLE II. Structure-activity Relationship of Pharmacokinetic Properties

Compound No. (Name)	Relative activity (%) compared to the key compound					
	Serum level at peak[a]		Urinary recovery[a]	Biliary recovery[a]	LD$_{50}$ (mg/kg)[b]	Ref.
	Mouse	Rat				
1 (Apalcillin)	100 (25–35 µg/ml)	100 (7–10 µg/ml)	100 (7–10%)	100 (45–55%)	1,450–1,950 mg/kg	4, 13
2	220	90	—	—	—	13
3	100	—	—	—	—	13
4	130	100–200	130–200	90–120	>5,000	13
5	285	130	—	—	—	13
6	—	85	—	—	—	13
7	70	—	115	—	—	13
9	100–200	100	310	30	5,000	13
14	50–70	60	—	—	—	13
15	80	—	—	—	—	13
16	55	—	—	—	—	13
17	40	<60	30	50	2,700	13
18	25	<50	30	70	—	13
19	120	70	150	30	—	13
20	70–100	100	60	—	—	13
21	40	20	50–60	—	—	13

22	30	<30	30-40	—	—	_13_
23	70-90	<30	220	—	—	_13_
24 (DL-threo)	—	—	105	—	—	_13_
25 (DL)	150-160	<40	170	—	—	_13_
26 (DL)	60	70	280	—	—	_13_
27 (DL)	90-150	60-170	140	—	—	_13_
28 (DL)	115	180	260-430	—	—	_13_
30	70	—	—	—	—	_13_
32	70	—	—	—	—	_13_
Carbenicillin	200 (50-70 µg/ml)	300 (30-50 µg/ml)	400 (30-50%)	30 (15-20%)	6,200-8,600	_4, 13_

See Table I for structure. a Administration: 50 mg/kg, s.c. b LD_{50} (mg/kg): mouse, i.p.

naphthyridine at R_1, and possessing phenyl at R_2, exhibited generally moderate antibacterial activities against GNB.

The potency ratios of *in vivo* antibacterial activities of these derivatives with apalcillin by parenteral administration were generally parallel with those of *in vitro* activities as far as tested. The *in vitro* activities of apalcillin were about 33 and 8 times as potent as those of carbenicillin against *P. aeruginosa* and *E. coli*, respectively. The *in vivo* efficacy of apalcillin was 4 to 10 times as potent as that of carbenicillin on *P. aeruginosa* and almost equal to carbenicillin on *E. coli*.

PHARMACOKINETIC STUDIES

These results are shown in Table II. The data were obtained with parenteral administration.

Displacement of R_1 with the monocyclic heteroaromatic group (2–7, 9) conferred serum levels comparable to or somewhat higher than the key compound, apalcillin (1). In contrast to the finding on antibacterial activities, OH introduction into the heteroaromatic nucleus did not influence the absorption. Introduction of 4-hydroxy-quinoline (14) or 4-hydroxy-1,5-naphthyridine (16–18) substituted into R_1 conferred poorer absorption than the 4-hydroxy-1,5-naphthyridine derivative, apalcillin.

When the phenyl group of apalcillin was displaced with the cyclohexadienyl (20), cyclohexenyl (21) or cyclohexanyl (22) group, peak serum levels were lowered in that order.

When R_2 was benzyl (23) or alkyl (25 and 26), peak serum levels were generally lower, but in some cases (27 and 28) better absorbability was observed. In the case of displacement of R_1 with an N-containing bicyclic heteroaromatic nucleus (30 and 32) other than naphthyridine as far as tested, peak serum levels higher than the key compound were not attained.

Serum levels of apalcillin were about one-half as high as those of carbenicillin in mice and one-half to one-third in rats. Urinary recovery of apalcillin was about one-fourth as much as that of carbenicillin but its biliary recovery was about three times as much as carbenicillin. Apalcillin is, therefore, a biliary excretion-type penicillin derivative as compared with other marketed penicillins.

PHYSICOCHEMICAL PROPERTIES

The physicochemical properties of apalcillin are shown in Table III. The molecular weight of the free form of apalcillin is 521.55.

It has been reported that substances having molecular weights higher than 500 are highly excreted into the bile in all species (*15*). This phenomenon may partly explain why apalcillin is a biliary excretion type penicillin.

The potent antipseudomonal activity of apalcillin is explained by the improved accessibility to the PBPs in inner membranes and a high affinity to them (*10, 11*).

TABLE III. Physicochemical Properties

Compound Name	Molecular weight (as free form)	Partition coefficient[a]	Serum protein binding rate (%)	Acid stability (T½)[b]	Ref.
Apalcillin	521. 55	−0. 18	98	+ (4. 7 hr)	4, 6, 7, 9, 13
Carbenicillin	378. 42	−1. 60	47	− (0. 4 hr)	1, 9, 13
Ampicillin	349. 42	−0. 50	20	+ (>6 hr)	1, 6, 13

[a] log P_{isobut}: isobutanol/water at pH 7.4. [b] At pH 2.0 at 37°C.

Activities against GNB can be explained by the partition coefficient value, but the broadening to *P. aeruginosa* cannot always be explained by this.

The binding extent of apalcillin with human serum protein is very high, being 98%, but not so high (82%) with mouse serum (*4, 6, 7*).

The *in vivo* potency ratio of apalcillin with carbenicillin is somewhat lower than the *in vitro* ratio, as mentioned before. This discrepancy seems to be explained at least partly by the differences in the serum protein binding rate and tissue distribution (*4, 6, 7*).

Apalcillin is rather acid-stable, but no serum levels were detected after oral administration. Therefore, it does not seem to be absorbed from the intestine.

The combination of the molecular weight, lipophilicity, and other physicochemical properties such as the shape, spatial disposition, and electronic character which were changed by the N-acylation of the α-amino group of ampicillin might influence the antibacterial activities and pharmacokinetic properties.

REFERENCES

1. Barker, B. M. and Prescott, F. 1973. Antimicrobial Agents in Medicine. Blackwell Scientific Public., Oxford, pp. 152.
2 Beecham Group Ltd. 1969. U.S. Patent, 3, 433, 784.
3. Benigni, F., Botre, C., and Riccieri, F. M. 1965. *Il Farmaco Ed. Sci.* 20, 885–890.
4. Irie, K., Okuda, T., Noguchi, H., Akakuri, N., Izawa, A., Yamamori, K., and Komatsu, T. 1978. *Chemotheraphy (Tokyo)*, 26 (S-2), 138–147.
5. Japan Society of Chemotherapy. 1978. *Chemotheraphy (Tokyo)*, 26 (S-2), 1–529.
6. Komatsu, T., Nagata, A., Iba, K., Ohbe, Y., Irie, K., and Miyawaki, H. 1978. *Curr. Chemother.*, 641–642.
7. Komatsu, T., Kisaki, Y., Irie, K., Okuda, T., Akakuri, N., Noguchi, H., Izawa, A., and Konno, M. 1978. *Chemotherapy (Tokyo)*, 26 (S-2), 154–158.
8. Korzybski, T., Kowszyk-Gindifer, Z., and Kurylowicz, W. 1978. Antibiotics-origin, Nature and Properties, American Society for Microbiology, Washington, D.C., p. 1963.

9. Noguchi, H., Eda, Y., Tobiki, H., Nakagome, T., and Komatsu, T. 1976. *Antimicrob. Agents Chemother.*, **9**, 262–273.
10. Noguchi, H. and Mitsuhashi, S. 1978. *Curr. Chemother.*, 635–638.
11. Noguchi, H., Matsuhashi, M., Takaoka, M., and Mitsuhashi, S. 1978. *Antimicrob. Agents Chemother.*, **14**, 617–624.
12. Price, K. E. 1977. *In* "Structure-activity Relationships among the Semisynthetic Antibiotics," ed. by D. Perlman, Academic Press, New York, pp. 52.
13. Sumitomo Chemical Co., Ltd., unpublished data.
14. Tobiki, H., Yamada, H., Nakatsuka, I., Shimago, K., Eda, Y., Noguchi, H., Komatsu, T., and Nakagome, T. 1980. *Yakugaku Zasshi* (*J. Pharm. Soc. Japan*), **100**, 38–48.
15. Williams, R. T. 1971. *In* "Fundamentals of Drug Metabolism and Drug Disposition," ed. by B. N. La Du, H. G. Mandel, and E. L. Way, The Williams & Wilkins Co., Baltimore, pp. 202–203.

PENICILLIN AND CEPHALOSPORIN HAVING
THE 2,3-DIOXOPIPERAZINE GROUP

Isamu SAIKAWA

*Research Laboratory, Toyama Chemical Co., Ltd.**

Carbenicillin (CPC) and sulbenicillin (SPC) have been clinically used as effective penicillins against *Pseudomonas aeruginosa*, but their antibacterial activities are not yet satisfactory.

Long *et al.* (*1*) have reported that ampicillin (APC) derivatives which introduced the acyl groups to an amino group of APC showed slight antibacterial activity against *P. aeruginosa*. Recently BLP-1654, mezlocillin and azlocillin having ureido groups at the α-position, have been reported as more effective penicillins against *P. aeruginosa*.

When we introduced piperazinylcarbonyl groups to an amino group of APC, they showed strong antibacterial activity against *P. aeruginosa* (*2*). Therefore many compounds having oxo groups at various positions on the piperazine ring were synthesized, and their antibacterial activities were compared (*3*).

Their antibacterial activities were in the following order:

Among them, the compound having 2,3-dioxopiperazine showed the strongest activity and this moiety was applied to penicillins and cephalosporins.

PIPERACILLIN (T-1220)

The compounds I that had the 4-alkyl-2,3-dioxopiperazinylcarbonyl group introduced into the amino group of APC were synthesized and the structure-activity relationships were investigated.

* Shimookui 2-4-1, Toyama 930, Japan.

TABLE I. Structure-activity Relationship of T-1220 Analogs

[I]

Compound				In vitro antibacterial				
	Structure		Molecular weight (as free form)	% of T-1220			ID$_{50}$	
Code No. (Name)	Type of comp.	R		S. aureus FDA209P	E. coli NIHJ	P. aeruginosa IFO3345	S. aureus	E. coli
T-1187	[I]	-CH$_3$	503.5	100 (0.78)^a	100 (<0.1)	100 (3.13)	1.56	2.9
T-1220 (Piperacillin)	[I]	-C$_2$H$_5$	517.6	100 (0.78)	100 (<0.1)	100 (3.13)	2.2	1.37
T-1221	[I]	-C$_4$H$_9$	545.6	100 (0.78)	100 (<0.1)	100 (3.13)	1.56	0.95
T-1213	[I]	-C$_8$H$_{17}$	601.7	200 (0.39)	100 (<0.1)	50.0 (6.25)	1.1	0.68
APC			349.4	780 (0.1)	<25.6 (0.39)	1.57 (200)	0.56	4.4
CPC			378.4	200 (0.39)	<12.8 (0.78)	6.26 (50)		

^{a} MIC (μg/ml). ^{b} Inoculum size: 1 loopful of 10^6 cells/ml. ^{c} Centrifugal ultrafiltration mouse). Infection: i.p. injection. Therapy: s.c. injection at 1 hr after infection. ^{g} s.c. injec-

[I]

The compounds I showed strong antibacterial activity against gram-positive and gram-negative bacteria, particularly against gram-negative bacilli such as *P. aeruginosa* and *Serratia marcescens*. The antibacterial activity of the compounds I was excellent in the compounds of R=C$_2$–C$_4$ alkyl, and against *Escherichia coli* and *S. marcescens* the antibacterial activity was relative to the increase in the carbon number of R (C$_1$→C$_8$).

It was found that the binding rate of the compounds I to human serum protein was elevated in accordance with the increase in the carbon number of R, and was correlated with the distribution coefficient. The protein binding rate of T-1220 [I: R=C$_2$H$_5$] was 25.3%, showing almost the same grade as that of APC.

The LD$_{50}$ (i.v. injection) in mice decreased remarkably in accordance with the

activity[b] (μg/ml)		Human serum protein binding (%)	Partition coefficient	Relative toxicity (%) compared to T-1220	In vivo antibacterial activity (%) of T-1220		Ref.
S. mar-cescens	P. aeru-ginosa				E. coli NIHJ	P. aeru-ginosa GN3315	
80	16	15.5[c]	4.3×10^{-3} [d]	80 (4,000)[e]	72.0 (0.25)[f]	88.5 (5.74)[g]	
27	6.25	25.3	8.7×10^{-3}	100 (5,000)	100 (0.18)	100 (5.08)[g]	3, 4
3.13	5.4	35.1	3.9×10^{-2}	36 (1,800)			
1.56	15.8	92.0	1.8×10^{0}	6 (300)			
>200	>200	22.9		92 (4,600)			
	70	52.3			40.9 (0.44)	19.0 (26.8)[g]	

method.   [d] $CHCl_3$/water at pH 7.0.   [e] LD_{50} (mg/kg), mice, ♂, i.v. injection.   [f] ED_{50} (mg/ tion at 0.5 and 4 hr after infection.

increase in the carbon number of R and LD_{50} of T-1220 having C_2 (ethyl) was 5,000 mg/kg, showing the highest value and low toxicity, the same as APC.

In the protective effects of T-1187 [I: R=CH_3], T-1220, and CPC against experimental infections of mice with E. coli NIHJ and P. aeruginosa GN3315, T-1220 showed the strongest therapeutic effect and T-1187 was the next strongest. The effects of both drugs were superior to the control drug, CPC. From these results, T-1220 was confirmed as the most excellent drug among those compounds.

The peak serum level in mice after subcutaneous injection of T-1220 was lower than that of CPC, and that in rats after intramuscular injection of T-1220 was almost the same as that of CPC.

In the excretion pattern in rats, CPC was excreted mainly in the urine, but T-1220 was excreted in the bile; that is, the excretion rate of T-1220 into bile was higher than that into urine. It was also reported that the absorption and excretion patterns of T-1220 were different among different animals (7).

When T-1220 was injected intramuscularly in humans at a dose of 1 g, the

TABLE II. Structure-activity Relationship of T-1551 Analogs

$$[\text{II}]$$

Compound				In vitro antibacterial		
	Structure		Molecular weight (as free form)	% of T-1551		
Code No. (Name)	Type of comp.	R_1	R_2	S. aureus FDA209P	E. coli NIHJ	P. aeruginosa IFO3345
T-1551 (Cefoperazone)	[II]	-OH	-S— (N—N ring, N-CH₃ tetrazole)	645.7	100 (1.56)[a]	100 (<0.1)	100 (3.13)
T-1543	[II]	-OH	-S— (N—N, S, CH₃ thiadiazole)	649.7	100 (1.56)	100 (<0.1)	12.5 (25)
T-1554	[II]	-OH	-OAc	633.6	100 (1.56)	100 (<0.1)	100 (3.13)
CEZ				454.5	>1,560 (<0.1)	<12.8 (0.78)	<1.57 (>200)

[a] MIC (μg/ml). [b] Inoculum size: 1 loopful of 10^6 cells/ml. [c] Centrifugal ultrafiltration i.p. injection. Therapy: s.c. injection at 1 hr after infection. [f] s.c. injection at 1 and 4 hr

maximum serum level was 33.4 μg/ml at 30 min and the urinary excretion rate was 66% within 6 hr (7).

The clinical application of T-1220 has been studied by Ueda et al. and T-1220 was recognized as a more useful drug, as well as a more effective one (9).

CEFOPERAZONE (T-1551)

The compounds II that had the 4-alkyl-2,3-dioxopiperazinylcarbonyl group introduced into the amino group of 7-(α-aminophenylacetamido)-3-substituted methyl-3-cephem-4-carboxylic acid were synthesized and the structure-activity relationships were investigated.

$$[\text{II}]$$

activity[b]				Human serum protein binding (%)	Acute toxicity (dose: 4 g/kg)	*In vivo* antibacterial activity (%) of T-1551		Ref.
ID_{50} (μg/ml)						E. coli K16	P. aeru-ginosa GN82	
S. aureus	E. coli	S. mar-cescens	P. aeru-ginosa					
1.50	<0.39	40	5.8	86.8[c]	3/3[d]	100 (1.45)[e]	100 (9.76)[f]	
1.17	<0.54	92	11.0	96.6	3/3	86.8 (1.67)	37.0 (26.4)[f]	5, 6
1.25	0.89	>100	5.6	72.4	3/3	43.4 (3.34)	24.8 (39.4)[f]	
<0.39	1.80	>200	>200	76.7		4.63 (31.3)		

method. [d] Mice, ♂, i.v. injection (survival No./tested No.). [e] ED₅₀ (mg/mouse). Infection: after infection.

In the course of these investigations, we found that phenylglycine derivatives [II: R_1=H] showed lower values in the LD_{50} test (i.v. injection) in mice than *p*-hydroxyphenylglycine derivatives [II: R_1=OH]. So we selected the following three compounds and further investigations were carried out.

T-1551 [II : R_1=OH , R_2=S—⟨N—N tetrazole N—N, CH₃⟩]

T-1543 [II : R_1=OH , R_2=S—⟨N—N thiadiazole S, CH₃⟩]

T-1554 [II : R_1=OH , R_2=OAc]

All compounds showed strong antibacterial activity against gram-positive and

TABLE III.   Structure-activity Relationship of Pharmacokinetic Properties

Compound	Relative activity (%) compared to T-1220 and T-1551				
Code No. (Name)	Serum level at peak		Urinary recovery (0–6 hr)	Biliary recovery (0–6 hr)	Ref.
T-1220 (Piperacillin)	100 (4.6 µg/ml)[a]	100 (7.2 µg/ml)[b]	100 (25.2%)[b]	100 (54.3%)[b]	
T-1551 (Cefoperazone)	100 (10.0)	100 (11.1)	100 (13.8)	100 (79.0)	7, 8
CPC	189 (8.7)	104 (7.5)	175 (44.2)	28.5 (15.5)	
CEZ	450 (45.0)	358 (39.7)	555 (76.6)	25.1 (19.8)	

[a] Mice, 20 mg/kg, s.c. injection.   [b] Rats, 20 mg/kg, i.m. injection.

gram-negative bacteria, particularly against gram-negative bacilli such as *P. aeruginosa* and *S. marcescens*, which were insensitive to cefazolin (CEZ). It was recognized that T-1551 had the strongest antibacterial activity of all. Against *Staphylococcus aureus* all compounds also showed strong antibacterial activity, but CEZ was more excellent.

In the test of LD_{50} (i.v. injection) on these compounds in mice, all mice administered a dose of 4,000 mg/kg survived, showing very low toxicity.

The binding rates of the three compounds to human serum protein were not less than 70%, showing a high binding rate the same as CEZ.

In the protective effects against experimental infections of mice with *E. coli* K16 and *P. aeruginosa* GN82, T-1551 showed the strongest therapeutic effect and was followed by T-1543 and T-1554, in that order. The effect of each compound was superior to that of CEZ.

The peak serum levels of T-1551 in mice and rats were lower than those of CEZ. But it is also reported that in monkeys and rabbits, T-1551 showed high and prolonged serum levels as compared with CEZ in a cross-over test (*8*). Moreover, when T-1551 was injected intramuscularly at a dose of 1 g in humans, the maximum serum level was 78 µg/ml after 1 hr and its biological half life was 120 min (*8*).

As for the excretion pattern in rats, CEZ was excreted mainly in the urine, but T-1551 was excreted in the bile as well as T-1220. It was reported that the excretion rates into urine in humans, when 1 g was injected intravenously, were 32.8% for T-1551 and 93.7% for CEZ within 6 hr in the cross over test (*12*).

The clinical application of T-1551 has been studied by Ueda *et al.* and T-1551 was recognized as a more useful drug, as well as a more effective one (*10*).

CONCLUSION

1-Ethyl-2,3-dioxopiperazine is the compound for a new moiety which has never been used as a medical drug. Especially, it must be emphasized that 1-ethyl-2,3-dioxopiperazine showed low toxicity in the test of acute toxicity in mice (4), and had almost no pharmacological action (11).

The antibacterial activities of piperacillin and cefoperazone having this moiety are almost similar, in the respect that these two compounds showed strong antibacterial activity against gram-negative bacilli including *P. aeruginosa* in comparison with the β-lactam antibiotics heretofore in use, and the *in vivo* effect was correlated with MIC values.

As an example of the same moiety being applied to both penicillin and cephalosporin, SPC-cefsulodin (SCE-129) having a sulfo group at the α-position of the side chain has been known. However, cefsulodin was a narrow spectrum antibiotic which showed strong antibacterial activity only against *P. aeruginosa*. Therefore, piperacillin-cefoperazone might be said to be unique new drugs that the common sense was broken.

From these results, 2,3-dioxopiperazine ring is expected to be of further wide application as a moiety for drugs such as antibiotics.

REFERENCES

1. Long, A. A. W. and Naylor, J. H. C. (Beecham Group Co., Ltd.) Br. Patent, 1, 224, 619 [*C.A.*, **74**, P141783, 1971].
2. Saikawa, I., Takano, S., Yoshida, C., Takashima, O., Momonoi, K., Yasuda, T., and Kasuya, K. 1977. *Yakugaku Zasshi* (*J. Pharm. Soc. Japan*), **97**, 883–889.
3. Saikawa, I., Takano, S., Yoshida, C., Takashima, O., Momonoi, K., Yasuda, T., Kasuya, K., and Komatsu, M. 1977. *Yakugaku Zasshi* (*J. Pharm. Soc. Japan*), **97**, 980–986.
4. Saikawa, I., Yasuda, T., Taki, H., Tai, M., Watanabe, Y., Sakai, H., Takano, S., Yoshida, C., and Kasuya, K. 1977. *Yakugaku Zasshi* (*J. Pharm. Soc. Japan*), **97**, 987–994.
5. Saikawa, I., Takano, S., Momonoi, K., Takakura, I., Kutani, C., Ochiai, H., Yoshida, C., Yasuda, T., and Taki, H. 1979. *Yakugaku Zasshi* (*J. Pharm. Soc. Japan*), **99**, 929–935.
6. Saikawa, I., Yasuda, T., Taki, H., Watanabe, Y., Tai, M., Matsubara, N., Takahata, M., and Fukuoka, Y. 1979. *Yakugaku Zasshi* (*J. Pharm. Soc. Japan*), **99**, 1073–1080.
7. Saikawa, I., Yasuda, T., Taki, H., Watanabe, Y., Matsubara, N., Nakagawa, M., and Kanagawa, S. 1977. *Chemotherapy* (*Tokyo*), **25**, 801–809.
8. Saikawa, I., Yasuda, T., Watanabe, Y., Taki, H., Matsubara, N., Hayashi, T., Matsunaga, K., and Takata, R. 1980. *Chemotherapy* (*Tokyo*), **28**, 163–172.

9. Ueda, Y., Saito, A., Shimada, J., Saikawa, I., and Yasuda, T. 1976. Abstr. 16th Intersci. Conf. Antimicrob. Agents Chemother., Chicago, No. 350.
10. Ueda, Y., Saito, A., Ohmori, M., Shiba, K., Yamaji, T., and Ihara, H. 1978. Abstr. 18th Intersci. Conf. Antimicrob. Agents Chemother., Atlanta, No. 158.
11. Yamanaka, Y., Kono, S., Tateishi, H., and Aratani, H. 1977. *Chemotherapy* (*Tokyo*), **25**, 769–782.
12. 27th Japanese Congress of Chemotherapy, Tokyo, New drug symposium (T-1551), 1979.

CEFSULODIN (SCE-129), CEFOTIAM (SCE-963), AND CEFMENOXIME (SCE-1365)

Kanji Tsuchiya

*Central Research Division, Takeda Chemical Industries, Ltd.**

The last two decades have witnessed a remarkable progress in the research on chemical modifications of cephalosporins, and some important cephalosporin derivatives have been developed. Cephalosporins, like penicillins, are inhibitors of bacterial cell wall synthesis and their human toxicity is rather low. Consequently these drugs have come to occupy a large share in chemotherapy against bacterial infections. On the other hand, due to increasing prescription of penicillins and cephalosporins, an increasing number of infections caused by penicillin- and cephalosporin-resistant bacteria have been observed in recent years. The mechanisms of resistance development against β-lactam antibiotics by these bacteria include, for example, (i) a barrier formation to prevent permeation of the bacterial outer membrane by an antibiotic; (ii) hydrolysis of the drugs by bacterial β-lactamases; and (iii) interaction of the drugs with enzymes and/or penicillin-binding proteins (PBPs) (*3, 4, 19, 24*). The present paper deals with cefsulodin (SCE-129), cefotiam (SCE-963), and cefmenoxime (SCE-1365), placing emphasis on their structure-activity relations and resistance to β-lactamases.

CEFSULODIN (SCE-129)

Pseudomonas aeruginosa is a species of clinically important pathogens frequently encountered in opportunistic infections and it is resistant to most penicillins and cephalosporins. Certain aminoglycoside antibiotics have been used in the treatment of *P. aeruginosa* infections, but the use of these antibiotics has a definite limitation because of their toxicities. Though some penicillins show a certain degree of antipseudomonal activity, the activity is relatively weak.

Sulbenicillin, α-sulfophenylacetylpenicillin, is one of the antipseudomonal penicillins originally discovered and developed by Takeda Chemical Industries, Ltd.,

* Jusohonmachi 2-17-85, Yodogawa-ku, Osaka 532, Japan.

TABLE I. Structure-activity Relationship of Antibacterial Activity of α-Sulfocephalosporin

Compound			MIC (μg/ml)				
No.	R_1	R_2	*P. aeruginosa* NCTC 10490	*E. coli*	*P. vulgaris* IFO 3049	*S. aureus* FDA 209 P	*S. aureus* 87 (PCGʳ)
1	⬡-CH-CO- | SO₃Na	-O-CO-CH₃	3. 13	25	12. 5	3. 13	3. 13
2	⬡-CH-CO- | SO₃Na	-N⁺◯ (pyridine)	0. 39	100	50	1. 56	3. 13
3	⬡-CH-CO- | SO₃Na (Cefsulodin ; SCE-129)	-N⁺◯-CO-NH₂	0. 39	25	50	3. 13	3. 13
4	⬡-CH-CO- | SO₃Na	-S⟨N-N⟩-CH₃ (thiadiazole)	100	25	6. 25	6. 25	12. 5
5	⬡-CH-CO- | SO₃Na	-S⟨N—N⟩ N-CH₃ (tetrazole)	100	25	6. 25	3. 13	12. 5
6	⟨S⟩-CH-CO- | SO₃Na	-N⁺◯	0. 78	>100	50	3. 13	3. 13
7	CH₃(CH₂)₃-CH-CO- | SO₃Na	-N⁺◯	3. 13	>100	100	0. 78	1. 56
8	⟨N⟩-CH-CO- | SO₃Na	-N⁺◯	12. 5	>100	>100	3. 13	12. 5
9	⟨N⁺CH₃⟩-CH-CO- | SO₃Na	-N⁺◯	50	>100	>100	25	25
10	⬡-CH-CO- | NH-SO₃Na	-N⁺◯-CO-NH₂	50	50	50	3. 13	3. 13
11	⬡-CH-CO- | COONa	-N⁺◯-CO-NH₂	50	50	100	12. 5	6. 25
12	⬡-CH-CO-NH- | SO₃Na (Sulbenicillin)	penicillin structure	3. 13	12. 5	1. 56	0. 78	12. 5

Medium: Trypticase soy agar (BBL); inoculum size: 10⁸ CFU/ml.

Osaka, Japan. The overwhelming majority of cephalosporins reported in the literature has shown only limited activity against *P. aeruginosa*. Therefore, attempts were made to introduce the α-sulfophenylacetyl moiety and other related moieties onto 7-aminocephalosporanic acid, and a number of cephalosporins having the α-sulfophenylacetyl side chain at the 7-position was prepared (*10, 11*).

The activities of cephalosporins with the D-α-sulfophenylacetyl side chain were much more potent than those of the corresponding L-isomers, as has been observed with other β-lactam antibiotics (*6, 21*). The most striking characteristic was the fact that some of the α-sulfophenylacetyl cephalosporins synthesized showed remarkable activity against *P. aeruginosa* but less activity against other gram-negative bacteria. Finally, cefsulodin, 7β-(D-α-sulfophenylacetamido)-3-(4-carbamoyl-1-pyridiniomethyl)ceph-3-em-4-carboxylate monosodium salt was selected for further development (Table I).

The antipseudomonal activity of cefsulodin was about 10 times as active as that of sulbenicillin (and carbenicillin) and was almost comparable to that of gentamicin. It showed also potent activities against both gentamicin-susceptible and

TABLE II. Comparative Activities of Cefsulodin, Sulbenicillin, and Gentamicin against *P. aeruginosa*

Compound	ID_{50} (μg/ml)[a]			
	SBPC^s-GM^s (128 strains)	SBPC^s-GM^r (54)	SBPC^r-GM^s (21)	SBPC^r-GM^r (15)
Cefsulodin	1.56	3.13	25	50
Sulbenicillin	25	50	>1,600	>1,600
Gentamicin	3.13	100	3.13	200

Compound	ED_{50} (mg/kg)[b]		
	SBPC^s-GM^s (U 31)[c]	SBPC^s-GM^r (TN 1352)[d]	SBPC^r-GM^s (GN 3345)[e]
Cefsulodin	31.3	6.02	77.7
Sulbenicillin	552	106	>2,400
Gentamicin	33.6	480	17.7

[a] The concentration required to inhibit the growth of clinical isolates by about 50% in number. [b] Antibiotics were administered subcutaneously at 0, 2, and 4 hr after infection. The ED_{50} values were indicated as the total dose. [c] *P. aeruginosa* U 31 has MICs of 6.25 μg/ml for cefsulodin, 50 μg/ml for sulbenicillin, and 1.56 μg/ml for gentamicin with an inoculum size of 10^6 CFU/ml. [d] *P. aeruginosa* TN 1352 has MICs of 3.13 μg/ml for cefsulodin, 25 μg/ml for sulbenicillin, and 100 μg/ml for gentamicin with an inoculum size of 10^6 CFU/ml. [e] *P. aeruginosa* GN 3345 has MICs of 12.5 μg/ml for cefsulodin, >800 μg/ml for sulbenicillin, and 3.13 μg/ml for gentamicin with an inoculum size of 10^6 CFU/ml.

-resistant *P. aeruginosa* (*7*, *25*, *26*) (Table II). The activity of cefsulodin was considered to be due mainly to the high permeability of the cephalosporin through the outer membrane of *P. aeruginosa* (*22*) and the stability of the cephalosporin to the β-lactamase produced by *P. aeruginosa* (*18*). Although cefsulodin exhibits an affinity for PBP 3 and PBP 1B obtained from *P. aeruginosa*, the binding affinity of cefsulodin for PBPs was much lower that those of other β-lactam antibiotics (*9*).

CEFOTIAM (SCE-963)

Investigations of the structure-activity relationships of cephalosporins in clinical use or with potent activities have taught our synthetic organic chemists that cephalosporins that show activity have "active hydrogen" on the α-carbon of the side chain acyl at the 7-position (*8*). It has also been known that the "intrinsic" antibacterial activity of β-lactam antibiotics can be correlated with the chemical reactivity of the β-lactam carbonyl (*5*).

In light of these speculations, it was assumed that, in a transition state of irreversible acylation of the enzyme by a cephalosporin molecule with an active α-hydrogen on the side chain acyl, the enzyme first abstracts the active hydrogen and then an intramolecular general-base catalysis occurs, whereby the reactivity of the β-lactam and hence the antibacterial activity would be enhanced (*8*). The whole picture of this mechanism can be depicted by the schematic model shown in Fig. 1.

Based on these ideas, various β-ketoacids were introduced in the side chain of cephalosporins because β-ketoacids are characterized by the possession of "active hydrogen." The compounds thus obtained in the early stage of our studies showed only moderate activities (Table III). A cephalosporin with the γ-methylthioacetoacetyl group, however, showed an activity as potent as that of cephalothin. Being encouraged by the progressive results, replacement of the chlorine of γ-chloroacetoacetyl cephalosporins by thiol compounds was tried, and during the course of these experiments, several new compounds having remarkable activities were obtained. Spectroscopic and physicochemical data indicated that the compounds no longer

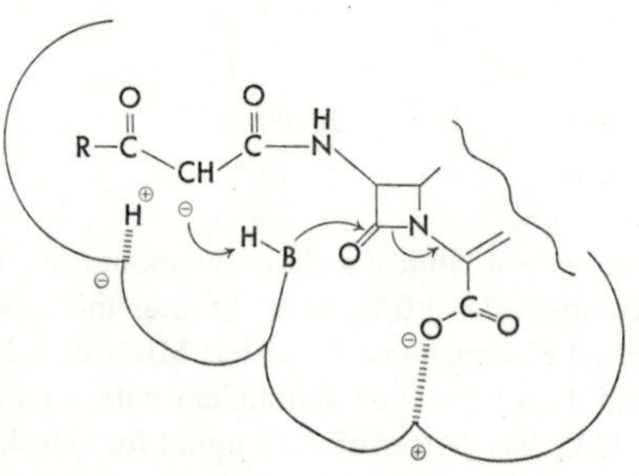

FIG. 1.   A proposed "intramolecular general-base catalysis" for irreversible acylation of the enzyme.
B denotes a nucleophile.

TABLE III. Structure-activity Relationship of Antibacterial Activity of β-Ketoacyl- and Aminothiazol-cephalosporins

Compound			MIC (μg/ml)					
No.	R₁	R₂	S. aureus FDA 209 P	E. coli NIHJ JC-2	E. coli T-7	K. pneumoniae DT	P. vulgaris IFO 3988	P. morganii IFO 3168
13	phenyl-CO-CH₂-CO-	-O-CO-CH₃	>100	>100	—	>100	—	—
14	furyl-CO-CH₂-CO-	-O-CO-CH₃	<0.78	50	—	25	—	—
15	thienyl-CO-CH₂-CO-	-O-CO-CH₃	100	100	—	>100	—	—
16	phenyl-CH₂-CO-CH₂-CO-	-O-CO-CH₃	<0.78	>100	—	>100	—	—
17	pyridyl-CO-CH₂-CO-	-O-CO-CH₃	1.56	>100	—	>100	—	—
18	CH₃-CO-CH₂-CO-	-O-CO-CH₃	3.13	50	—	25	—	—
19	furyl-CO-CH₂-CO-	-S-thiadiazolyl-CH₃	<0.78	25	—	25	—	—
20	CH₃-CO-CH₂-CO-	-S-thiadiazolyl-CH₃	<0.78	25	—	12.5	—	—
21	CH₃-CO-CH₂-CO-	-S-tetrazolyl-CH₃	<0.78	6.25	—	3.13	—	—
22	CH₃-S-CH₂-CO-CH₂-CO-	-S-tetrazolyl-CH₃	<0.78	1.56	—	1.56	—	—
23	thiazolone-CH₂-CO-	-O-CO-CH₃	0.78	6.25	>100	6.25	25	100
24	thiazolone-CH₂-CO-	-S-thiadiazolyl-CH₃	0.2	1.56	>100	1.56	6.25	50

TABLE III. (continued)

No.	R₁	R₂	S. aureus FDA 209 P	E. coli NIHJ JC-2	E. coli T-7	K. pneu- moniae DT	P. vul- garis IFO 3988	P. mor- ganii IFO 3168
25	[structure: O=, S, HN, CH₂-CO-]	[structure: N—N tetrazole, -S-, CH₃]	<0.2	0.78	50	1.56	1.56	50
26	[structure: H₂N, S, N, CH₂-CO-]	-O-CO-CH₃	0.78	1.56	50	0.39	0.39	50
27	[structure: H₂N, S, N, CH₂-CO-]	[structure: N—N, S, -S-, CH₃]	0.39	1.56	25	0.39	0.78	3.13
28	[structure: H₂N, S, N, CH₂-CO-]	[structure: N—N tetrazole, -S-, CH₃]	0.39	0.39	6.25	0.1	0.39	3.13
29	[structure: H₂N, S, N, CH₂-CO-] (Cefotiam ; SCE-963)	[structure: N—N tetrazole, -S-, CH₂-CH₂-N(CH₃)₂]	0.39	0.2	1.56	≤0.2	0.78	≤0.2
30	[structure: N=N, N, N-CH₂-CO-] (Cefazolin)	[structure: N—N, S, -S-, CH₃]	0.39	1.56	100	1.56	6.25	100

Medium: Trypticase soy agar (BBL); inoculum size: 10^8 CFU/ml.

possessed β-ketoacid moieties in the side chain, but had been transformed into 2-aminothiazol-4-ylacetyl cephalosporins.

Cefotiam, 7β-[2-(2-aminothiazol-4-yl)acetamido]-3-[[[1-(2-dimethylaminoethyl)-1H-tetrazol-5-yl]thio]methyl]ceph-3-em-4-carboxylic acid was finally selected (13–15) (Table III). Cefotiam showed excellent in vitro and in vivo antibacterial activities against a wide range of gram-positive and gram-negative bacteria (27) (Table IV). The cephalosporin also showed excellent permeability through the outer membrane of E. coli (21) and high affinities for PBPs 1A, 1B, and 3 of Escherichia coli (12). Furthermore, cefotiam showed a unique distribution pattern in the organs in both animals and humans. The cefotiam levels in the liver and the biliary excretion rate were rather high, although it was principally excreted in the urine (28) (Table V).

CEFMENOXIME (SCE-1365)

Although cefotiam did show potent and broad antibacterial activities, some of the gram-negative bacteria still remained resistant to the drug. Up to date (2, 20, 31), several researchers have performed the introduction of various substituents onto the

TABLE IV.   Comparative Activities of Cefotiam, Cefazolin, Cephaloridine, and Cephalothin against Gram-negative Bacteria

Compound	ID_{50} (μg/ml)[a]								
	E.coli (98 strains)	K. pneumoniae (89)	H. influenzae (64)	P. mirabilis (52)	P. vulgaris (52)	P. morganii (54)	P. rettgeri (44)	C. freundii (52)	E. cloacae (54)
Cefotiam	0.1	0.2	0.78	0.2	12.5	0.78	0.05	3.13	1.56
Cefazolin	1.56	1.56	12.5	3.13	>100	>100	6.25	>100	>100
Cephaloridine	3.13	3.13	12.5	6.25	>100	>100	25	>100	>100
Cephalothin	6.25	3.13	6.25	3.13	>100	>100	100	>100	>100

Compound	ED_{50} (mg/kg)[b]					
	E. coli O-111[c]	E. coli T-7[d]	P. mirabilis[e] GN 4336	P. vulgaris[f] GN 4712	P. morganii[g] GN 4794	P. rettgeri[h] TN 338
Cefotiam	0.0607	5.63	1.81	27.6	6.54	0.157
Cefazolin	1.84	48.9	10.6	89.3	64.3	1.72
Cephalothin	13.1	>800	26.5	276	>800	69.3

[a] The concentration required to inhibit the growth of clinical isolates by about 50% in number. [b] Cephalosporins were administered subcutaneously at 0 hr after infection. [c] E. coli O-111 has MICs of 0.05 μg/ml for cefotiam, 1.56 μg/ml for cefazolin, and 1.56 μg/ml for cephalothin with an inoculum size of 10^6 CFU/ml. [d] E. coli T-7 has MICs of 0.78 μg/ml for cefotiam, 25 μg/ml for cefazolin, and 100 μg/ml for cephalothin with an inoculum size of 10^6 CFU/ml. [e] P. mirabilis GN 4336 has MICs of 1.56 μg/ml for cefotiam, 12.5 μg/ml for cefazolin, and 25 μg/ml for cephalothin with an inoculum size of 10^6 CFU/ml. [f] P. vulgaris GN 4712 has MICs of 1.56 μg/ml for cefotiam, 100 μg/ml for cefazolin, and 100 μg/ml for cephalothin with an inoculum size of 10^6 CFU/ml. [g] P. morganii GN 4794 has MICs of 3.13 μg/ml for cefotiam, >100 μg/ml for cefazolin, and >100 μg/ml for cephalothin with an inoculum size of 10^6 CFU/ml. [h] P. rettgeri TN 338 has MICs of <0.025 μg/ml for cefotiam, 6.25 μg/ml for cefazolin, and 0.78 μg/ml for cephalothin with inoculum size of 10^6 CFU/ml.

TABLE V. Comparative Pharmacokinetic Properties of Cephalosporins

Animal	Compound[a]	Peak level (μg/ml or g)			Percent excretion	
		Plasma	Kidney	Liver	Urine	Bile
Mice	Cephalothin[b]	11.5	14.9	0	29.9	—[f]
	Cephaloridine	25.5	56.2	11.4	71.0	—
	Cefazolin	41.3	63.0	7.7	68.7	—
	Cefotiam	12.8	65.3	39.8	49.0	—
	Cefmenoxime	22.9	63.5	14.1	65.8	—
	Cefotaxime (a)[c]	28.7	10.8	1.2	40.5	—
	(b)[d]	26.1	0.3	—	27.8	—
	(c)[e]	7.2	30.9	—	36.0	—
Rats	Cephalothin	19.2	21.3	1.7	20.6	0.44
	Cephaloridine	26.3	73.5	3.4	82.0	0.62
	Cefazolin	44.5	71.1	20.5	83.0	11.8
	Cefotiam	14.6	91.3	28.4	53.0	32.9
	Cefmenoxime	66.7	122	27.3	52.5	32.6
	Cefotaxime (a)	43.4	17.4	1.6	48.4	1.27
	(b)	36.5	0	—	25.2	0.63
	(c)	41.1	51.1	—	75.6	2.54
Dogs	Cephalothin	21.3	36.0	5.9	41.9	0.16
	Cephaloridine	39.2	128	11.0	89.3	0.14
	Cefazolin	35.8	93.3	18.9	55.7	1.55
	Cefotiam	30.7	90.2	91.5	75.9	2.95
	Cefmenoxime	22.7	281	63.6	72.1	4.02
	Cefotaxime (a)	34.0	76.8	4.6	57.4	0.23
	(b)	30.5	53.9	0.3	52.3	0.11
	(c)	40.7	121	12.8	16.7	0.26

[a] A single dose of 20 mg/kg of cephalosporin was administered subcutaneously to mice and intramuscularly to rats and dogs. [b] As cephalothin activity. [c] As cefotaxime activity. [d] Cefotaxime. [e] Deacetylcefotaxime. [f] Not tested.

α-carbon of the acyl side chain at the 7-position to obtain cephalosporins with various properties. It appeared, therefore, interesting to find out if further chemical modification of cefotiam could lead to compounds with further enhanced activities or resistance to hydrolysis by β-lactamases (8).

Introduction of the amino, α-hydroxyl, α-methyl, α,α-dimethyl, and other groups into the 2-aminothiazol-4-ylacetyl side chain led to cephalosporins with

TABLE VI.   Structure-activity Relationship of Antibacterial Activity of Aminotiazol-cepha-
losporins

Compound			MIC (μg/ml)				
No.	R_1	R_2	S. aureus 1840 (PCase)	E. coli T-7 (PCase)	S. marcescens TN 24 (PCase, CSase)	P. vulgaris GN 4413 (CSase)	E. cloacae TN 1282 (CSase)
31			1. 56	1. 56	25	>100	6. 25
32			3. 13	25	12. 5	>100	100
33			50	>100	>100	>100	>100
34			12. 5	3. 13	50	>100	25
35			3. 13	0. 78	0. 78	0. 78	6. 25
36			3. 13	0. 39	0. 2	1. 56	6. 25
37			3. 13	0. 78	0. 2	0. 39	1. 56
38			3. 13	1. 56	3. 13	1. 56	3. 13
39			3. 13	6. 25	3. 13	12. 5	6. 25
40			50	0. 39	0. 78	0. 025	0. 78
41			3. 13	6. 25	6. 25	6. 25	>100
42			1. 56	3. 13	100	>100	100

Medium: Trypticase soy agar (BBL); inoculum size: 10^8 CFU/ml. PCase, penicillinase; CSase, cephalosporinase.

TABLE VII. Comparative Activities of Cefmenoxime, Cefotaxime, Cefuroxime, and Cefotiam

ID$_{50}$ (µg/ml)[a]

Compound	E. coli (104 strains)	K. pneu-moniae (75)	H. influ-enzae (69)	P. mira-bilis (107)	P. vul-garis (78)	P. mor-ganii (81)	P. rett-geri (40)	P. incon-stans (32)	S. mar-cescens (105)	C. freundii (80)	E. cloacae (79)
Cefmenoxime	0.1	0.1	0.013	0.05	0.1	0.025	0.013	0.1	0.2	0.39	0.2
Cefotaxime	0.1	0.05	0.013	0.025	0.05	0.05	0.013	0.05	0.39	0.39	0.39
Cefuroxime	6.25	3.13	0.78	1.56	>100	25	0.39	3.13	50	12.5	12.5
Cefotiam	0.1	0.2	0.78	0.2	12.5	0.39	0.1	0.2	6.25	1.56	1.56

ED$_{50}$ (mg/kg)[b]

Compound	E. coli O-111	E. coli[d] T-7	K. pneu-moniae[d] DT	K. pneu-moniae[e] S 22	P. mira-bilis[f] GN 4336	P. vul-garis[g] GN 4712	P. mor-ganii[i] TN 373	P. rett-geri[j] TN 338	S. mar-cescens[k] TN 66	C. freundii[l] TN 549	E. clo-acae[m] TN 618
Cefmenoxime	0.016	0.490	0.189	0.322	0.049	0.202	0.097	0.256	0.580	0.271	0.069
Cefotaxime	0.017	0.259	0.445	0.349	0.079	0.534	1.17	1.43	0.241	0.278	0.064
Cefuroxime	0.550	10.3	12.2	14.8	7.11	368	20.9	32.2	33.7	3.72	4.00
Cefotiam	0.066	0.952	5.25	5.62	3.61	51.9	58.8	9.72	6.12	1.34	0.126

[a] The concentration required to inhibit the growth of clinical isolates by about 50% in number. [b] Cephalosporins were administered subcutaneously at 0 hr after infection. [c] E. coli O-111 has MICs of 0.013 µg/ml for cefmenoxime, 0.025 µg/ml for cefotaxime, 1.56 µg/ml for cefuroxime, and 0.025 µg/ml for cefotiam with an inoculum size of 10^6 CFU/ml. [d] E. coli T-7 has MICs of 0.2 µg/ml for cefmenoxime, 0.2 µg/ml for cefotaxime, 12.5 µg/ml for cefuroxime, and 0.39 µg/ml for cefotiam with an inoculum size of 10^6 CFU/ml. [e] K. pneumoniae DT has MICs of 0.025 µg/ml for cefmenoxime, 0.025 µg/ml for cefotaxime, 0.78 µg/ml for cefuroxime, and 0.1 µg/ml for cefotiam with an inoculum size of 10^6 CFU/ml. [f] K. pneumoniae S 22 has MICs of 0.1 µg/ml for cefmenoxime, 0.1 µg/ml for cefotaxime, 3.13 µg/ml for cefuroxime, and 0.78 µg/ml for cefotiam with an inoculum size of 10^6 CFU/ml. [g] P. mirabilis GN 4336 has MICs of 0.1 µg/ml for cefmenoxime, 0.05 µg/ml for cefotaxime, 3.13 µg/ml for cefuroxime, and 0.78 µg/ml for cefotiam with an inoculum size of 10^6 CFU/ml. [h] P. vulgaris GN 4712 has MICs of 0.1 µg/ml for cefmenoxime, 6.25 µg/ml for cefotaxime, 25 µg/ml for cefuroxime, and 0.39 µg/ml for cefotiam with an inoculum size of 10^6 CFU/ml. [i] P. morganii TN 373 has MICs of 0.025 µg/ml for cefmenoxime, 0.025 µg/ml for cefotaxime, 25 µg/ml for cefuroxime, 0.006 µg/ml for cefmenoxime, 0.006 µg/ml for cefotiam with an inoculum size of 10^6 CFU/ml. [j] P. rettgeri TN 338 has MICs of 0.006 µg/ml for cefmenoxime, 0.025 µg/ml for cefotaxime, 50 µg/ml for cefuroxime, and 3.13 µg/ml for cefotiam with an inoculum size of 10^6 CFU/ml. [k] S. marcescens TN 66 has MICs of 0.2 µg/ml for cefmenoxime, 0.2 µg/ml for cefotaxime, 6.25 µg/ml for cefuroxime, and 6.25 µg/ml for cefotiam with an inoculum size of 10^6 CFU/ml. [l] C. freundii TN 549 has MICs of 0.2 µg/ml for cefmenoxime, 0.2 µg/ml for cefotaxime, and 0.78 µg/ml for cefotiam with an inoculum size of 10^6 CFU/ml. [m] E. cloacae TN 618 has MICs of 0.2 µg/ml for cefmenoxime, 0.2 µg/ml for cefotaxime, 12.5 µg/ml for cefuroxime, and 0.39 µg/ml for cefotiam with an inoculum size of 10^6 CFU/ml.

various degrees of the activity as shown in Table VI (*17*). Finally, cefmenoxime, 7β-[2-(2-aminothiazol-4-yl)-(*Z*)-2-methoxyiminoacetamido]-3-[(1-methyl-1H-tetrazol-5-yl)thiomethyl]ceph-3-em-4-carboxylic acid was obtained (*16*) (Table VI). At almost the same time, two other research groups succeeded in synthesizing compounds with the same side chain structure, and all these compounds were found to exhibit further extended antibacterial spectra and activities exceeding the spectra of cefotiam (*1*, *23*) and other previously reported cephalosporins.

Cefmenoxime, cefotaxime, and ceftizoxime are unique in that these cephalosporins lack the active hydrogen on the α-carbon of the side chain acyl, and still show potent antibacterial activities like cefuroxime does. The potent antibacterial activity of the cephalosporins with a *syn*-methoxyimino group on the side chain acyls appears to be accounted for by the general-base-catalysis mechanism (*8*). Cefmenoxime is highly resistant to hydrolysis by β-lactamases.

Cefmenoxime exhibits a potent and extraordinarily extended antibacterial activity against a wide range of gram-positive and gram-negative bacteria. It should be noted that the spectral advantage of cefmenoxime encompasses the so-called "problem" pathogenic bacteria such as indole-positive *Proteus, Serratia marcescens, Citrobacter freundii,* and *Enterobacter cloacae,* both *in vitro* and in experimental infections in mice (*29*) (Table VII), and cefmenoxime has a high stability to hydrolysis by various β-lactamases (*17*). The potent antibacterial activity of cefmenoxime also suggested that the cephalosporin might have a high permeability into bacterial cells (*29*), and this was confirmed with *S. marcescens* (Suginaka, H. *et al.*, personal communication). The affinity of cefmenoxime for PBPs of *E. coli* was the highest for PBP 3 and decreased in the order of PBPs 1A, 1B, and 2 (*29*). Furthermore, cefmenoxime exhibits, like cefotiam, a unique pharmacokinetic profile excreted into the bile at a high percentage and no active metabolite has been found in the specimens from both humans and animals administered cefmenoxime (*30*) (Table V).

REFERENCES

1. Bucourt, R., Heymes, R., Luts, A., Penasse, L., and Perronnet, J. 1977. *C. R. Acad. Sci.*, **284**, D, 1847–1849.
2. Cherry, P. C., Cook, M. C., Foxton, M. W., Gregson, M., Gregory., and Webb, G. B. 1977. *In* "Recent Advances in the Chemistry of β-Lactam Antibiotics," ed. by J. Elks, The Chemical Society, London, pp. 145–152.
3. Costerton, J. W. and Cheng, K.-J. 1975. *J. Antimicrob. Chemother.*, **1**, 363–377.
4. Davis, J. 1979. *Rev. Infect. Dis.*, **1**, 23–27.
5. Gorman, M. and Ryan, C. W. 1972. *In* "Cephalosporins and Penicillins, Chemistry and Biology," ed. by E. H. Flynn, Academic Press, New York and London, pp. 532–582.
6. Gourevitch, A., Wolfe, S., and Levine, J. 1961. *Antimicrob. Agents Chemother.*, 576–580.

7. Kondo, M. and Tsuchiya, K. 1978. *Antimicrob. Agents Chemother.*, **14**, 151–153.
8. Morita, K., Nomura, H., Numata, M., Ochiai, M., and Yoneda, M. 1980. *Phil. Trans. Roy. Soc. Lond. B*, **289**, 181–190.
9. Noguchi, H., Matsuhashi, M., and Mitsuhashi, S. 1979. *Eur. J. Biochem.*, **100**, 41–49.
10. Nomura, H., Fugono, T., Hitaka, T., Minami, I., Azuma, T., Morimoto, S., and Masuda, T. 1974. *J. Med. Chem.*, **17**, 1312–1315.
11. Nomura, H., Minami, I., Hitaka, T., and Fugono, T. 1976. *J. Antibiot.*, **29**, 298–306.
12. Nozaki, Y., Imada, A., and Yoneda, M. 1979. *Antimicrob. Agents Chemother.*, **15**, 20–27.
13. Numata, M., Yamaoka, M., Minamida, I., Kuritani, M., and Imashiro, Y. 1978. *J. Antibiot.*, **31**, 1245–1251.
14. Numata, M., Minamida, I., Yamaoka, M., Shiraishi, M., and Miyawaki, T. 1978. *J. Antibiot.*, **31**, 1252–1261.
15. Numata, M., Minamida, I., Yamaoka, M., Shiraishi, M., Miyawaki, T., Akimoto, H., Naito, K., and Kida, M. 1978. *J. Antibiot.*, **31**, 1262–1271.
16. Ochiai, M., Aki, O., Morimoto, A., Okada, T., and Matsushita, Y. 1977. *Chem. Pharm. Bull.*, **25**, 3115–3117.
17. Ochiai, M., Morimoto, A., Okada, T., Matsushita, Y., Aki, O., Kida, M., and Okonogi, K. 1978. Abstr. 18th Intersci. Conf. Antimicrob. Agents Chemother., No. 150.
18. Okonogi, K., Kida, M., and Yoneda, M. 1979. *Chemotherapy (Tokyo)*, **27** (S-2), 65–73.
19. Richmond, M. H. 1979. *Rev. Infect. Dis.*, **1**, 30–36.
20. Ryan, C. W., Simon, R. L., and Van Heyningen, E. M. 1969. *J. Med. Chem.*, **12**, 310–313.
21. Spencer, J. L., Flynn, E. H., Roeske, R. W., Siu, F. Y., and Chauvette, R. R. 1966. *J. Med. Chem.*, **9**, 746–750.
22. Suginaka, H., Shimatani, M., Kotani, S., Ogawa, M., Hama, M., and Kosaki, G. 1979. *FEMS Microbiol. Lett.*, **5**, 177–179.
23. Takaya, T., Takasugi, H., Tsuji, K., and Chiba, T. 1976. Japan Patent. Appl., 53-137988.
24. Tipper, D. J. 1979. *Rev. Infect. Dis.*, **1**, 39–53.
25. Tsuchiya, K., Kondo, M., and Nagatomo, H. 1978. *Antimicrob. Agents Chemother.*, **13**, 137–145.
26. Tsuchiya, K. and Kondo, M. 1978. *Antimicrob. Agents Chemother.*, **14**, 557–568.
27. Tsuchiya, K., Kida, M., Kondo, M., Ono, H., Takeuchi, M., and Nishi, T. 1978. *Antimicrob. Agents Chemother.*, **14**, 557–568.
28. Tsuchiya, K., Kondo, M., Kita, Y., Noji, Y., Takeuchi, M., and Fugono, T. 1978. *J. Antibiot.*, **31**, 1272–1282.

29. Tsuchiya, K., Kondo, M., Kida, M., Nakao, M., Iwahi, T., Nishi, T., Noji, Y., Takeuchi, M., and Nozaki, Y. 1981. *Antimicrob. Agents Chemother.*, **19**, 56–65.
30. Tsuchiya, K., Kita, Y., Yamazaki, I., Kondo, M., Noji, Y., and Fugono, T. 1980. *J. Antibiot.*, **33**, 1532–1544.
31. Whick, W. E. and Preston, D. A. 1972. *Antimicrob. Agents Chemother.*, **1**, 221–234.

CEFOTAXIME

E. Schrinner,[*1] M. Limbert,[*1] R. Heymes,[*2] and W. Dürckheimer[*1]

Hoechst AG[*1] *and Roussel Uclaf*[*2]

Cefotaxime sodium (CTX), also known as HR 756, is a new injectable cephalosporin highly active *in vitro* and *in vivo*. It possesses a broad antibacterial spectrum including many species of clinically important gram-positive and gram-negative bacteria. Its MICs especially against Enterobacteriacae are in many cases more than 100 times lower than those of classical cephalosporins like cefazolin (CEZ) and broad spectrum penicillins like ampicillin.

CTX, unlike many other cephalosporins, also shows a high inhibitory potency against *Enterobacter*, the indol-positive *Proteae, Serratia*, and *Haemophilus influenzae*. CTX is the first broad spectrum cephalosporin to be described with a therapeutic relevant activity against *Pseudomonas aeruginosa (2, 3)*.

The wide spectrum of CTX and its high activity is based on its high affinity to important cell wall synthesizing enzymes, on its exceptional stability to β-lactamases of gram-positive and most gram-negative bacteria (*1, 6*) and furthermore on its relatively good penetration through the bacterial cell envelope.

The *in vitro* characteristics of CTX were confirmed by *in vivo* experiments in animals but more importantly by its high efficacy in widespread clinical trials. CTX has been used successfully in a variety of infectious diseases (*4, 7*).

CTX is the most prominent representative of a series of semisynthetic cephalosporin derivatives listed in Tables I and II. Table III shows the *in vitro* activity of these antibiotics against some strains of clinically important bacterial species and Table IV shows the *in vivo* effects in the model of experimental septicemia in mice.

The MIC values in Table III demonstrate the high potency of CTX against these

[*1] D-6230, Frankfurt 80, West Germany.

[*2] F-93230, Romainville, West Germany.

The synthesis of the compounds discussed and chemotherapeutic studies were done in a joint venture in the laboratories of Hoechst AG and Roussel Uclaf. Besides the authors, the following scientists were involved this work: Drs. Bormann, Blumbach, Ehlers, Klesel, Lutz, and Seeger.

TABLE I. Modification of the 7-Side Chain

Code No.	R_1	R_2	R_3	R_4
Cefotaxime	NH_2	H	$N^{\parallel}\!\!\diagdown_{OCH_3}$	H
II	NH_2	H	$H_3CO\diagup^{N^{\parallel}}$	H
III	NH_2	H	$N^{\parallel}\!\!\diagdown_{OC_2H_5}$	H
IV	NH_2	H	$N^{\parallel}\!\!\diagdown_{OCH_2C_2H_5}$	H
V	NH_2	H	$N^{\parallel}\!\!\diagdown_{O\emptyset}$	H
VI	NH_2	H	$N^{\parallel}\!\!\diagdown_{OH}$	H
VII	NH_2	H	$O^{\parallel}$	H
VIII	CH_3CONH	H	$N^{\parallel}\!\!\diagdown_{OCH_3}$	H
IX	H	H	$N^{\parallel}\!\!\diagdown_{OCH_3}$	H
X	NH_2	Cl	$N^{\parallel}\!\!\diagdown_{OCH_3}$	H
XI	NH_2	Br	$N^{\parallel}\!\!\diagdown_{OCH_3}$	H
XII	NH_2	H	$N^{\parallel}\!\!\diagdown_{OCH_3}$	C_2H_5

microorganisms. CTX is active not only against usually cephalosporin-sensitive bacteria but also against resistant strains producing β-lactamases (*Escherichia coli* TEM, *Klebsiella aerogenes* 1082E, *Proteus vulgaris* 867).

TABLE II.   Modification of the Cephem Nucleus

Code No.	R_1	R_2	n	m
Cefotaxime	$-CH_2-OAc$	H	0	0
XIII	$-CH_2-OAc$	H	1	0
XIV	$-CH_2-OAc$	H	0	1
XV	$-CH_2OH$	H	0	0
XVI	$-CH_3$	H	0	0
XVII	$-CH_2-S-$ (tetrazole with CH_3)	H	0	0
XVIII	$-CH_2-S-$ (quinoline)	H	0	0
XIX	$-CH_2-S-$ (pyridine)	H	0	0
XX	$-CH_2-OAc$	CH_3	0	0

CTX shows a marked protective effect in the model of experimental septicemia in white mice (Table IV). In infections induced by *Streptococcus pyogenes* A77 and a strain of *E. coli* and *Salmonella typhimurium*, CTX protected 100% of the animals after subcutaneous administration of 2×1.953, 3.906, and 15.625 $\mu g/20$ g mouse, respectively.

The two reference compounds, CEZ and cefuroxime (CXM), showed, with exception of the gram-positive bacteria, much lower antibacterial *in vitro* activity than CTX (Table III). In some cases CTX exceeds the activity of CXM and CEZ more than 100 times.

Both CEZ and CXM are inactive against *P. aeruginosa* ATCC 9027, *K. aerogenes* 1082E, and *P. vulgaris* 867. In the mouse protection test CEZ and CXM showed antibacterial activity only in concentrations far above those of CTX (Table IV).

TABLE III. Antibacterial *In Vitro* Activity, MIC (μg/ml)[a]

Code No.	S. aureus SG 511	S. pyogenes A 77	P. aeruginosa ATCC 9027	E. coli TEM[b]	E. coli 1507E	E. cloacae 1321E	K. aerogenes 1522E	K. aerogenes 1082E[b]	P. vulgaris 867[b]
Cefotaxime	0.781	0.008	12.5	0.078	0.019	0.019	0.039	3.906	6.25
II	50.0	0.25	>1,000.0	50.0	12.5	25.0	12.5	>1,000.0	>1,000.0
III	0.625	0.004	25.0	1.25	0.313	0.625	0.313	3.125	3.125
IV	0.313	0.008	50.0	2.5	2.5	1.25	5.0	7.813	c
V	0.625	0.008	31.25	6.25	0.781	0.781	0.781	500.0	62.5
VI	0.156	0.002	62.5	0.039	0.031	0.039	0.031	250.0	100.0
VII	0.625	0.004	>100.0	62.5	0.078	0.078	0.078	>1,000.0	500.0
VIII	2.5	0.125	>100.0	7.813	7.813	7.813	3.906	250.0	100.0
IX	25.0	0.5	>100.0	1,000.0	250.0	>1,000.0	500.0	>1,000.0	c
X	1.563	0.006	25.0	1.25	1.25	5.0	1.25	1.563	3.125
XI	5.0	0.008	50.0	3.906	1.953	1.953	1.953	7.813	c
XII	>100.0	6.25	>100.0	62.5	15.625	62.5	62.5	>1,000.0	c
XIII	12.5	0.031	500.0	0.039	0.039	0.039	0.062	1.25	0.195
XIV	25.0	1.25	25.0	0.781	0.195	0.195	0.195	>1,000.0	100.0
XV	6.25	0.008	1,000.0	1.25	0.625	0.313	0.156	7.813	3.125
XVI	50.0	0.062	>100.0	0.781	0.781	0.391	0.781	3.125	c
XVII	1.25	0.008	50.0	0.156	0.019	0.039	0.078	12.5	12.5
XVIII	0.625	0.004	62.5	0.625	0.313	0.313	0.313	7.813	10.0
XIX	1.25	0.015	>100.0	1.25	1.25	1.25	0.625	250.0	c
XX	6.25	0.156	>100.0	7.813	3.906	3.906	3.125	>1,000.0	c
Cefazolin	0.078	0.031	>1,000.0	15.625	1.25	3.125	1.563	1,000.0	1,000.0
Cefuroxime	0.313	0.004	500.0	6.25	0.781	2.5	2.5	>1,000.0	500.0

[a] Determined in the serial dilution test in Mueller-Hinton Broth (Difco); inoculum: 5×10^5 CFU/ml. [b] β-Lactamase producers.

c Not determined.

TABLE IV. Antibacterial *In Vivo* Activity in Experimental Mouse Septicemia[a]

Code No.	ED$_{100}$ (2 × μg/ml)		
	S. typhimurium	*E. coli* O 78	*S. pyogenes* A77
Cefotaxime	15.625	3.906	1.953
II	1,000.0	>1,000.0	62.5
III	500.0	b	3.906
IV	250.0	b	31.25
V	b	b	15.625
VI	125.0	1.953	3.906
VII	62.5	b	15.625
VIII	b	b	31.25
IX	b	b	b
X	500.0	125.0	7.813
XI	b	b	31.25
XII	b	b	>1,000.0
XIII	500.0	7.813	15.625
XIV	2,000.0	b	250.0
XV	b	b	b
XVI	b	b	15.625
XVII	500.0	31.25	15.625
XVIII	b	b	31.25
XIX	b	62.5	15.625
XX	b	b	>125.0
Cefazolin	1,000.0	250.0	15.625
Cefuroxime	500.0	250.0	7.813

[a] Challenge of the mice by intraperitoneal injection of 0.3 ml of the suspension of bacteria (approx. 10×lethal dose); 10 animals per dose; treatment of the animals simultaneously and 4 hr after infection.   [b] Not determined.

ANTIBACTERIAL *IN VITRO* AND *IN VIVO* ACTIVITY OF CTX DERIVATIVES

1. Side Chain Modifications (Table I)

The superiority of the *in vitro* activity of CTX is strongly influenced by the substitution of the oximino group in the α-position of the 7-side chain and its stereochemistry. CTX is only highly active in the *syn* configuration of this substituent. Its *anti* configuration (II), which is thermodynamically more stable, shows a low antibacterial activity. With the exception of *S. pyogenes* A77 none of the test strains is inhibited by compound II in concentrations below 10 μg/ml. Compound II is nearly inactive in the *in vivo* protection test.

Modifications of the methoximino group by higher lipophilic substituents leads to compounds III and IV, which showed nearly the same activity against *Staphylococcus aureus* SG 511 and *S. pyogenes* A77, but their inhibitory effects against gram-negative organisms were much lower than those of CTX. Their activity against the β-lactamase-producing bacteria indicate no influence on β-lactamase stability. Against *K. aerogenes* 1082E the two substances act on the same level as CTX.

The *in vivo* data reflect the difference in the *in vitro* activities between CTX and compounds III and IV.

Compound V with a phenylated *syn*-oximino group is, *in vitro* and *in vivo*, comparable to compounds III and IV, but this modification leads to a marked loss of β-lactamase stability, as shown by the high MIC values against *K. aerogenes* 1082E and *P. vulgaris* 867.

Compound VI, the free oxime, is an antibiotic with an increased activity against gram-positive bacteria. Against two strains of *E. coli* and one strain each of *Enterobacter cloacae* and *K. aerogenes* it has nearly the same effects as CTX. Surprising is the loss of activity against *Pseudomonas, P. vulgaris*, and the other β-lactamase producing strains. Compound VI is also highly active in the *in vivo* test model in infections with gram-positive and gram-negative bacteria and exceeds CEZ and CXM.

Compound VII, a α-keto derivative, represents a modification of CTX which is as active as the parent compound *in vitro* against non-β-lactamase producing microorganisms.

Compounds VIII and IX demonstrate the importance of the amino group of the thiazole ring for the antibacterial activity of CTX. Acetylation or removal of this group leads to much lower antibacterial effects both *in vitro* and *in vivo*.

Compounds X and XI with a chlorine or bromine substituent in the aminothiazol ring are antibiotics with reasonably good antibacterial activity and, as the MIC values for β-lactamase producers indicate, have high β-lactamase stability. With the exception of its activity against *S. aureus* SG 511, they surpass the *in vitro* activity of CEZ and CXM. N-ethylation of the 7-amido group in CTX to compound XII results in an almost complete loss of antibacterial activity.

2. Modifications of the Cephem Nucleus (Table II)

Cephalosporins can be modified not only in the 7-position but also in the cephem nucleus itself, and especially in the 3-position by nucleophilic exchange of the acetoxy group.

The S-sulfoxide XIII or the R-sulfoxide XIV (chiral specification according to Cahn, Ingold, and Prelog) of CTX possesses an extraordinarily high *in vitro* activity against *E. coli, Enterobacter*, and *Klebsiella*. Especially, compound XIII shows nearly the same effect against Enterobacteriaceae as CTX itself, but in contrast to the key compound the sulfoxides XIII and XIV show rather poor activity against *S. aureus* and only limited effects against *P. aeruginosa*.

The low MIC values of compound XIII for the β-lactamase-producing microorganisms demonstrate the high β-lactamase stability of this substance. Compound XIII is the first example of a β-oriented β-lactam sulfoxide with high antibacterial *in vitro* and *in vivo* activity.

The desacetyl derivative of CTX (XV) possesses the same antibacterial spectrum, with the exception of that against *P. aeruginosa*, and at least the same stability to β-lactamases as CTX itself. Desacetyl-CTX (XV) is the main metabolite in humans. Therefore its antibacterial activity is of special importance. Against *Streptococci* and *P. cepacia*, compound XV exhibits *in vitro* nearly the same activity as CTX. Against most common Enterobacteriaceae it possesses approximately one-tenth the activity of the parent compound, but is still somewhat more active than CXM, CEZ, or cefoxitin (8).

The MICs of compound XV for most of the test strains in Table III are also on the average 10 times lower than those of the key compound. Against *S. pyogenes* A77 and *P. vulgaris* 867 it is as active as CTX or even more active. In spite of this marked reduction of antibacterial activity the desacetylated CTX also was shown in this study to be at least as active as CXM or CEZ against gram-negative bacteria and *Streptococci*.

Compound XVI, the desacetoxy-CTX, shows properties similar to those of XV. The substitution of the acetoxy group is a well known method to improve the antibacterial properties of cephalosporins. This exchange in the CTX series by mercaptoheterocycles leads to compounds XVII, XVIII, and XIX. They all are broad spectrum antibiotics with much higher activity than CEZ and CXM. None of these derivatives markedly surpasses the broad spectrum and high intrinsic activity of CTX.

Esterification of the carboxy group of CTX leads to compound XX, which possesses a reasonable antibacterial activity. In the model of experimental septicemia no *in vivo* effect of this CTX-ester could be demonstrated.

PROTEIN BINDING AND PHARMACOKINETICS

CTX is bound reversibly to human serum proteins to approximately 50%. Most modifications of the molecule in the 7-acyl-side chain or the cephem nucleus lead to no significant alteration. Only compound XV has a lower (15%) and compound XVII a higher (76%) protein binding.

In humans 1 g CTX produces after a 15-min infusion a peak level of 93 μg/ml. The terminal half-life was 75 ± 7 min (5). It can be concluded from animal experiments that no one derivative of CTX, described in this paper, shows a pharmacokinetic behavior more favorable than that of the key compound. All these derivatives show insufficient enteral absorption.

REFERENCES

1. Fu, K. P. and Neu, H. C. 1978. *Antimicrob. Agents Chemother.*, **14**, 322–326.
2. Hamilton-Miller, J. M. T., Brumfitt, W., and Reynolds, A. V. 1978. *J. Antimicrob. Chemother.*, **4**, 437–444.
3. Heymes, R., Lutz., A., and Schrinner, E. 1977. *Infection*, **5**, 259–260.
4. Kafetzis, D. A., Kanarios, J., Sinaniotis, C. A., and Papadatos, C. J. 1979. Abstr. 19th Intersci. Conf., Boston, No. 873.
5. Lüthy, R., Münch, R., Blaser, J., Bhend, H., and Siegenthaler, W. 1979. *Antimicrob. Agents Chemother.*, **16**, 127–133.
6. Mirelman, D. and Nuchamowitz, Y. 1980. *Antimicrob. Agents Chemother.*, **17**, 115–119.
7. Shah, P. M., Helm, E. B., and Stille, W. 1979. *Med. Welt*, **30**, 298–301.
8. Wise, R., Wills, P. J., Andrews, J. H., and Bedford, K. A. 1980. *J. Antimicrob. Chemother.*, **17**, 84–86.

CEFTIZOXIME

Hiroshi NAKANO and Minoru NISHIDA

Fujisawa Pharmaceutical Co., Ltd.*

The purpose of this brief review is to present the structure-activity relationships of a selected number of the semisynthetic cephalosporins related to ceftizoxime (FK 749) in view of their *in vitro* antibacterial activities.

Since cefazolin (*5*) was successfully marketed in 1971, Fujisawa has made continuous efforts to seek a new broad spectrum cephalosporin antibiotic with increased stability toward β-lactamases. Then, nocardicin A (*6*) was isolated from the fermentation broth of *Nocardia uniforms* subsp. *tsuyamanesis* ATCC 21809. This was a new monocyclic-β-lactam antibiotic with a unique, novel acyl side chain. This finding gave us an important clue in developing an extensive new family of cephalosporins bearing the 7-(α-oxyiminoaryl)acetyl side chain, as shown in structural type (I) in which the aryl group (R), oxime O-substituent (R_1), and 3-substituent (R_2) are varied. Two isomeric configurations, *syn*(Z) and *anti*(E), exist in the oxyimino ether group.

Nocardicin A   I

Similar to the *"syn-anti"* structure-activity relationship for nocardicins, *syn* isomers of the oxyimino cephems (I) always had much more excellent antibacterial activity than *anti* isomers. Therefore, we will discuss here the *in vitro* activity of the cephalosporins (I) with the *syn*-configuration.

---

* Kashima 2-1-6, Yodogawa-ku, Osaka 532, Japan.

MODIFICATION OF THE 7-ACYL SIDE CHAIN

Our initial efforts were directed to the selection of the aryl moiety in structural type (I). The structure-activity-relationships of the 7-acyl group are conveniently dealt with by first keeping the 3-substituent (R_2) constant as hydrogen. Table I shows the antibacterial activity of 3-hydrogen cephems (1–6) with various kinds of 7-(2-methoxy-iminoaryl)acetyl side chains. Clearly, the thiazole analog (4) tends to show the best gram-negative activity.

Our next synthetic attempt was focused on what kind of functional groups and which position of the 2-methoxyiminoacetyl moiety on the thiazole ring were most favorable. As listed in Table II, a cephem (7) with a 2-(2-amino-4-thiazolyl)-2-meth-oxyiminoacetyl side chain exhibits both a very superior potency and spectrum of antibacterial activities against gram-positive and gram-negative bacteria, including opportunistic pathogens. The data in Table II also indicate that when one of the hydrogens in the amino group is replaced by various substituents (8–12), activities against all bacteria are dramatically decreased. The 2-hydroxy analog (13) is much less active. The activity of the 4-thiazolyl isomer (7) is much better than that of the 5-thiazolyl isomer (14) with respect to the position of the 2-methoxyiminoacetyl moiety on the thiazole ring. The 4-amino-2-thiazolyl isomer was too unstable for its activity to be determined.

In the following stage of this program, we systematically investigated the effect of changing the oxime O-substituent (R_1) in the 2-amino-4-thiazolyl series on the antibacterial activity. Some of the derivatives in this category are given in Table III. The data on the effect of alkyl chain length on antibacterial activity in Table III indicate that extension of the chain causes a significant increase in gram-positive activity, but that the increased lipophilic nature of the higher homologous members adversely influences the gram-negative activity. The activity in the methylene homo-log series tends to a constant MIC value with a total of three or four carbon atoms. The highest gram-negative activity is shown by a compound which contains one carbon atom ($R_1 = CH_3$). In comparing the activity of the homolog (17: $R_1 = CH_2CH_2CH_3$), congeners (22–24) with hydrophilic function in the oxime ether exhibit similar or better activity against gram-negative bacteria but only poor activity against gram-positive bacteria. An exception is the hydroxyimino analog (15: $R_1 = H$), which is four to eight times more active against gram-positive bacteria and equally active against gram-negative bacteria, except for opportunistic pathogens, in comparison with the activity of ceftizoxime. Similar results in the 7-acyl structure-activity rela-tionships described in the 3-hydrogen series were also observed in the 3-substituents such as the acetoxymethyl, carbamoyloxymethyl, and heterocyclic thiomethyl groups listed in Table IV.

TABLE I. Effect of Changing the Aromatic Group on Antibacterial Activity

$$R-\underset{\underset{N-OCH_3}{\|}}{C}-CONH-\text{(cephem nucleus, COOH)}$$

Compound	R	MIC (μg/ml)[a]								
		S. aureus		E. coli		K. pneumoniae	P. mirabilis	P. vulgaris	P. aeruginosa	S. marcescens
		6	33[b]	32	28[c]	20	18	1	NCTC10490	35
1	(m-hydroxyphenyl)	12.5	50	1.56	0.39	0.20	0.39	0.20	50	12.5
2	(2-furyl)	12.5	50	3.13	1.56	0.39	0.78	0.39	200	>100
3	(2-thienyl)	6.25	25	12.5	1.56	0.39	3.13	0.78	800	>100
4	(thiazolyl)	12.5	100	0.78	0.39	0.05	0.05	0.10	400	50
5	(thiazolyl)	12.5	—	1.56	1.56	0.39	0.39	1.56	800	—
6	(thiadiazolyl)	25	50	6.25	6.25	0.39	3.13	1.56	800	>100

[a] The MICs were determined by the agar dilution method using heart infusion agar (Difco). Incubation: 37°C, 20 hr, inoculum of 10^6 CFU/ml. [b] Penicillinase producer. [c] Cephalosporinase producer.

TABLE II. Effect on Antibacterial Activity of Functional Groups and Position of 2-Methoxyiminoacetyl Moiety on the Thiazole Ring

Com-pound	X	MIC (μg/ml)[a]								
		S. aureus		E. coli		K. pneumoniae	P. mirabilis	P. vulgaris	P. aeruginosa	S. marcescens
		6	33[b]	32	28[c]	20	18	1	NCTC 10490	35
7	NH_2	3.13	12.5	0.05	0.05	≦0.025	≦0.025	≦0.025	0.39	1.56
8	$NHCH_3$	3.13	12.5	25	6.25	0.78	1.56	0.78	6.25	>100
9	NHCHO	3.13	12.5	1.56	1.56	0.39	0.20	0.39	200	50
10	$NHCOCH_3$	6.25	25	25	12.5	3.13	6.25	6.25	100	>100
11	$NHSO_2CH_3$	100	>100	50	25	6.25	3.13	3.13	>800	>100
12	$NHC(=NH)NH_2$	12.5	50	50	6.25	3.13	12.5	12.5	>800	>100
13	OH	50	100	>100	25	12.5	12.5	12.5	>800	>100
14	NH_2 (5-Thiazolyl isomer)	25	100	100	50	3.13	12.5	25	>800	>100

a-c See Table I.

TABLE III.   Effect on Antibacterial Activity of Changing the Oxime Ether Group

Compound	R_1	S. aureus		E. coli		K. pneumoniae	P. mirabilis	P. vulgaris	P. aeruginosa	S. marcescens
		6	33[b]	32	28[c]	20	18	1	NCTC 10490	35
15	H	0.78	1.56	0.05	0.10	≦0.025	≦0.025	0.10	6.25	12.5
7	CH_3	3.13	12.5	0.05	0.05	≦0.025	≦0.025	≦0.025	0.39	1.56
16	CH_2CH_3	3.13	6.25	0.39	0.10	≦0.025	≦0.025	≦0.025	≦1.56	0.78
17	$CH_2CH_2CH_3$	0.78	3.13	0.39	0.10	≦0.025	0.10	0.10	≦1.56	3.13
18	$CH(CH_3)_2$	1.56	6.25	0.39	0.20	0.05	0.10	≦0.025	≦1.56	3.13
19	$CH_2CH(CH_3)_2$	0.78	3.13	1.56	0.20	0.10	0.20	0.10	≦1.56	6.25
20	$CH_2(CH_2)_3CH_3$	0.78	3.13	0.78	0.39	0.10	0.78	0.10	≦1.56	6.25
21	$CH_2(CH_2)_4CH_3$	0.78	3.13	1.56	0.39	0.05	0.78	0.10	≦1.56	12.5
22	CH_2CH_2OH	12.5	50	0.10	0.10	≦0.025	≦0.025	≦0.025	3.13	12.5
23	CH_2COOH	12.5	100	0.20	0.20	0.10	≦0.025	0.05	3.13	6.25
24	$CH_2CH_2NH_2$	100	>100	0.10	0.10	0.05	0.20	0.39	25	3.13

MIC (µg/ml)[a]

a–c See Table I.

TABLE IV.   Effect on Antibacterial Activity of the Substituents at the 3-Position in the Cephem Nucleus

Compound	R_2	MIC (μg/ml)[a]								
		S. aureus		E. coli		K. pneumoniae	P. mirabilis	P. vulgaris	P. aeruginosa	S. marcescens
		6	33[b]	32	28[c]	20	18	1	NCTC 10490	35
7	H	3.13	12.5	0.05	0.05	≦0.025	≦0.025	≦0.025	0.39	1.56
25	CH_2OCOCH_3	3.13	6.25	0.10	0.05	≦0.025	≦0.025	0.05	1.56	3.13
26	CH_2OCONH_2	1.56	6.25	0.05	0.05	≦0.025	≦0.025	≦0.025	1.56	6.25
27	CH_2S-thiadiazole-S	0.78	1.56	0.20	0.10	≦0.025	0.05	≦0.025	1.56	1.56
28	CH_2S-triazole-CH_3	1.56	3.13	0.10	0.05	≦0.025	0.05	≦0.025	1.56	0.78
29	CH_2S-triazole-CH_2COOH	12.5	25	0.20	0.39	0.20	≦0.025	0.05	6.25	3.13
30	CH_3	50	100	0.78	0.20	0.05	0.10	0.20	100	50
31	Cl	12.5	25	0.10	0.20	0.10	≦0.025	0.05	50	50
32	OCH_3	50	—	0.39	0.39	0.10	0.10	0.39	12.5	—

a-e See Table I.

MODIFICATION AT THE 2- AND 3-POSITIONS

After this investigation of the 7-acyl side chain, we studied the influence of substituents in the 3-position of the cephem nucleus in the 2-(2-amino-4-thiazolyl)-2-methoxyiminoacetyl series. Table IV presents the antibacterial activity of the selected derivatives that have the same 3-substituent as cephalosporin antibiotics under clinical use. The 3-acetoxymethyl (25: cefotaxime), carbamoyloxymethyl (26), and heterocyclic thiomethyl (27 and 28: SCE 1365) analogs have activity similar to ceftizoxime, though the 1,3,4-thiazolylthiomethyl analog (27) has much better gram-positive activity than the others. The N-carboxymethyltetrazolylthiomethyl analog (29) is less active than the N-methyltetrazolylthiomethyl analog (28), but was observed to have high and extended blood levels in the pharmacokinetic profile.

The 3-methyl (30), 3-chloro (31), and 3-methoxy (32) analogs are less active than the others. Especially the gram-positive activity of the above three analogs is very poor, although gram-negative activity is still attractive. Therefore, we intended to structurally modify a cephem nucleus to enhance the gram-positive activity of the 3-methyl analog (30). By contrast introduction of a methyl group into the 2-position of the 3-methyl analog (30) resulted in a significant decrease in the activity of the 2,3-dimethyl analog (33). Removal of the 3-methyl group from the dimethyl analog (33) resulted in a dramatic enhancement of activity; the α-2-methyl analog (34: FR 13374) (3) is as active as ceftizoxime against gram-negative bacteria, but slightly less active than ceftizoxime against gram-positive bacteria and opportunistic pathogens. Interestingly, the enantiomer, the β-2-methyl analog (35), is remarkably less active than that of the α-methyl enantiomer (34). Further replacement of the methyl group by hydrogen in the 2-methyl analog successfully led to ceftizoxime, and an improvement of the activity of FR 13374 against gram-positive bacteria and opportunistic pathogens. The *in vitro* data for the above cephems are summarized in Table V.

MODIFICATION OF THE β-LACTAM NUCLEUS

Any modification of the nucleus seems to result in compounds with reduced antibacterial activity in the 7-oxyiminoarylacetyl series. Table VI shows examples of the effect of modifying the β-lactam nucleus. The cephem nucleus can be found to be the most favorable combinations of the 2-amino-4-thiazolyl-2-methoxyiminoacetyl side chain and the related β-lactam nuclei.

Thus, ceftizoxime (FK 749) was selected as a clinical candidate for further evaluation (1, 2, 4, 7).

TABLE V. Effect on Antibacterial Activity of Hydrogen and Methyl Group at the 2- and 3- Positions in the Cephem Nucleus

| Com-pound | R₂ | R₃ | MIC (μg/ml)[a] | | | | | | | | |
| | | | S. aureus | | E. coli | | K. pneumoniae | P. mirabilis | P. vulgaris | P. aeruginosa | S. marcescens |
			6	33[b]	32	28[c]	20	18	1	NCTC 10490	35
30	CH₃	H	50	100	0.78	0.20	0.05	0.10	0.20	100	50
33	CH₃	CH₃(α)	>100	—	6.25	3.13	0.39	0.39	3.13	50	—
34	H	CH₃(α)	6.25	25	0.10	0.10	≦0.025	≦0.025	≦0.025	12.5	6.25
35	H	CH₃(β)	12.5	50	0.78	1.56	3.13	0.20	0.20	800	100
7	H	H	3.13	12.5	0.05	0.05	≦0.025	≦0.025	≦0.025	0.39	1.56

a-c See Table I.

TABLE VI. Effect on Antibacterial Activity of Modifying the β-Lactam Nucleus

$$H_2N \underset{S}{\overset{N}{\diagdown}} \text{--C--CO--NH--}\beta\text{- lactam ring}$$
$$\overset{\|}{N}\text{--OCH}_3$$

Compound	β-Lactam nucleus	S. aureus		E. coli		K. pneumoniae	P. mirabilis	P. vulgaris	P. aeruginosa	S. marcescens
						MIC (μg/ml)[a]				
		6	33[b]	32	28[c]	20	18	1	NCTC 10490	35
36		>100	>100	25	12.5	6.25	6.25	12.5	200	>100
37		>100	>100	>100	100	25	50	50	>800	>100
38		12.5	>100	0.20	1.56	0.10	0.05	0.20	100	25
39		100	>100	0.78	0.20	0.10	0.10	0.20	25	12.5
40		>100	>100	3.13	0.78	0.39	0.78	0.78	50	12.5
41		1.56	—	25	>100	25	12.5	50	25	—
42		>100	—	>100	>100	100	25	100	>800	—
43		6.25	—	6.25	6.25	1.56	3.13	3.13	100	—

a–c See Table I.

REFERENCES

1. Kamimura, T., Matsumoto, Y., Okada, N., Mine, Y., Nishida, M., Goto, S., and Kuwahara, S. 1979. *Antimicrob. Agents Chemother.*, **16**, 540–548.
2. Kojo, H., Nishida, M., Goto, S., and Kuwahara, S. 1979. *Antimicrob. Agents Chemother.*, **16**, 549–553.
3. Mine, Y., Murakawa, T., Kamimura, T., Takaya, T., Nishida, M., Goto, S., and Kuwahara, S. 1977. Abstr. 17th Intersci. Conf. Antimicrob. Agents Chemother., No. 147.
4. Murakawa, T., Sakamoto, H., Fukada, S., Nakamoto, S., Hirose, T., Ito, N., and Nishida, M. 1980. *Antimicrob. Agents Chemother.*, **17**, 157–164.
5. Nakano, H. 1977. *In* "Pharmacological and Biochemical Properties of Drug Substances," ed. by M. E. Goldberg, American Pharmaceutical Association, Washington, Vol. 1, pp. 155–182.
6. Nakano, H., Imanaka, H., Nishida, M., and Kamiya, T. 1978. *In* "Future Trends in Therapeutics," ed. by F. G. McMahon, Futura Publishing Co., Inc., New York, Vol. 15, pp. 209–244.
7. Nishida, M., Kamimura, T., Okada, N., Matsumoto, Y., Mine, Y., Murakawa, T., Goto, S., and Kuwahara, S. 1979. *J. Antibiot.*, **32**, 1319–1327.

CEFMETAZOLE (CS-1170)

Hideo NAKAO and Shinichi SUGAWARA

*Central Research Laboratories, Sankyo Co., Ltd.**

The discovery of a new family of β-lactam antibiotics the "cephamycins," from culture filtrates of streptomycetes by Lilly's (*6*) and Merck's (*10*) groups followed by ourselves (*1*) and the development of cefoxitin (*4, 9, 13*) by Merck stimulated our efforts to synthesize hundreds of cephamycin derivatives to obtain more active compounds. By modifications at the 3-position, the 7β-acyl group and the 7α-methoxy group of cephamycin we have decided on cefmetazole (*7, 8, 11*) as the most effective and suitable candidate for clinical application.

Structure-activity relationships of cefmetazole analogs on antibacterial activities and pharmacokinetic properties in mice are described in this chapter.

MODIFICATION OF THE 7β-ACYL GROUP

There are two routes in general for obtaining 7α-methoxy-cephalosporins. One is an acyl exchange of naturally occurring cephamycin C and the other is chemical methoxylation at the 7-position of a cephalosporin nuclues. By these methods we have synthesized many 7β-substituted-thioacetamido-7α-methoxy-cephalosporins. Similar to the cephalosporin series, lipophilic acyl derivatives were active against gram-positive bacteria and hydrophilic acyl derivatives were relatively active against gram-negative bacteria. Among these, the most active compound against both gram-positive and gram-negative bacteria is 7β-[(cyanomethyl)thio]acetamido-7α-methoxy-3-[(1-methyl-1H-tetrazol-5-yl)thio]methyl-3-cephem-4-carboxylic acid (cefmetazole) (*7, 8*). When the (cyanomethylthio)acetyl was replaced by other (substituted-thio)acetyl groups, the activity against gram-negative bacteria was generally decreased except for the 2-carboxyethyl congener (*7*). This compound showed similar *in vivo* antibacterial activity against gram-negative bacteria and an excretion pattern similar to cefmetazole. The (cyanomethyl)oxyacetyl analog (11) was four times less active than

* Hiromachi 1-2-58, Shinagawa-ku, Tokyo 140, Japan.

cefmetazole against both gram-positive and gram-negative bacteria. While the methylthioacetyl analog (9) had one-half the activity of cefmetazole, the trifluoromethyl analog (10, SKF-73678 (2, 5, 12)) showed antibacterial activity similar to cefmetazole. We have noticed that biliary excretion of the compound was rather high in mice. Introduction of the methyl (2) or ethyl (3) group at the cyanomethyl portion also resulted in very greatly enhanced biliary excretion.

MODIFICATION AT THE 3-POSITION

In the cephalosporin series, when the substituent on the methylene at the 3-position is a leaving group such as an acetoxy, heterocyclicthio, or pyridinium group, the antibacterial activity can be enhanced compared to that of the hydrogen, halogen or hydroxy group. Besides, the cephalosporins with a vinyl group, which is substituted with an electron-withdrawing group, in the 3-position often show a potent activity.

In the case of the cefmetazole series, the carbamoyloxymethyl group was replaced by various substituents. As anticipated, the 3-methyl (14), 3-chloro (15), and 3-hydrogen (16) congeners were inactive. Surprisingly, the 3-tetrazolylvinyl analog (22) did not show any activity against gram-negative bacteria even though the corresponding 7α-hydrogen compound was highly active (3). The 3-acetoxymethyl analog (13) was as active as the 3-carbamoyloxymethyl compound (12). Among heterocyclicthiomethyl congeners, the N-methyltetrazolyl analog (cefmetazole) was the most active compound, being two to eight times more active than any other substituents at the 3-position of 7β-cyanomethylthioacetyl cephamycins. The presence of a good leaving group on the methylene at the 3-position is essential for a potent, broad antibacterial activity.

From the data on urinary and fecal recoveries of some selected congeners of the series in mice, we have judged the excretion pattern of cefmetazole to be better balanced than any others.

MODIFICATION OF THE 7α-METHOXY GROUP

As analogs of cefmetazole, the 7α-ethoxy (24), propyloxy (25), methylthio (26), and cyano (27) derivatives were synthesized by a procedure similar to the methoxylation of the cephalosporin nucleus. None of these were active against bacteria. On the other hand, the corresponding 7α-hydrogen analog (23) showed a remarkable activity against tested organisms except for β-lactamase-producing *Escherichia coli*. Urinary excretion of this compound was at a level similar to cefmetazole; however, like other cephalosporins no bioactivity was recovered from feces probably due to the lack of stability against β-lactamases present in intestinal flora in mice. The *in vivo* efficacy of this compound was similar to cefmetazole in the case of β-lactamase-nonproducing *E. coli* but was ten times less active in the case of *Proteus vulgaris*.

TABLE I. Structure-activity Relationships of Cefmetazole Analogs on Antibacterial Activities and Pharmacokinetic Properties

Core structure: cephem nucleus with R_1-NH and R_3 substituents on the β-lactam, R_2 at the 3-position, and $COOH$. For Cefmetazole (CMZ), $R_2 = CH_2S$–(1-methyltetrazol-5-yl, $N{=}N{-}N$ with CH_3).

No. (Name)	Structure R₁	R₂	R₃	MIC (μg/ml)ᵃ S. aureus Sᵇ	Rᶜ	E. coli Sᵈ	Rᵉ	P. vul-garisᶠ	ED₅₀ (mg/kg)ᵍ E. coli	P. vul-garis	Recovery (%)ʰ Urine	Feces
Cefmetazole (CMZ)	$NCCH_2SCH_2CO$	CH₂S-tetrazole(CH_3)	OCH_3	0.2	0.8	0.8	0.8	1.5	2.7	9.5	59.2	15.1
1	$NCCH_2CH_2SCH_2CO$			0.1	0.8	1.5	6.2	3.1			49.3	26.3
2	$NCCH(CH_3)SCH_2CO$			0.4	0.8	1.5	3.1	0.8			20.1	60.4
3	$NCCH(C_2H_5)SCH_2CO$			0.2	0.4	6.2	6.2	0.8				
4	$NCC(CH_3)_2SCH_2CO$			0.4	0.8	6.2	12.5	1.5				
5	$H_2NCOCH_2SCH_2CO$			0.8	3.1	3.1	3.1	12.5				
6	$HOOCCH_2SCH_2CO$			25	25	3.1	3.1	6.2		15.6	55.2	6.0
7	$HOOCCH_2CH_2SCH_2CO$			6.2	12.5	0.8	0.8	0.8	2.0		68.9	14.7
8	$HOCH_2CH_2SCH_2CO$			0.8	1.5	1.5	1.5	6.2	6.3		71.5	5.1
9	CH_3SCH_2CO			0.4	0.4	1.5	1.5	0.4			61.9	17.2
10	CF_3SCH_2CO			0.8	1.5	3.1	3.1	12.5			28.8	35.1
11	$NCCH_2OCH_2CO$			0.8	3.1	1.5	1.5	6.2				
12	$NCCH_2SCH_2CO$	CH_2OCONH_2		0.8	3.1	1.5	1.5	6.2				
13	$NCCH_2SCH_2CO$	CH_2OCOCH_3	CH_3	0.2	0.8	1.5	1.5	6.2			49.3	31.5
14	$NCCH_2SCH_2CO$		CH_3	>200	>200	>200	>200	>200				
15			Cl	200	>200	>200	>200	>200				

No.	Structure									
16	H	>200	>200	100	100	200				
17	CH₂S—(tetrazole)—N—C₂H₅	0.2	0.8	1.5	1.5	1.5				
18	CH₂S—(tetrazole)—N—CH₂CO₂H	3.1	6.2	25	25	1.5				
19	CH₂S—(tetrazole)—N—C₆H₅	0.2	0.4	50	100	0.8				
20	CH₂S—(thiadiazole)—CH₃	0.8	1.5	12.5	12.5	3.1				
21	CH₂N⁺(pyridinium)—CONH₂	0.2	0.8	6.2	6.2	25				
22	CH=CH—(triazole)—N—CH₃	12.5	>200	>200	>200	>200				
23	H / CH₂S—(tetrazole)—N—CH₃	0.1	0.4	0.8	12.5	3.1	3.1	81.3	58.0	—
24	OC₂H₅	6.2	12.5	50	50	50				

TABLE I. (continued)

No. (Name)	Structure R_1	Structure R_2	Structure R_3	MIC (μg/ml)[a] S. aureus S^b	MIC S. aureus R^c	MIC E. coli S^d	MIC E. coli R^e	MIC P. vul-garis[f]	ED$_{50}$ (mg/kg)[g] E. coli	ED$_{50}$ P. vul-garis	Recovery (%)[h] Urine	Recovery Feces
25			OC_3H_7	200	200	>200	>200	200				
26			SCH_3	25	100	>200	>200	>200				
27			CN	25	50	100	100	100				
Cefoxitin	(thiophene)–CH_2CO	CH_2OCONH_2	OCH_3	0.8	1.5	3.1	3.1	3.1	6.2	12.5	63.0	9.3
Cefazolin	(tetrazolyl, N=N/N–N)–CH_2CO	CH_2S–(5-methyl-1,3,4-thiadiazolyl, N–N, S, CH_3)	H	0.1	0.4	0.8	12.5	12.5	4.9	157	73.0	—

[a] The MICs were determined by the 2-fold serial dilution method on nutrient agar; incubation at 37°C, 18 hr; inoculum size, one loopful of 10^7 CFU/ml. [b] *Staphylococcus aureus* 209 P JC. [c] *S. aureus*, a penicillinase-producing strain. [d] *E. coli* NIHJ JC-2. [e] *E. coli*, a clinical isolate. [f] *P. vulgaris*, a cephalosporinase-producing strain. [g] Bacterial suspension was challenged by i.p., drugs were administered by two doses of s.c. at zero and 4 hr after infection in ddY mice. [h] Urinary and fecal recoveries were recorded after 24 hr, the drug was administered subcutaneously at 50 mg/kg in mice.

CONCLUSION

Based upon more detailed studies of the *in vitro* and *in vivo* antibacterial activities we were convinced that cefmetazole is a major advance over presently available β-lactam antibiotics. The positive features of cefmetazole such as its broader spectrum, high susceptibility of most frequently isolated hospital pathogens (*e.g., Escherichia, Klebsiella, Proteus, Staphylococcus, etc.*), sharp bactericidal activity, and extreme resistance to β-lactamases, together with the good pharmacokinetics in humans and good safety, provided the foundation for the development of cefmetazole in clinical application.

REFERENCES

1. Arai, M., Ito, Y., Nakahara, M., Kayamori, H., and Sugawara, S. 1974. Japan Patent Provisional Publication, 49-42893.
2. DeMarinis, R. M., Uri, J. V., and Weisbach, J. A. 1976. *J. Antibiot.*, **29**, 973–975.
3. Hashimoto, T., Kawano, Y., Natsume, S., Tanaka, T., Watanabe, T., Nagano, M., Sugawara, S., and Miyadera, T. 1978. *Chem. Pharm. Bull.*, **26**, 1803–1811.
4. Miller, A. K., Celozzi, E., Kong, Y., Pelak, B. A., Hendlin, D., and Stapley, E. O. 1974. *Antimicrob. Agents Chemother.*, **5**, 33–37.
5. Miyadera, T., Hashimoto, T., Nakao, H., Shimizu, B., and Sugawara, S. 1977. *Annu. Rep. Sankyo Res. Lab.*, **29**, 143–146.
6. Nagarajan, R., Boeck, L. D., Gorman, M., Hamill, R. L., Higgens, C. E., Hoehn, M. M., Stark, W. M., and Whitney, J. G. 1971. *J. Am. Chem. Soc.*, **93**, 2308–2310.
7. Nakao, H., Yanagisawa, H., Shimizu, B., Kaneko, M., Nagano, M., and Sugawara, S. 1976. *J. Antibiot.*, **29**, 554–558.
8. Nakao, H., Yanagisawa, H., Ishihara, S., Nakayama, E., Ando, A., Nakazawa, J., Shimizu, B., Kaneko, M., Nagano, M., and Sugawara, S. 1979. *J. Antibiot.*, **32**, 320–329.
9. Onishi, H. R., Daoust, D. R., Zimmerman, S. B., Hendlin, D., and Stapley, E. O. 1974. *Antimicrob. Agents Chemother.*, **5**, 38–48.
10. Stapley, E. O., Jackson, M., Hernandez, S., Zimmerman, S. B., Currie, S. A., Mochales, S., Mata, J. M., Woodruff, H. B., and Hendlin, D. 1972. *Antimicrob. Agents Chemother.*, **2**, 122–131.
11. Sugawara, S., Tajima, M., Igarashi, I., Utsui, Y., Ohya, S., and Nakahara, M. 1978. *Chemotherapy (Tokyo)*, **26** (S-5), 81–98.
12. Uri, J. V., Actor, P., Guarini, J. R., Phillips, L., Pitkin, D., DeMarinis, R. M., and Weisbach, J. A. 1978. *J. Antibiot.*, **31**, 82–91.
13. Wallick, H. and Hendlin, D. 1974. *Antimicrob. Agents Chemother.*, **5**, 25–32.

SOME CEPHAMYCIN DERIVATIVES

Masaru IWANAMI

Central Research Laboratories, Yamanouchi Pharmaceutical Co., Ltd.*

A key limitation of early cephalosporins was their incomplete gram-negative spectrum. Recently, however, cephamycin derivatives have been known to have an expanded gram-negative spectrum, because of the marked resistance to hydrolysis by β-lactamases (*1–5*). In our laboratory, several kinds of cephamycin derivatives have been prepared and their activity was examined. Some of our results are reported here.

IN VITRO COMPARISON OF CEPHAMYCINS WITH CORRESPONDING CEPHALOSPORINS

The antimicrobial activity of representative 3-(1-methyltetrazolylthiomethyl) cephamycin derivatives prepared in our laboratory was compared with the corresponding 7α-hydrogen cephalosporin derivatives.

The mean MIC values against gram-positive and gram-negative bacteria were taken for each of five microorganisms, including *Staphylococcus aureus, Bacillus subtilis, Proteus morganii, Serratia marcescens, etc.*, and the compounds having the same 7β-side chain are connected with an arrow, which indicates the change in activity upon 7α-substitution (Fig. 1).

Figure 1 shows that the introduction of the hydroxy group into the pyridine ring enhances the effect of the 7α-methoxy group and the methoxy analog shows better activity against gram-negative organisms compared to its 7α-hydrogen congener. Usually, in each pair of 7β-substituents, 7α-methoxy substitution increases its activity against gram-negative organisms 2–9 times over the hydrogen congeners. On the other hand, the methoxy substitution decreases its activity against gram-positive organisms 1/2–1/6 times relative to the hydrogen congeners. However, an unusual effect of the 7α-methoxy group was observed in the presence of the

* Azusawa 1-1-8, Itabashi-ku, Tokyo 174, Japan.

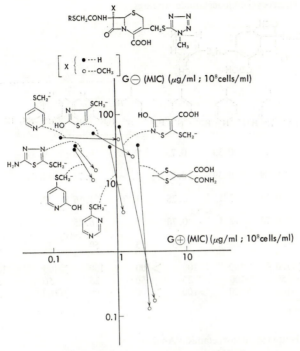

FIG. 1.   *In vitro* comparison of cephamycins with the corresponding cephalosporins.

isothiazolylthioacetamido or 1,3-dithietancarboxamido group at the 7α-position.

These methoxy analogs show over 200 times greater activity against gram-negative organisms than the hydrogen congeners.

7β-HETROCYCLICTHIOACETAMIDO TYPE SIDE CHAIN

Several kinds of 7α-methoxy-7β-heterocyclicthioacetamido cephalosporin derivatives having a functional group, such as the hydroxy or amino group, as substituents on the heterocyclic ring were prepared.

The MIC values of the representative compounds are shown in Table I. Cefazolin (CEZ), cefoxitin (CFX), and cefmetazole (CMZ) served as standards in this and following tables.

These compounds tend to show a more expanded gram-negative spectrum than that of CEZ. In this spectrum, *P. morganii, P. rettgeri, S. marcescens, etc.* are representatives of resistant gram-negative bacteria.

Among them, the 3-hydroxy-5-isothiazolylthioacetamido derivative showed the best gram-negative activity, which is better than that of CFX or CMZ.

TABLE I. MIC of Heterocyclicthioacetamide Analogs

Organism	R						
S. aureus ATCC 6633	0.78	0.39	0.78	0.78	0.78	0.39	12.5
E. coli NIHJ	0.39	0.39	0.78	1.56	0.78	1.56	12.5
E. coli Ebara (R)	0.78	3.13	0.78	1.56	1.56	3.13	6.25
K. pneumoniae V-17 (R)	0.78	12.5	0.78	25	6.25	25	12.5
P. morganii Kono	25	50	12.5	25	50	50	50
P. rettgeri Y-1	>100	>100	100	>100	100	>100	100
S. marcescens	50	>100	25	50	25	50	50
E. aerogenes	>100	>100	>100	>100	100	>100	50

MIC (μg/ml) 10^8 cells/ml.

TABLE II. MIC of Isothiazolylthioacetamido Analogs

Organism	R_1 OCH$_3$	NH$_2$	OH	OH	OH	OH
	R_2 –CN	–CN	–CN	H	–COOH	–CH$_3$
S. aureus ATCC 6633	0.19	0.39	1.56	0.78	6.25	1.56
E. coli NIHJ	12.5	1.56	0.78	0.19	0.19	0.78
E. coli Ebara (R)	12.5	3.13	0.78	0.19	0.19	0.78
K. pneumoniae V-17 (R)	50	25	25	0.39	0.19	25
P. morganii Kono	>100	100	12.5	6.25	0.78	12.5
P. rettgeri Y-1	>100	>100	50	12.5	0.78	50
S. marcescens	>100	>100	25	3.13	0.39	25
E. aerogenes	>100	>100	>100	50	12.5	>100

MIC (μg/ml) 10^8 cells/ml.

							CEZ	CFX	CMZ
3.13	1.56	1.56	0.39	0.78	3.13	0.78	0.19	1.56	0.78
3.13	3.13	0.78	0.78	0.78	3.13	0.19	3.13	1.56	0.78
3.13	6.25	3.13	6.25	1.56	1.56	0.19	25	0.78	0.78
1.56	3.13	12.5	3.13	1.56	3.13	0.39	100	12.5	0.78
25	100	50	50	25	25	6.25	>100	25	6.25
>100	>100	>100	>100	>100	100	12.5	>100	50	50
25	100	>100	50	100	25	3.13	>100	50	6.25
>100	>100	>100	>100	>100	100	50	>100	100	>100

OH $-CONH_2$	OH $-CH_2OH$	OH $-CH_2NH_2$	OH $-NH_2$	OH	CEZ	CFX	CMZ
6.25	3.13	6.25	3.13	0.78	0.19	1.56	0.78
0.39	0.78	1.56	0.78	6.25	3.13	1.56	0.78
1.56	1.56	1.56	0.78	6.25	25	0.78	0.78
0.78	0.78	1.56	1.56	50	100	12.5	0.78
3.13	12.5	12.5	12.5	>100	>100	25	6.25
12.5	25	12.5	12.5	>100	>100	50	50
6.25	12.5	12.5	6.25	>100	>100	50	6.25
>100	>100	>100	>100	>100	>100	100	>100

TABLE III. MIC of 1,3-Dithietane Analogs

	R₁	CN	COCH₃	COOH	←				COOH
Organism	R₂	–CONH₂	–CONH₂	–CONH₂	H	CH₃	OCH₃	SCH₃	COCH₃
	X	←						-S-(N—N tetrazole CH₃)	
S. aureus ATCC 6633		0.78	3.13	6.25	1.56	1.56	3.13	1.56	3.13
E. coli NIHJ		0.78	1.56	0.09	0.19	0.09	0.09	0.09	0.19
E. coli Ebara (R)		3.13	1.56	0.09	0.78	0.39	0.19	0.39	0.39
K. pneumoniae V-17 (R)		1.56	1.56	0.09	0.39	0.79	0.09	0.09	0.39
P. morganii Kono		12.5	6.25	0.39	1.56	1.56	0.19	0.39	0.39
P. rettgeri Y-1		12.5	25	0.19	1.56	3.13	0.39	0.78	1.56
S. marcescens		6.25	6.25	0.39	0.78	0.78	0.78	0.39	1.56
E. aerogenes		>100	>100	12.5	50	100	>100	>100	>100

MIC (μg/ml) 10^8 cells/ml.

Accordingly, various isothiazole analogs were prepared and thier activity was examined to find more active compounds. Table II shows the results.

In this series, the requirement for the hydroxy group at R_1 is assured by first keeping R_2 constant as the cyano group and by changing the R_1 group, and then the effect of the R_2 group on the activity is explored by keeping R_1 as the hydroxy group. The activity against gram-negative organisms increased in the order of ⬡ ≪ CN<CH₂OH, CONH₂<H≪COOH. Especially, the 4-carboxy-3-hydroxyisothiazol-5-ylthioactamido derivative showed the strongest and most expanded gram-negative spectrum, against such as indole positive species as *Proteus, Serratia, Enterobacter, etc.*

7β-1,3-DITHIETANE TYPE SIDE CHAIN

When we studied the reaction of this isothiazole derivative (I), we knew that it rearranges easily into its tautomer: the 1,3-dithietane derivative (II) in a dilute sodium hydrogencarbonate solution.

The 1,3-dithietane derivative (II) thus formed exhibited excellent antibacterial activity against gram-negative organisms, comparable to the original isothiazole derivative (I).

——————————— COOH ———————→									
SO$_2$CH$_3$	SO$_2$NH$_2$	CN	COOH	⟨◯⟩	CONH$_2$	CONH$_2$ ————→ (thiadiazole) OAC	CEZ	CFX	CMZ
6.25	3.13	3.13	6.25	1.56	12.5	12.5	0.19	1.56	0.78
0.19	0.19	0.19	0.19	0.39	0.78	0.78	3.13	1.56	0.78
0.78	0.39	0.39	0.19	1.56	1.56	0.78	25	0.78	0.78
0.39	0.19	0.19	0.19	0.78	0.78	0.78	100	12.5	0.78
3.13	3.13	0.78	0.39	0.39	6.25	3.13	>100	25	6.25
3.13	0.78	0.78	0.19	6.25	12.5	1.56	>100	50	50
0.78	0.78	0.39	0.39	12.5	1.56	1.56	>100	50	6.25
>100	>100	3.13	1.56	25	100	>100	>100	100	>100

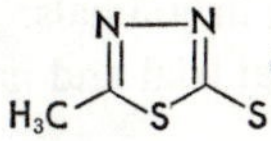

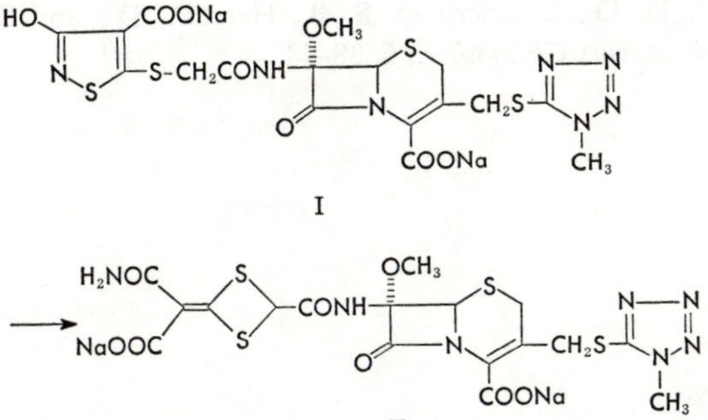

FIG. 2.   Rearrangement of isothiazole derivative (I) into 1,3-dithietane derivative (II).

Thus, new cephamycin derivatives having the 1,3-dithietane group in the 7β-side chain were prepared and their activity was examined. The results are shown in Table III.

The requirement for the carboxy group is assured by keeping R_2 constant as the carboxamide group and by changing the R_1 group, and then the effect of the R_2 group on activity is explored by keeping R_1 as the carboxy group.

The activity against gram-negative organisms increased in the order of ⬡ ≪ SO_2CH_3, SO_2NH_2, $COCH_3$, $SCH_3 ≦ CN$, $COOH$, $OCH_3 ≦ CONH_2$.

Most of these compounds showed good MIC values against gram-negative organisms, as shown in Table III. The great influence of the 3-substituents is also shown in Table III Clearly, 1-methyltetrazolylthiomethyl analogs tend to show the best MIC values.

Among these compounds, 7β-[4-(carbamoylcarboxymethylene)-1,3-dithietan-2-yl]-carboxamido-7α-methoxy-3-(1-methyltetrazol-5-yl)thiomethyl-$Δ^3$-cephem-4-carboxylic acid (YM-09330) was selected in view of its low toxity, good protection in mice, and good pharmacokinetics in animals. As a result of these data, this compound (YM-09330) is under clinical trial and has been successful so far.

REFERENCES

1. Daust, D. D., Onishi, H. R., Wallick, H., Hendlin, D., and Stapley, E. O. 1973. *Antimicrob. Agents Chemother.*, **3**, 254–261.

2. Mahoney, D. F., Koppel, G. A., and Turner, J. R., 1976. *Antimicrob. Agents Chemother.*, **10**, 470–475.

3. Miller, T. W., Goegelman, R. T., Weston, R. G., Putter, I., and Wolf, F. J. 1972. *Antimicrob. Agents Chemother.*, **2**, 132–135.

4. Nagarajan, R., Boeck, L. D., Gorman, M., Hamill, R. L., Higgens, C. E., Hoehn, M. M., Stark, W. M., and Whitney, J. G. 1971. *J. Am. Chem. Soc.*, **93**, 2308–2310.

5. Onishi, H. R., Daust, D. D., Zimmerman, S. B., Hendlin, D., and Stapley, E. O. 1974. *Antimicrob. Agents Chemother.*, **5**, 38–48.

A NEW 1-OXACEPHEM (6059-S)

Tadashi Yoshida and Wataru Nagata

Shionogi Research Laboratories, Shionogi & Co., Ltd.*

The structural modification of the naturally occurring penem and cephem has increasingly developed more potent and clinically useful antibiotics (*13*). In the past decade, research efforts on a different line have also increased (*4*), exemplified by the synthesis of new nuclear analogs having a common β-lactam functionality. The discovery of new families of β-lactam antibiotics from natural sources such as clavulanic acid, nocardicin and thienamycin greatly encourages investigators to challenge new fields of chemistry for antibiotics with unique biological activity.

The 1-oxacephem-4-carboxylic acid structure is an example of this class, which was first reported as racemic form from two laboratories in 1974 (*3, 14*). Christensen and his coworkers in the Merck Company showed that the *in vitro* antibacterial activity of 1-oxacephalothin was comparable to that of cephalothin (*3*) but the activity of cefamandole was improved to some degree by 1-oxa-1-dethia displacement (*5*). In 1977, optically active 3-methyl-1-oxacephem derivatives were prepared in the Beecham laboratories (*2*) and in our laboratories (*10*), and an interesting antibacterial activity of these compounds was found. It was clearly demonstrated that the replacement of 1-thia to 1-oxa in the cephem nucleus generally resulted in a 4- to 16-fold increase in the antibacterial activity of cephalosporin and cephamycin derivatives (*10, 11, 15*). Such a favorable antibacterial shift was observed mainly in the gram-negative activity and appeared to depend on the type of side chain structure (*15*). However, it was accompanied by the unfavorable property that the 1-oxa congeners were consistently more hydrolyzable by β-lactamase than the corresponding cephalosporins (*15*). The purpose of our research efforts was concentrated on conferring β-lactamase stability and a complete gram-negative spectrum and to improve the pharmacokinetic characteristics. By an extensive survey of the structure-activity relationships, we discovered a biologically attractive compound named 6059-S (LY-127935 or moxalactam) as a candidate for clinical evaluation (*11, 16*). The progress

---

* Sagisu 5-12-4, Fukushima-ku, Osaka 553, Japan.

TABLE I. Structure-activity Relationship of Antibacterial Activity

(A)

$$R_1-CONH \quad \begin{array}{c} R_3 \\ \text{(β-lactam structure with X, } R_2\text{, COOH)} \end{array}$$

$R_2 = A \left(-CH_2S- \text{(triazole)} \dfrac{N-N=N}{CH_3} \right)$

$R_2 = B \left(-CH_2S- \text{(thiadiazole)} S \dfrac{N-N}{CH_3} \right)$

$R_2 = C (-CH_2OCOCH_3)$

Code No.	Structure R_1	R_2	R_3	X	S. aureus 209P JC-1	E. coli NIHJ JC-2	K. pneu- moniae SRL-1	Kleb- siella sp. 363	P. vul- garis CN-329	E. cloacae 233	S. mar- cescens 13880	P. aeru- ginosa PS-24	E. coli EC-14	P. aeru- ginosa PS-24
					\[In vitro antibacterial activity[a] — % of key compound (6059-S)\]								\[In vivo antibacterial activity[b] — % of 6059-S\]	
6059-S														
a	HO–⟨CH–COOH⟩	A	CH$_3$O	O	100 (6.25)[b]	100 (0.1)	100 (0.1)	100 (0.1)	100 (0.2)	100 (0.1)	100 (0.39)	100 (25)	100 (0.10)	100 (8.9)
b	HO–⟨CH–COOH⟩	A	CH$_3$O	S	50	12	25	25	50	12	25	100	8	49
c	HO–⟨CH–COOH⟩	A	H	O	100	25	25	0.1	50	12	50	<25	20	<30
d	HO–⟨CH–COOH⟩	A	H	S	50	3	3	0.2	12	1.6	3	<25	2	NT[d]
e	HO–⟨CH–COOH⟩	B	CH$_3$O	O	50	12	50	50	50	25	50	50	28	19
f	HO–⟨CH–COOH⟩	C	CH$_3$O	O	50	12	25	25	25	25	50	100	14	18

Side chain													
g phenyl–CH(COOH)–	A	CH$_3$O	O	200	200	200	400	400	200	200	100	67	16
h HO–C$_6$H$_4$–CH$_2$–	A	CH$_3$O	O	3,200	50	100	50	25	0.1	12	<25	67	32
i HO–C$_6$H$_4$–CH$_2$–	A	H	O	6,400	25	50	<0.1	1.6	0.2	<0.4	<25	NT	NT
Cefazolin (CEZ)				6,400 (0.39)	6 (6.25)	6 (1.56)	<0.1 (>100)	0.2 (100)	<0.1 (>100)	<0.4 (>100)	<25 (>100)	22 (0.45)	NT
Sulbenicillin (SPC)				400 (1.56)	1.6 (6.25)	6 (1.56)	<0.1 (>100)	12 (1.56)	0.8 (12.5)	3 (12.5)	50 (50)	2.4 (4.1)	22 (40)

(B)

In vitro activity

ID$_{50}$ (µg/ml)

Compound	S. aureus	E. coli	Klebsiella sp.	Indole-positive Proteus	Entero-bacter sp.	S. marcescens	P. aerugi-nosa	B. fragilis ss fragilis
a								
6059-S	5.7	0.15	0.15	0.14	0.15	0.33	16.8	0.6
CEZ	0.34	2.0	2.0	>100	>100	>100	>100	12.8
CMZ	1.0	0.95	0.86	3.5	>100	10.8	>100	4.8
CMD	0.41	1.3	0.95	6.3	2.3	>100	>100	NT
SPC	2.1	8.5	>100	1.5	6.1	20.0	27.6	NT

a Relative activity (%) was compared to the antibacterial activity of 6059-S against standard strains.   The agar dilution MIC values (µg/ml) were determined by using an inoculum of one loopful of 10^6 cells per ml and indicated in parentheses.   b Compounds were administered subcutaneously 1 hr and 5 hr after intraperitoneal infection.   ED$_{50}$ values were expressed in mg/kg per injection and indicated in parentheses.   Relative activity (%) was compared to the activity of 6059-S.   c The concentration required to inhibit the growth of clinical isolates by 50% in number.   d Not tested.

in chemistry allowed a straightforward and industrially feasible synthesis for the preparation of this new 1-oxacephem (9).

IN VITRO ANTIBACTERIAL ACTIVITY

At the beginning of our studies, a number of 1-oxa congeners of 3-methyl-cephalosporins were prepared with various side chain structures at the 7β-position, and the MIC values against diverse organisms were carefully compared between each pair of structural analogs. The phenylmalonylamino derivative of 1-oxacephem was qualified for further modification by the following observations (15): (1) it had the greatest antibacterial shift with a 16-fold increase upon S→O replacement; (2) its wide-ranging gram-negative spectrum including that against Proteus, Enterobacter, Serratia, and a highly sensitive Pseudomonas; and (3) its antibacterial shift equally favored to both β-lactamase producing and -nonproducing gram-negative organisms. Then modification at C-3' was made for 7β-phenylmalonylamino-1-oxacephems and introduction of (1-methyltetrazolyl)thiomethyl (c in Table I) greatly improved the antibacterial potency with an approximately 100-fold increase (15) as observed in the case of cephalosporins (13). Comparing the gram-negative activity between c and d in Table I, a remarkable increase in antibacterial activity was indicated, except for against the penicillinase producing strains e.g., Klebsiella sp. 363, which even showed an unfavorable shift. Substitution of the methoxy group at the 7α-position of c, which converts to 6059-S (a), was quite sufficient to resume the susceptibility of this resistant strain and also to exhibit a significant antibacterial shift against every gram-negative organism, especially Pseudomonas aeruginosa and Enterobacter sp. A substantial improvement in gram-negative activity was also observed between two 1-thia congeners d to b. A similar effect of the methoxy group was reported in the case of arylmalonylpenicillin (1). It has been clearly demonstrated that the 7α-methoxy and the side chain α-carboxyl groups in 6059-S (a) work together complementarily for complete protection from hydrolysis by every type of β-lactamase and contribute to such a complete gram-negative spectrum (15). The unsubstituted analog i is easily hydrolyzed by β-lactamase and has very poor activity except against E. coli and Klebsiella, which produce no β-lactamase. The sensitivity of penicillinase-producing Klebsiella was restored by the 7α-methoxy group (h) but not by an arylmalonyl side chain (c). On the contrary, Enterobacter and Serratia produce inducible cephalosporinase and are specifically sensitive to the arylmalonyl analog c. An incorporation of the side chain carboxyl function greatly sacrifices gram-positive activity but is indispensable for absolute effectiveness against gram-negative bacteria.

IN VIVO ANTIBACTERIAL ACTIVITY

The p-hydroxy function on the phenyl ring in the side chain of 6059-S brings about an increased peak plasma level and lower serum protein binding, as indicated by the comparison between a and g in Tables II and III. As the unsubstituted analog g

TABLE II. Structure-activity Relationship of Pharmacokinetic Properties

Compound		Relative activity (%) compared to 6059-S			Relative toxicity (%)[c] compared to 6059-S
Code No.	Name	Plasma level at peak[a]	Urinary recovery[b]	Biliary recovery[b]	
a	6059-S	100 (34. 4)	100 (74. 3)	100 (21. 7)	100 (6, 000)
b		99			
c		124			
d		106			
e		67			
f		51			
g		66	57	89	
h		43	77	157	
	CEZ	185 (63. 6)	108 (80. 0)	74 (16)	146 (4, 100)

[a] A dose of 20 mg/kg was injected subcutaneously into mice. Numbers in parentheses represent average concentrations in μg/ml at 15 min after injection. [b] A dose of 10 mg/kg was injected subcutaneously into rats. Numbers in parentheses represent the average percentage of a compound excreted for 24 hr after dosing. [c] A compound was administered intravenously into mice. LD_{50} (mg/kg)-values are shown in parentheses.

TABLE III. Structure-activity Relationship of Physicochemical Properties

Compound		Molecular weight (as free form)	Partition[a] coefficient	Serum[b] protein binding rate (%)	Acid stability
Code No.	Name				
a	6059-S	520. 5	−0. 59	57	+
b		536. 5	0. 44	89	+
c		490. 5	0. 44	54	+
d		506. 5	1. 47	82	+
e		520. 5	0. 19	70	+
f		464. 4	0. 12	59	+
g		504. 5	−0. 02	88	+
h		476. 5	0. 61	64	+
	CEZ	454. 5	NT	87	+
	CPC	378. 4	NT	71	−

[a] The experimental value (log Pu) was obtained for 6059-S as a free acid form. The values for compounds except for 6059-S were theoretically calculated from the additivity of the f value and/or π value (Kubota and Ezumi, unpublished data). [b] Human serum albumin solution (50 mg/ml) was employed instead of human serum.

significantly reduces the urinary recovery in comparison to a, the introduction of the *p*-hydroxy group appears to give metabolic stability to this compound. These pharmacological advantages may be responsible for the excellent *in vivo* antibacterial activity. The ED_{50} values of 6059-S against experimental infection of mice with *E. coli* and *P. aeruginosa* were found to be significantly lower than those of the unsubstituted analog g, although the *p*-hydroxy function tends to diminish *in vitro* activity. When the substituent of 6059-S at the C-3' position is modified to e and f, the *in vivo* activity strikingly decreased in response to the lower *in vitro* activity and plasma levels.

Finally, the complete gram-negative spectrum together with its more preferable pharmacokinetic properties led us to choose 6059-S as a clinical candidate. The agar dilution MIC distribution (ID_{50}) of 6059-S against clinical isolates is shown in Table I-B. Clinically important gram-negative pathogens except for *P. aeruginosa* were equally inhibited by less than 1 µg/ml. The superiority of 6059-S to the reference β-lactam antibiotics is evident. 6059-S is outstanding in its potent activity against *Bacteroides fragilis*. The pharmacokinetics of 6059-S were studied in normal volunteers, and a long duration of serum levels and high urinary recovery were demonstrated (*7, 6, 12*). The mean serum half-lives ranged from 1.3 to 2.3 hr for the β-phase of i.v. injection and from 2.3 to 2.8 hr for i.m. injection. Such a favorable balance of the activity and pharmacology of 6059-S has been found to reflect well on its clinical effectiveness (*8*).

Acknowledgments
We are very grateful to many colleagues in the Shionogi Research Laboratories for their collaboration in this study, especially Dr. M. Narisada, Dr. M. Yoshioka, Dr. S. Matsuura, Dr. M. Mayama, Dr. T. Kubota, and Dr. K. Ezumi. Thanks are also due to Dr. H. Otsuka, the managing director of this laboratory, for his encouragement throughout this work.

REFERENCES

1. Bentley, P. H. and Clayton, J. P. 1977. *In* "Recent Advances in the Chemistry of β-Lactam Antibiotics," ed. by J. Elks, The Chemical Society, Burlington House, London, pp. 68–72.
2. Brain, E. G., Branch, C. L., Eglington, A. J., Nayler, J. H. C., Osborne, N. F., Pearson, M. J., Smale, T. C., Southgate, R., and Tolliday, P. 1977. *In* "Recent Advances in the Chemistry of β-Lactam Antibiotics," ed. by J. Elks, The Chemical Society, Burlington House, London, pp. 204–213.
3. Cama, L. D. and Christensen, B. G. 1974. *J. Am. Chem. Soc.*, **96**, 7582–7584.
4. Cooper, R.D.G. 1980. *In* "Topics in Antibiotics Chemistry," ed. by P. Sammes, Ellis Horwood Ltd., Chichester, Vol. 3, pp. 40–203.
5. Firestone, R. A., Fahey, J. L., Maciejewicz, N. C., Patel, G. S., and Christensen, B. G. 1977. *J. Med. Chem.* **20**, 551–556.
6. Israel, K. S., Black, H. R., Griffith, R. S., Brier, G. L., and Wolny, J. D. 1980.

In "Current Chemotherapy and Infectious Diseases," ed. by J. D. Nelson and C. Grassi, Am. Soc. Microbiol, Washington, D. C., Vol. I, pp. 107–108.

7. Kurihara, J., Matsumoto, K., Uzuka, Y., Shishido, H., Nagatake, T., Yamada, H., Yoshida, T., Oguma, T., Kimura, Y., and Tochino, Y. 1980. *In* "Current Chemotherapy and Infectious Diseases," ed. by J. D. Nelson and C. Grassi, Am. Soc. Microbiol., Washington, D. C., Vol. I, pp. 110–111.

8. Matsumoto, K., Uzuka, Y., Nagatake, T., and Shishido, H. 1980. *In* "Current Chemotherapy and Infectious Diseases," ed. by J. D. Nelson and C. Grassi, Am. Soc. Microbiol., Washington, D. C., Vol. I, pp. 112–113.

9. Nagata, W. 1980. *Phil. Trans. Roy. Soc. Lond. B*, **289**, 225–230.

10. Narisada, M., Onoue, H., and Nagata, W. 1977. *Heterocycles*, **7**, 839–849.

11. Narisada, M., Yoshida, T., Onoue, T., Ohtani, M., Okada, T., Tsuji, T., Kikkawa, I., Haga, N., Satoh, H., Itani, H., and Nagata, W. 1979. *J. Med. Chem.*, **22**, 757–759.

12. Parsons, J. N., Romano, J. M., and Levison, M. E. 1980. *Antimicrob. Agents Chemother.*, **17**, 226–228.

13. Webber, J. A. and Ott, J. L. 1977. *In* "Structure-activity Relationships among the Semisynthetic Antibiotics," ed. by D. Perlman, Academic Press, New York, pp. 161–237.

14. Wolfe, S., Ducep, J. B., Tin, K. C., and Lee, S. L. 1974. *Can. J. Chem.*, **52**, 3996–3999.

15. Yoshida, T. 1980. *Phil. Trans. Roy. Soc. Lond. B*, **289**, 231–237.

16. Yoshida, T., Matsuura, S., Mayama, M., Kameda, Y., and Kuwahara, S. 1980. *Antimicrob. Agents Chemother.*, **17**, 302–312.

PS-SERIES β-LACTAM ANTIBIOTICS

Yasuo FUKAGAWA, Kazuhiko OKAMURA, Norio SHIBAMOTO, and Tomoyuki ISHIKURA

Central Research Laboratories, Sanraku-Ocean Co., Ltd.*

A new family of β-lactam antibiotics (called the olivanate family) have recently been reported which includes thienamycin (6), N-acetylthienamycin (5), epithienamycins A, B, C, and D (1), MM 4550, MM 13902, MM 17880 (4), PS-5 (8, 16), PS-6, and PS-7 (14) (Table I). These new β-lactam compounds that are produced by several species of *Streptomyces* share a common chemical structure of 7-oxo-1-azabicyclo-[3.2.0]hept-2-ene(conventionally called 1-carbapenem or heptem). In clear contrast to known types of penicillin and cephalosporin compounds, they have not only potent antimicrobial activity against both gram-positive and gram-negative bacteria, but also marked inhibitory activity against β-lactamases that are essentially responsible for the defense mechanism of pathogens resistant to β-lactam drugs.

Because of unavailability of thienamycin, N-acetylthienamycin, epithienamycins, and MM-series compounds, this paper largely deals with PS-5, PS-6, PS-7, NS-5 (deacetylated PS-5), and PS-5 S-oxide. The first three PS-series compounds were produced by fermentation using *Streptomyces cremeus* subsp. *auratilis* (8, 14), whereas NS-5 and PS-5 S-oxide were chemically prepared from PS-5 (9, 15).

ANTIMICROBIAL ACTIVITY

The antimicrobial spectra of PS-5, PS-6, PS-7, NS-5, and PS-5 S-oxide are summarized in Table II, using ampicillin and cefazolin as reference β-lactam compounds (9, 12, 13, 15).

The results in Table II together with the antimicrobial data of thienamycin (7), epithienamycins (1), and MM-series compounds (4) reported in the literature clearly show that the β-lactam compounds of the olivanate family generally have a broad antimicrobial spectrum against both gram-positive and gram-negative bacteria. It

---

* Johnan 4-9-1, Fujisawa 251, Japan.

TABLE I. β-Lactam Compounds of the Olivanate Family

	n	R	R'	R''	
	0	–H	–CH$_3$	–COCH$_3$	PS-5
	0	–CH$_3$	–CH$_3$	–COCH$_3$	PS-6
	0	–H	–CH$_3$	–H	NS-5 (synthetic)
	1	–H	–CH$_3$	–COCH$_3$	PS-5 S-oxide (synthetic)
		–CH$_3$	–OH	–H	Thienamycin
		–CH$_3$	–OH	–COCH$_3$	N-acetylthiena-mycin
		–OH	–CH$_3$	–COCH$_3$	Epithienamycin C
		–OH	–CH$_3$		Epithienamycin D
		H	–CH$_3$		PS-7
		OSO$_3$H			MM 17880
		–OH			Epithienamycin A
	0	–OH			Epithienamycin B
	0	–OSO$_3$H			MM 13902
	1	–OSO$_3$H			MM 4550

is in good contrast with common penicillin and cephalosporin compounds possessing very weak activity against gram-negative bacteria.

Among the PS-series compounds tested, NS-5 exhibits the highest antimicrobial activity againt *Pseudomonas* (about 10 times more active than PS-5). The free amino group (basicity) of the S side chain seems to be one of the important factors for action against *Pseudomonas*. The excellent antipseudomonal activity of thienamycin and N-formidoylthienamycin has also been reported (7).

Although the length and nature of the alkyl side chain at the 6-position are likely to be less influential, PS-5 with the ethyl group gives smaller MIC values on all the test microorganisms than PS-6 with the isopropyl group. A more or less significant change in antimicrobial activity probably results from the hydroxylation of PS-5 to epithienamycin C, the epimerization of epithienamycin C to epithienamycin A or to N-acetylthienamycin and the sulfation of epithienamycin A to MM 17880.

TABLE II. Antimicrobial Spectra of PS-5, PS-6, PS-7, NS-5, and PS-5 S-oxide

Microorganism	PS-5	PS-6	PS-7	NS-5	PS-5 S-oxide	APC	CEZ
Bacillus subtilis ATCC 6633	0.1	0.78	0.39	0.05	6.25	0.05	0.1
Sarcina lutea	0.1	0.39	0.20	0.024	0.78	<0.013	0.78
Staphylococcus aureus FDA 209P	0.024	0.10	0.39	0.0008	25	<0.013	0.1
Smith	0.20	0.20	0.39	0.003		0.05	0.2
Russell	0.20	0.20	0.39	0.024		25	0.2
S. epidermidis	0.20	0.39	0.20	0.05		0.024	0.2
Alcaligenes faecalis A1	0.78	1.56	0.78	1.56	>100	3.13	3.13
Citrobacter freundii GN346	3.13	12.5	3.13	6.25	>100	>400	>400
Comamonas terrigena B-996	0.024	0.1	0.05	0.05		0.05	0.39
Enterobacter aerogenes E-19	6.25	25	3.13	6.25	>100	>400	>400
E. cloacae 45	6.25	25	3.13	12.5		>400	>400
E. sp. E-8	3.13	6.25	1.56	6.25		6.25	3.13
Escherichia coli K 12	3.13	6.25	0.78	6.25	>100	3.13	1.56
RGN823	3.13	6.25	1.56	3.13		>400	200
Klebsiella pneumoniae K13	6.25	6.25	3.13	6.25		>400	400
Proteus mirabilis P-6	12.5	12.5	6.25	12.5	>100	3.13	6.25
P. rettgeri P-7	12.5	6.25	1.56	12.5		>400	>400
P. vulgaris GN76	25	12.5	12.5	12.5		>400	>400
Providencia sp. P-8	6.25	6.25	1.56	6.25	>100	>400	100
Pseudomonas aeruginosa IFO 3445	25	50	12.5	3.13		>400	>400
NCTC 10490	25	50	6.25	0.78		>400	>400
Serratia marcescens S-18	6.25	25	1.56	12.5	>100	200	>400
T55	6.25	50	3.13	12.5		50	>400

The presence of a double bond in the S side chain (PS-7) slightly reduces the antibacterial activity against gram-positive organisms, while the activity against gram-negative bacteria is improved comparatively well. This tendency is also confirmed between MM 17880 and MM 13902 (4).

Oxidation of the sulfur atom in the S side chain (PS-5 S-oxide) leads to a drastic reduction of the antimicrobial activity against all the test organisms except for *Sarcina lutea*. A similar observation is reported on MM 4550 (4), suggesting that the sulfur atom is critically important for the antimicrobial activity.

INHIBITORY ACTIVITY AGAINST β-LACTAMASES

One of the possibly useful advantages of the olivanate compounds over traditional penicillin and cephalosporin compounds will be found in their potent inhbitiory (partially destructive) activity against various types of β-lactamases from gram-positive and gram-negative bacteria. Clavulanate, a fermentation product of *Streptomyces clavuligerus*, is also known to be a specific β-lactamase inhibitor with least antimicrobial activity (11).

Typical penicillinase from *Bacillus licheniformis* 749/C cannot attack PS-5 even at an extremely high enzyme concentration, but the β-lactamase activity measured with benzylpenicillin as the substrate is diminished by PS-5 to extents depending on the period of preincubation and the concentration of the inhibitor (3). The rate of inactivation of *B. licheniformis* 749/C β-lactamase by PS-5 follows first-order kinetics. Although no precise mechanism of inactivation has yet been elucidated, a part of the enzyme activity inhibited by PS-5 cannot be restored even by dialysis and substrate dilution, which indicates that the inactivation of the β-lactamase by the inhibitor is partially irreversible (destructive).

Cephalosporinase (type Ic) from *Proteus vulgaris* P-5 is inhibited by PS-5, too. In contrast with *B. licheniformis* 749/C penicillinase, this cephalosporinase hydrolyzes PS-5 at a very slow rate, while the β-lactamase activity is simultaneously inactivated by the inhibitor in a partially irreversible manner (10).

PS-5 also inactivates β-lactamases from *Bacillus cereus* 569, *Citrobacter freundii* GN346, *P. vulgaris* GN76, and *Streptomyces* sp. E750-3 in irreversible manners, with concomitant partial hydrolysis of the inhibitor by the enzymes. A similar mode of inhibition is described in the system of *Escherichia coli* RTEM β-lactamase with clavulanate (2).

Although the least data are available on the inhibition of β-lactamases by the PS-series compounds other than PS-5, PS-7 seems to have a higher affinity to some of the enzymes than PS-5. There is no substantial difference in the β-lactamase inhibitory activity between PS-5 and PS-6 except that PS-6 is less effective than PS-5.

ANTIMICROBIAL SYNERGISM WITH TRADITIONAL β-LACTAM COMPOUNDS

Table III summarizes the synergistic effects of PS-5 and PS-7 combined with ampi-

TABLE III. Synergism of PS-5 and PS-7 with Ampicillin and Cefazolin

Microorganism	MIC (μg/ml)				Relative synergism index[a]			
	PS-5	PS-7	APC	CEZ	With APC	PS-5 CEZ	With APC	PS-7 CEZ
C. freundii GN346	1.56	1.56	1,600	3,200	16	128	2	4
E. aerogenes E19	3.13	3.13	200	800	4	16	1	2
E. cloacae 45	3.13	3.13	1,600	1,600	4	4	1	2
E. coli RGN823	3.13	1.56	>3,200	12.5		2		2
K. pneumoniae K13	3.13	3.13	>3,200	12.5		2		2
P. vulgaris GN76	12.5	6.25	800	400	8	16	32	64
Proteus sp. P22	12.5	12.5	3,200	3,200	8	16	256	512
P. aeruginosa IFO 3445	6.25	3.13	100	800	4	2	2	1
NCTC 10490	6.25	3.13	100	400	2	2	4	1
S. marcescens S-18	3.13	3.13	100	>3,200	4	>64	8	>128
T-55	3.13	3.13	25	3,200	1	64	1	128

[a] Relative synergism index = MIC of APC or CEZ/MIC of APC or CEZ in the presence of 0.5 μg/ml of PS-5 or PS-7. Two-fold dilution series of the drug(s) singly or in combination were assayed by the standardized disc-agar diffusion method (inoculum size 10^6 cells/ml).

cillin and cefazolin on *in vitro* antimicrobial activity. The clear synergism of PS-5, but not of PS-7, is noted with *C. freundii* GN346, whereas the reverse is observed with *Proteus* sp. P22. A large portion of the synergistic effect seems to be ascribed to the inhibitory activity against β-lactamases.

It has very recently been reported that the combination of PS-5 with cefoxitin shows significant synergism when the MIC is determined in the presence of 1 μg/ml of PS-5 (about 1/5 of the MIC of PS-5) on 19 cefoxitin-resistant clinical isolates of *Enterobacter cloacae* (type Ia β-lactamase producers) in spite of the fact that cefoxitin is not attacked by this type of β-lactamase (*17*).

REFERENCES

1. Cassidy, P. J., Stapley, E. O., Goegelman, R., Miller, T. W., Arison, B., Albers-Schönberg, G., Zimmerman, S. B., and Birnbaum, J. 1977. Abstr. 17th Intersci. Conf. Antimicrob. Agents Chemother., New York, No. 81.
2. Fisher, J., Charnas, R. L., and Knowles, J. R. 1978. *Biochemistry*, **17**, 2180–2184.
3. Fukagawa, Y., Takei, T., and Ishikura, T. 1980. *Biochem. J.*, **185**, 177–188.
4. Hood, J. D., Box, S. J., and Verrall, M. S. 1979. *J. Antibiot.*, **32**, 295–304.
5. Kahan, J. S., Kahan, F. M., Goegelman, R., Stapley, E. O., and Hernandez, S. 1977. Ger. Offen. 2652681.

6. Kahan, J. S., Kahan, F. M., Goegelman, R., Currie, S. A., Jackson, M., Stapley, E. O., Miller, T. W., Miller, A. K., Hendlin, D., Mochales, S., Hernandez, S., Woodruff, H. B., and Birnbaum, J. 1979. *J. Antibiot.*, **32**, 1–12.

7. Kropp, H., Sundelof, J. G., Kahan, J. S., Kahan, F. M., and Birnbaum, J. 1980. *Antimicrob. Agents Chemother.*, **17**, 993–1000.

8. Okamura, K., Hirata, S., Koki, A., Hori, K., Shibamoto, N., Okumura, Y., Okabe, M., Okamoto, R., Kouno, K., Fukagawa, Y., Shimauchi, Y., Ishikura, T., and Lein, J. 1979. *J. Antibiot.*, **32**, 262–271.

9. Okamura, K., Hirata, S., Okumura, Y., Fukagawa, Y., Shimauchi, Y., Ishikura, T., Kouno, K., and Lein, J. 1979. Japan Kokai 73788/1979.

10. Okamura, K., Sakamoto, M., and Ishikura, T. 1980. *J. Antibiot.*, **33**, 293–302.

11. Reading, C. and Cole, M. 1977. *Antimicrob. Agents Chemother.*, **11**, 852–857.

12. Sakamoto, M., Iguchi, H., Okamura, K., Hori, S., Fukagawa, Y., Ishikura, T., and Lein, J. 1979. *J. Antibiot.*, **32**, 272–279.

13. Sakamoto, M., Shibamoto, N., Iguchi, H., Okamura, K., Hori, S., Fukagawa, Y., Ishikura, T., and Lein, J. 1980. *J. Antibiot.*, **33**, 1138–1145.

14. Shibamoto, N., Koki, A., Nishino, M., Nakamura, K., Kiyoshima, K., Okamura, K., Okabe, M., Okamoto, R., Fukagawa, Y., Shimauchi, Y., Ishikura, T., and Lein, J. 1980. *J. Antibiot.*, **33**, 1128–1137.

15. Yamada, K., Shimauchi, Y., and Ishikura, T. 1979. Japan Kokai 135790/1979.

16. Yamamoto, K., Yoshioka, T., Kato, Y., Shibamoto, N., Okamura, K., Shimauchi, Y., and Ishikura, T. 1980. *J. Antibiot.*, **33**, 796–803.

17. Yokota, T. 1980. Abstr. Papers for the 28th Annual Meeting of Japan Society of Chemotherapy, Tokyo, pp. 38–39.

β-LACTAMASE STABLE β-LACTAM ANTIBIOTICS

L. D. Cama and B. G. Christensen

*Merck Sharp & Dohme Research Laboratories**

The β-lactam antibiotics play an important role in antibacterial chemotherapy because of their high efficacy combined with a lack of toxicity. The classical β-lactam antibiotics such as the penicillins and the early cephalosporins (cephalothin, cephaloridine, cephalexin), though effective against both gram-positive and gram-negative organisms, are characterized by a lack of activity against many bacteria which produce β-lactamases.

Since 1971 a number of new β-lactam antibiotics have appeared which show remarkable stability to β-lactamases when compared to the classical β-lactam antibiotics. All of these have unusual structural features which contribute to their stability to these enzymes. The first of the new β-lactam antibiotics were the cephamycins (1) (*38, 51*). With the discovery of cephamycin C (1a), one had a β-lactam antibiotic which demonstrated good activity against many cephalosporinase-producing gram-negative bacteria. Replacement of the 7β-aminoadipoyl group by thienylacetyl gave cefoxitin (2a) (*32*) which shows a large increase in gram-positive activity analogous to the corresponding change in going from cephalosporin C to cephalothin (*16*) as well as a smaller increase in activity against gram-negative organisms including β-lactamase-producing organisms.

A comparison of the structures of cephalothin (2b) and cefoxitin (2a) shows two unusual features: (1) a carbamoyloxymethyl at C-3 instead of acetoxymethyl; and (2) a methoxy at C-7α. It was of interest to see which of these groups was responsible for the improved activity of cefoxitin over cephalothin.

Replacing the acetoxy group of cephalothin by a carbamoyloxy group was achieved by treatment of deacetyl cephalothin (*28*) with chlorosulfonylisocyanate, followed by hydrolysis of the chlorosulfonyl group to give 7β-thienylacetamido-3-carbamoyloxy-deacetoxycephalosporanic acid (2c). This compound shows an *in vitro* antibacterial spectrum essentially identical with that of cephalothin (*50*), demonstrat-

* Rahway, New Jersey 07065, U.S.A.

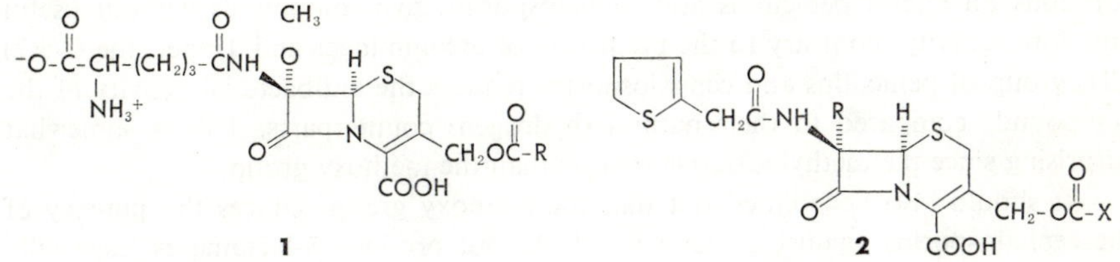

1a, R=NH$_2$
 b, R=CH$_3$
 c, R=C(OCH$_3$)=CHC$_6$H$_4$OH-p
 d, R=C(OCH$_3$)=CHC$_6$H$_4$OSO$_3^-$-p

 e, R=C(OCH$_3$)=CH—⬡—OH
                      |
                      OH

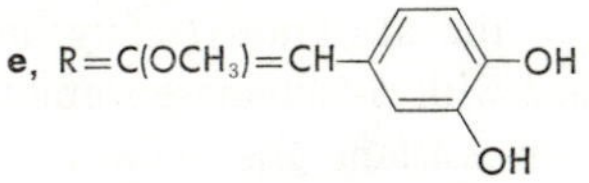

2a, R=OCH$_3$, X=NH$_2$
 b, R=H,   X=CH$_3$
 c, R=H,   X=NH$_2$
 d, R=OCH$_3$, X=CH$_3$

FIG. 1.   Some cephalosporin and cephamycin antibiotics

TABLE I.   β-Lactamase Stability of 7α-Substituted Cephalosporins

7α-Substituent	H	OCH$_3$	OCH$_2$CH$_3$	SCH$_3$	CHOH
% destruction	>96%	16%	0%	20%	0%

ing that the carbamoyloxy group is not responsible for stability to β-lactamases. 7α-Methoxycephalothin (2d) was also prepared (12). Compound 2d is markedly stable to β-lactamase producers and has an antibacterial spectrum superior to that of cephalothin (50) and comparable in vitro to cefoxitin (2a). In vivo in mice and rhesus monkeys, compound 2a is better than compound 2d presumably because the carbamoyloxy group is stable to serum esterases while the acetyl group is not (50).

The discovery that the 7α-methoxy group is responsible for the improved antibacterial properties of a cephalosporin molecule, along with a prediction by Stromminger and Tipper (52) that 6α-methyl penicillins may be more active antibiotics than the 6αH analogs, stimulated the synthesis of a large number of C-6(7)-substituted penicillins and cephalosporins with varying substituents such as alkoxy (2, 12, 33, 34, 46), alkyl (4, 22, 30, 42), acyl (3, 42), methylthio (29, 34), acetoxy (45), hydroxy (47), alkoxyformamido (13), and cyano (55).

Substitution at C-7α in the cephalosporin series increases stability to β-lactamase, as shown in Table I. Under conditions where >96% of cephalothin is destroyed by the β-lactamase from E. coli MK-2885, the C-7 substituted analog is destroyed to the indicated extent, indicating greater stability toward β-lactamase is achieved by substitution at the C-7α position with groups larger than H.

Antibacterial activity decreases rapidly with the size of the C-6(7) group (50, 56) and except for the methoxy group on the cephalosporin nucleus, all other substitutions on C-6(7) penicillins and cephalosporins give compounds without useful antibiotic activity; contrary to the prediction of Stromminger and Tipper, the C-6(7) CH_3 group of penicillins and cephalosporins reduces the antibacterial activity of the compounds compared to their natural (hydrogen) counterparts. This is somewhat surprising since the methyl group is smaller than the methoxy group.

It should also be pointed out that the methoxy group reduces the potency of the cephalosporins against bacteria which do not produce β-lactamases (especially the gram-positive ones) (50). Thus, the 7α-methoxy group appears to achieve a good balance of steric and electronic factors retaining antibacterial activity combined with β-lactamase stability to the cephalosporins. The reasons for its not having a similar effect on the penicillins are not apparent. The cephamycins then are a new class of broad spectrum β-lactam antibiotics which have the attributes (safety and good pharmacokinetics) of the cephalosporins combined with β-lactamase stability which makes them effective against many cephalosporin-resistant gram-negative bacteria and *Bacteroides fragilis*.

Cefoxitin is currently marketed in Europe and the United States. Table II lists other cephamycins which are at earlier stages of development. These new cepha- mycins are reported to have *in vitro* activities 2 to 8 times higher than cefoxitin. None are active against *Pseudomonas* species and all have activity similar to cefoxitin against anaerobes such as *B. fragilis*.

It has been shown above that the 7α-methoxy group confers stability to β- lactamases to the cephalosporins; however, this is not the only way to achieve this property.

A number of cephalosporins not having a 7α-methoxy substituent listed in Table III also have considerable stability to β-lactamases. An examination of their structure shows a common feature, the presence of a *syn*-methoxyimino side chain. Molecular models show that the OCH_3 group of the side chain can occupy the same space near the β-lactam carbonyl that is occupied by the 7α-methoxy group in cepha- mycins, albeit only some of the time because of the greater degrees of freedom that the methoxyimino side chain has available to it.

In general, these cephalosporins appear to have higher *in vitro* and *in vivo* anti- bacterial activity against many β-lactamase-producing strains when compared to the cephamycins. Some of these, however, are less active against anaerobes such as *B. fragilis*. Some of these compounds have good antipseudomonal activity *in vitro*.

A novel modification of the methoxyimino side chain has recently been reported (23). The antibiotic GR 20263 has a 2,2-dimethylacetic acid group in place of the methyl of the methoxyimino side chain. This compound is reported to have an ex- ceptionally broad spectrum of activity including against *P. aeruginosa*. It is stable to a wide range of β-lactamases and appears to be superior to the cephalosporins listed in Table II.

The demonstration of clinical utility of the semi-synthetic cephamycin derivatives led to a reexamination of the concept of nuclear modification. Earlier workers, most notably the Lowe (37) and Woodward (25) groups, had explored this field, but lack

TABLE II. Structure and *In Vitro* Activity of Cephamycins[a]

General structure (cephem nucleus): R–C(=O)–NH, 7α-OCH₃, CH₂X at 3-position, COOH at 4-position.

Code No. or Name	Structure R	Structure X	*In vitro* antibacterial activity[b] MIC (µg/ml)							
			S. aureus 2868	E. coli 2391	K. pneumoniae 2826	S. marcescens 2854	P. morganii 2833	E. cloacae 2646	P. aeruginosa 2835	B. fragilis 3249
CS-1170	CNCH₂SCH₂–	O=C–NH₂	1.56	100	NA	12.5	3.12	NA	>100	NA
			(0.8)[c]	(3.1)	(0.8)	(3.1)	(3.1)	(0.8)	NA	
SKF-73678	CF₃SCH₂–	–S–Tet[b]	(0.4)	(3.1)	(0.4)	(3.1)	(1.6)	(0.8)	NA	NA
SQ-14359	(thienyl)CH–HN–C(=O)–NH₂	–S–Tet	1	64	<0.5	32	4	>128	>128	16
YM-09330	(COOH)(C(=O)NH₂)C=C(thienyl)	–S–Tet	8	16	<0.06	8	1	128	>128	16
CFX	(thienyl)–CH₂–	OC–NH₂ (O=C)	2	128	1	32	16	>128	>128	16

[a] Biological activities reported in Tables II and III were determined by Koupal, L. and Weissberger, B., Merck Sharp & Dohme Research Laboratories, Rahway, whose kind permission to allow their publication is gratefully acknowledged.   [b] All test strains are known β-lactamase producers and mouse virulent.   [c] Tet= (1-methyl-tetrazol-5-yl, N=N–N(CH₃)–N ring)   [d] MIC in parenthesis from ref. 53.

TABLE III. Structure and *In Vitro* Activity of Methoxyimino Cephalosporin

Code No. or Name	Structure R	X	Y	*In vitro* antibacterial activity[a] MIC (μg/ml) S. aureus 2868	E. coli 2891	K. pneumoniae 2826	S. marcescens 2854	P. morganii 2833	E. cloacae 2646	P. aeruginosa 2835	B. fragilis 3249
Cefuroxime	(furanyl)C=N–OCH$_3$	CH$_2$–OCNH$_2$	H	1.56	100	NA	NA	6.5	NA	>100	NA
HR-756	(aminothiazolyl)C=N–OCH$_3$	CH$_2$OCCH$_3$	H	2	4	<0.06	4	1.0	128	32	64
SCE-1365	''	CH$_2$S–(triazolyl N–CH$_3$)	H	2	2	<0.0075	8	0.125	32	16	4
FR-13374	''	H	CH$_3$	4	16	<0.06	4	4	64	>128	8
FK-749	''	H	H	4	8	<0.06	8	0.5	128	32	1

[a] All test strains are known β-lactamase producers and mouse virulent.

GR-20263

of interesting biological activity of these analogs deterred further work in this area. The Merck group developed total syntheses of the penicillins, cephalosporins and cephamycins (21, 43). Specifically, these syntheses were convergent routes designed to make a large variety of nuclear analogs available. The cephalosporin-cephamycin total synthesis may be represented sequentially to illustrate the diversity of final products available via simple modification of the basic scheme.

Of all the nuclear variants thus prepared, the 1-oxacephalosporins have stimulated the most interest. 1-Oxacephalothin (8), the first reported member of this series, was shown to possess twice the activity of its natural sulfur counterpart, cephalothin. A representatively potent compound synthesized by the Merck group was 1-oxacefamandole (11). Assuming that a 2–3-mm increase in zone size represents a doubling of potency, this compound is up to five times as active as cefamandole. Presumably, the smaller size of the oxygen atom and its smaller dihedral angle contributes to a higher degree of ring strain in the azetidinone portion of the oxacephalosporins, thus accounting for their increased potency.

Recently, the Shionogi group (39) has published a series of papers confirming the original observation that 1-oxacephalosporins are more active than cephalosporins. A compound, designated 6059S, has been investigated extensively. Its in vitro potency (40) is shown in Table V. The presence of the 7α-methoxy group, as in cefoxitin, confers β-lactamase stability upon 6059S. This compound is currently undergoing extensive clinical evaluation.

Based upon the improved potency of the 1-oxacephalosporins, other groups (19, 20) have also looked extensively at novel nuclei. However, the discovery of the natural products, clavulanic acid (26), nocardicin (24), and thienamycin has diverted many medicinal chemists to other goals.

Scheme.   Convergent cephem total synthesis.

6059S

TABLE IV. Comparative Activities of Cefamandole and Oxacefamandole

Organism	X=O	S
S. aureus	28.5	24
B. subtilis	34.5	31.5
P. vulgaris	30.5	27
S. gallinarum	11.5	0
V. percolans	25	23.5
E. coli	23	18
K. pneumoniae	20	15.5
A. aerogenes	19.5	0

Zone diam. (mm, at 10 μg/ml)

TABLE V. *In vitro* Potency (50% MIC, μg/ml) of 60595

Compound	S. aureus	H. influenzae	E. coli	K. pneumoniae	P. vulgaris	B. fragilis	P. aeruginosa
60595	6.2	0.1	0.1	0.1	0.1	6.2	12.5
Cefoxitin	3.1	0.2	3.1	1.6	3.1	6.2	>100
Cefotaxime	1.6	—	0.1	0.05	>100	50	25

Thienamycin (6a) is a novel β-lactam antibiotic isolated from *Streptomyces cattleya*. It is unusually potent and has remarkable stability to β-lactamase-producing bacteria (*31*). It has three structural features (*1*) not found in the classical β-lactam antibiotics, the penicillins, and cephalosporins: (i) an α-hydroxyethyl side chain instead of a β-amido side chain at C-6; (ii) an unusual cysteamine side chain at position 2; and (iii) a highly strained nucleus consisting of an unsaturated five-membered ring fused to a β-lactam in which a methylene replaces the sulfur at position 1.

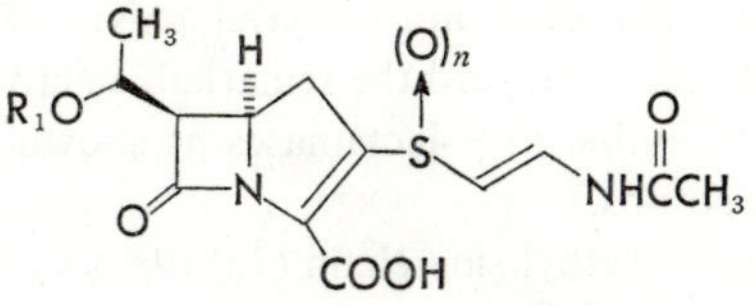

3a, R₁=SO₃H, n=0
 b, R₁=SO₃H, n=0
 c, R₁=H, n=0

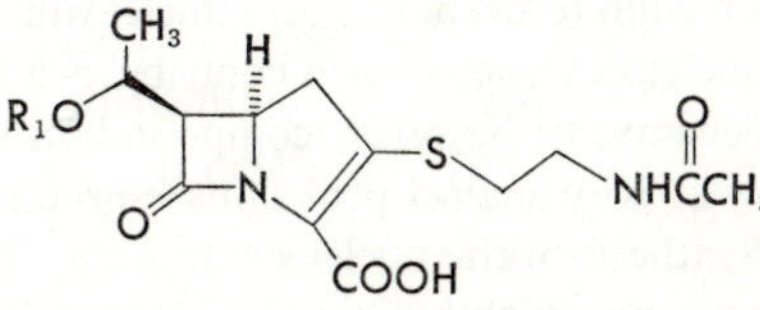

4a, R₁=SO₃H
 b, R₁=H

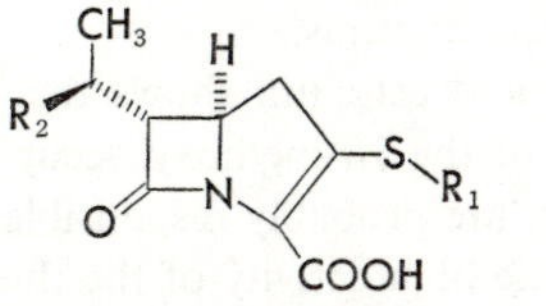

5a, R₁=CH₂ CH₂NHAc, R₂=OH
 b, R₁=CH=CH NHAc, R₂=OH
 c, R₁=CH₂CH₂NHAc, R₂=H
 d, R₁=CH₂CH₂NHAc, R₂=CH₃

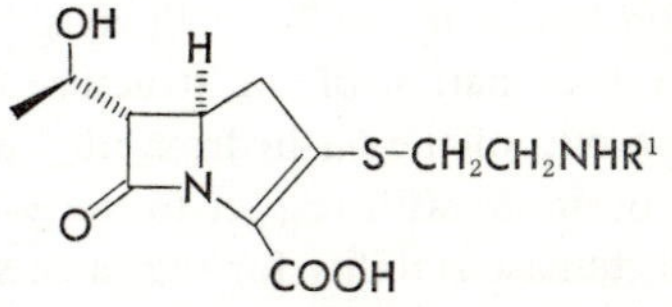

6a, R₁=H
 b, R₁=Ac

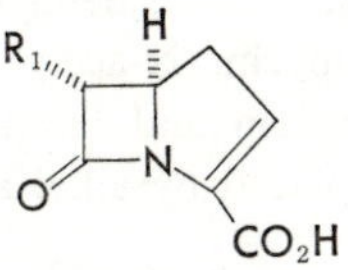

7a, R₁=H

 b, R₁=H

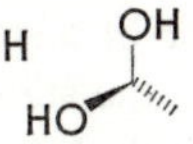

Fig. 2.   Carbazenem antibiotics.

Other structurally related β-lactam antibiotics, the epithienamycins (3b, 3c, 4, 5a, 5b) (*14, 15, 48, 49*), the olivanic acids (3, 4, 5a, 5b) (*5, 6, 17*), PS-5 (5c) (*41*), and PS-6 (5d) (*27*) have been reported recently from other *Streptomyces* species. All are less active than thienamycin (6a).

Introduction of the hydroxyethyl side chain at the C-6(7) position of a penicillin (cephalosporin) (*18*) or of a cysteamine side chain at position 3 of a cephalosporin (*7*) did not increase the activity of these nuclei. It appeared, therefore, that the nucleus of thienamycin, 1-carba-2-penem-3-carboxylic acid (7a), may be primarily responsible for the high antibiotic activity of thienamycin.

Synthesis of compound 7a (*9*) confirmed these expectations. Compound 7a has antibiotic activity comparable to ampicillin. This result should be compared with the penicillin or cephalosporin nuclei which have almost no antibacterial activity (54). The nucleus of thienamycin contributes a major factor toward the remarkable activity of thienamycin; however, compound 7a is susceptible to β-lactamases as shown by its low activity against penicillinase-producing strains.

Synthesis of the nucleus with an α (R) hydroxyethyl side chain (7b) (9, 44) gives a compound which has activity comparable to that of the parent thienamycin against both gram-positive organisms and the Enterobacteriaceae gram-negative organisms including β-lactamase producers. Against *Pseudomonas* species it is about one-third as active, though it has activity against carbenicillin-resistant strains. Thus, the 6α-(R)-hydroxyethyl side chain appears to confer the stability to the β-lactamases in a fashion similar to the 7α-methoxy side chain of the cephamycins.

An examination of the structure of thienamycin and cefoxitin shows that the methyl group of the 6α-hydroxyethyl and the methyl of the 7α-methoxy occupying similar positions with respect to the β-lactam carbonyl are probably responsible for the β-lactamase stability for the same steric reasons, the high activity of the thienamycin nucleus counteracts any steric inhibition of activity induced by the hydroxyethyl side chain. The hydroxy group of the side chain is probably involved in binding of the molecule on the active site as seen from the lower activity of compound 5a compared to compound 6b which differs only in the stereochemistry of the hydroxy group on the side chain (14).

The amino group of the cysteamine side chain is also responsible for the antipseudomonal activity of thienamycin. N-acetyl thienamycin (6b) lacks the antipseudomonal activity of thienamycin and has a lower overall potency (14). The cysteamine side chain can be replaced by alkyl and aryl side chains with retention of good activity (10).

However promising the potency, breadth of spectrum and β-lactamase stability of thienamycin appeared, it was evident from the outset that the antibiotic could only be regarded as a lead because of a stability problem. At dilute concentrations, thienamycin appeared to approach the stability of some of the penicillin family (31). As concentrations increased, stability decreased rapidly. Because of the lack of oral absorption, concentrations of antibiotics suitable for parenteral administration were deemed too unstable. Accordingly, a search for a thienamycin analog which was equivalent biologically, but stable at high concentrations, was immediately launched. While an empirical drug derivatization program might well lead to such an entity,

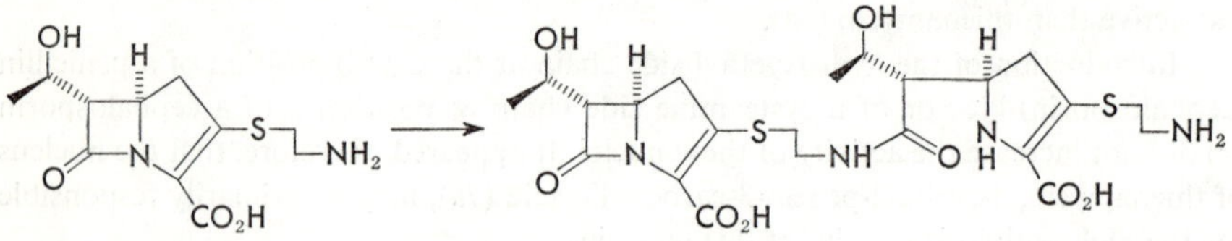

FIG. 3. Intermolecular dimerization of thienamycin.

a basic understanding of the mode of decomposition could well lead to a more rational design. Two observations seemed quite important in the understanding of this problem: the isolation of a degradation product with a net negative charge upon decomposition and the decline of twice the rate of loss of hydroxylamine extinguishable UV absorbance. These findings were suggestive that a bimolecular reaction leading to a dimer (8) was occurring. Simultaneous with these findings was the evolving understanding of a structure-activity relationship of thienamycin derivatives devised as a result of an intensive empirical analog program. It became apparent that what was needed was to convert the amine of the cysteamine side chain into a nonnucleophilic basic function.

Amidines possess both properties. They would appear to be relatively nonnucleophilic and they are also even more basic than amines. Although many amidines were prepared, the parent N-formimidoylthienamycin (36) appeared to possess the highest antibacterial activity. Indeed (Table VI), it is even more active than the parent antibiotic, and more importantly, shows an enhanced high concentration stability.

Finally, the solid state stability of the crystalline product suggests an acceptable shelf-life for a commercial drug. Accordingly, N-formidoylthienamycin was selected for clinical trial and given the code designation MK-0787.

TABLE VI.   Antibacterial Activity of Thienamycin and MK-0787

Compound	MIC (μg/ml)/ED$_{50}$ mg/kg/dose (s.c.)			
	S. aureus 2985	*E. coli* 2891	*K. pneumoniae* 2888	*E. cloacae* 2646
MK-0787	0.01/0.06	0.2/0.65	0.64/0.64	0.64/0.65
Thienamycin	0.02/0.26	0.4/1.6	1.3/1.6	0.64/4.9

Compound	MIC (μg/ml)/ED$_{50}$ mg/kg/dose (s.c.)			
	P. morganii 2883	*S. marcescens* 2548	*P. aeruginosa* 40	*B. fragilis* 3286
MK-0787	3.1/0.94	0.8/3.8	1.6/0.74	3.1/0.95
Thienamycin	3.1/6.25	1.6/11.7	3.1/1.56	12.5/4.65

MK-0787

It can be seen from Table VI that MK-0787 is remarkably potent, especially against pseudomonads. In contrast to most β-lactam antibiotics having good anti-pseudomonas activity, MK-0787 is exceptionally active against gram-positive strains including *Enterococci*. This consistency of potency occurs across a broad spectrum of bacteria *in vivo* as well. Combined with its β-lactamase stability and bactericidal nature, MK-0787 has become the standard against which all antibiotics must be measured.

REFERENCES

1. Albers-Schonberg, G., Arison, B. H., Hensens, O. D., Hirshfield, J., Hoogsteen, K., Kaczka, E., Rhodes, R. E., Kahan, J. S., Kahan, F. M., Ratcliffe, R. W., Walton, E., Ruswinkle, L. J., Morin, R. B., and Christensen, B. G. 1978. *J. Am. Chem. Soc.*, **100**, 6491–6499.
2. Applegate, H. E., Dolfini, J. E., Puar, M. S., Slusarchyk, W. A., Toeplitz, B., and Gougoutas, J. Z. 1974. *J. Org. Chem.*, **39**, 2794–2796.
3. Bohme, E. H. W., Applegate, H. E., Ewing, J. B., Funke, P. T., Puar, M. S., and Dolfini, J. E. 1973. *J. Org. Chem.*, **38**, 230–236.
4. Bohme, E. H. W., Applegate, H. E., Toeplitz, B., Dolfini, J. E., and Gougoutas, J. Z. 1971. *J. Am. Chem. Soc.*, **93**, 4324–4326.
5. Brown, A. G., Corbett, D. F., Eglington, J. A., and Howarth, T. T. 1979. *J. Antibioti.*, **32**, 961–963.
6. Brown, A. G., Corbett, D. F., Eglington, A. J., and Howarth, T. T. 1977. *J. Chem. Soc. Chem. Commun.*, 523–525.
7. Cama, L. D. Unpublished results, Merck Sharp & Dohme Research Laboratories, Rahway, New Jersey.
8. Cama, L. D. and Christensen, B. G. 1974. *J. Am. Chem. Soc.*, **96**, 7582–7584.
9. Cama, L. D. and Christensen, B. G. 1978. *J. Am. Chem. Soc.*, **100**, 8006–8007.
10. Cama, L. D. and Christensen, B. G. Manuscripts submitted for publication.
11. Cama, L. D., Firestone, R. A., and Christensen, B. G. 1976. Abstr. 10th ACS Middle Atlantic Regional Meeting, Philadelphia, Pa.
12. Cama, L. D., Leanza, W. J., Beattie, T. R., and Christensen, B. G. 1972. *J. Am. Chem. Soc.*, **94**, 1408–1410.
13. Campbell, M. M. and Johnson, G. 1974. *J. Chem. Soc. Chem. Commun.*, 479–480.
14. Cassidy, P. J., Albers-Schonberg, G., Goegelman, R. T., Arison, B., Stapley, E. O., and Birnbaum, J. *J. Antibiot.*, in preparation.
15. Cassidy, P. J., Goegelman, R., Miller, T. W., Arison, B., Albers-Schonberg, G., Zimmerman, S. B., and Birnbaum, J. 1977. Abstr. 17th Intersci. Conf. Antimicrob. Agents Chemother., No. 81.
16. Chauvette, R. R., Flynn, E. H., Jackson, B. G., Lavagnino, E. R., Morin, R. B., Mueller, R. A., Pioch, R. P., Roeske, R. W., Ryan, C. W., Spencer, J. L., and Van Heyningen, E. 1962. *J. Am. Chem. Soc.*, **84**, 3401–3402.

17. Corbett, D. F., Eglington, A. J., and Howarth, T. T. 1977. *J. Chem. Soc. Chem. Commun.*, 953–954.

18. DiNinno, F., Beattie, T. R., and Christensen, B. G. 1977. *J. Org. Chem.*, **42**, 2960–2965.

19. Doyle, T. W., Conway, T. T., Lim, G., and Luh, B.-Y. 1979. *Can. J. Chem.*, 227–232.

20. Finklestein, J., Holden, K. G., and Perchonock, C. D. 1978. *Tetrahedron Lett.*, 1629–2632.

21. Firestone, R. A., Maciejewicz, N. S., Ratcliffe, R. W., and Christensen, B. G. 1974. *J. Org. Chem.*, **39**, 437–440.

22. Firestone, R. A., Schelechow, N., Johnston, D. B. R., and Christensen, B. G. 1972. *Tetrahedron Lett.*, 375–378.

23. Harper, P. B., Kirby, S. M., O'Callaghan, C. H. 1979. Abstr. 11th Int. Congress of Chemother, and 19th Intersci. Conf. Antimicrob. Agents Chemother., No. 559.

24. Hashimoto, M., Komori, T., and Kamiya, T. 1976. *J. Antibiot.*, **29**, 890–901.

25. Heusler, K. 1972. *In* "Cephalosporins and Penicillins," ed. by E. H. Flynn, Academic Press, New York, pp. 270–279.

26. Howarth, T. J., Brown, A. G., and Kind, T. J. 1974. *J. Chem. Soc. Chem. Commun.*, 266–271.

27. Japanese Patent JA-160424. Sanraku Ocean Co.

28. Jeffery, J. D'A., Abraham, E. P., and Newton, G. G. F. 1961. *Biochem. J.*, **81**, 591–596.

29. Jen, T., Frazee, J., Hoover, J. R. E. 1973. *J. Org. Chem.*, **38**, 2857–2859.

30. Johnston, D. B. R., Schmitt, S. M., Firestone, R. A., and Christensen, B. G. 1972. *Tetrahedron Lett.*, 4917–4920.

31. Kahan, J. S., Kahan, F. M., Goegelman, R., Currie, S. A., Jackson, M., Stapley, E. O., Miller, T. W., Miller, A. K., Hendling, D., Mochales, G., Hernandez, S., Woodruff, H. B., and Birnbaum, J. 1979. *J. Antibiot.*, **32**, 1–12.

32. Karady, S., Pines, S. H., Weinstock, L. M., Roberts, F. E., Brenner, G. S., Hoinowski, A. M., Cheng, T. Y., and Sletzinger, M. 1972. *J. Am. Chem. Soc.*, **94**, 1410–1411.

33. Koppel, G. A. and Koehler, R. E. 1973. *Tetrahedron Lett.*, 1943–1946.

34. Koppel, G. A. and Koehler, R. E. 1973. *J. Am. Chem. Soc.*, **95**, 2403–2404.

35. Kropp, H., Sundelof, J. G., Kahan, J. S., Kahan, F. M., and Birnbaum, J. Submitted for publication.

36. Leanza, W. J., Wildonger, K. J., Miller, T. W., and Christensen, B. G. 1979. *J. Med. Chem.*, **22**, 1435–1436.

37. Lowe, G. 1975. *Chem. Ind.*, 459–464.

38. Nagarajan, R., Boeck, L. D., Gorman, M., Hamill, R. L., Higgins, C. E., Hoehn, M. M., Stark, W. M., and Whitney, J. G. 1971. *J. Am. Chem. Soc.*, **93**, 2308–2310.

39. Narisada, M., Yoshida, T., Ononi, H., Ohtani, M., Okoda, T., Tsuji, T., Kik-

kowa, I., Hoga, N., Satoh, H., Itoni, H., and Nagata, W. 1979. *J. Med. Chem.*, **22**, 757–759.

40. Neu, H. C., Aswapokee, N., Fu, K. P., and Aswapokee, P. 1979. *Antimicrob. Agents Chemother.*, **16**, 141–149.
41. Okamura, K., Hirata, S., Okamura, Y., Fukagawa, Y., Shimauchi, Y. Kouno, K., Ishikura, T., and Leiu, J. 1978. *J. Antibiot.*, **31**, 480–482.
42. Rasmusson, G. H., Reynolds, G. F., and Arth, G. E. 1973. *Tetrahedron Lett.*, 145–148.
43. Ratcliffe, R. W. and Christensen, B. G. 1973. *Tetrahedron Lett.*, 4645–4656.
44. Shih, D. H., Hannah, J., and Christensen, B. G. 1978. *J. Am. Chem. Soc.*, **100**, 8004–8006.
45. Slusarchyk, W. A., Applegate, H. E., Funke, P., Koster, W., Puar, M. S., Young, M., and Dolfini, J. E. 1973. *J. Org. Chem.*, **38**, 943–950.
46. Spitzer, W. A. and Goodson, T. 1973. *Tetrahedron Lett.*, 273–276.
47. Spitzer, W. A., Goodson, T., Jr., Chaney, M. O., and Jones, N. D. 1974. *Tetrahedron Lett.*, 4311–4314.
48. Stapley, E. O., Cassidy, P., Currie, S. A., Daoust, D., Goegelman, R., Hernandez, S., Jackson, M., Mata, J. M., Miller, A. K., Monaghan, R. L., Tunac, J. B., Zimmerman, S. B., and Hendlin, D. 1977. Abstr. 17th Intersci. Conf. Antimicrob. Agents Chemother., No. 80.
49. Stapley, E. O., Cassidy, P. J., Zimmerman, S. B., Tunac, J., Monaghan, R. L., Jackson, M., Hernandez., S., Mata, J. M., Currie, S. A., Daoust, D., and Hendlin, G. *J. Antibot.*, in preparation.
50. Stapley, E. O., Daoust, D. R., Hendlin, D., Miller, A. K., Zimmerman, S. B., Birnbaum, J., Cama, L. D., and Christensen, B. G. 1979. In "Microbial Drug Resistance," ed. by S. Mitsuhashi, Japan Sci. Soc. Press, Tokyo/Univ. Park Press, Baltimore, Vol. II, pp. 405–417.
51. Stapley, E. O., Jackson, J., Hernandez, S., Zimmerman, B. S., Currie, S. A., Mochales, S., Mata, J. M., Woodruff, H. B., and Hendlin, D. 1972. *Antimicrob. Agents Chemother.*, **2**, 122–131.
52. Strominger, J. L. and Tipper, D. J. 1965. *Am. J. Med.*, **39**, 708–721.
53. Uri, J. V., Actor, P., Guarini, J. R., Phillips, L., Pitkin, D., Memarinis, R. M., and Weisback, J. A. 1978. *J. Antibiot.*, **31**, 82–91.
54. Walton, E. Unpublished results, Merck Sharp & Dohme Research Laboratories, Rahway, New Jersey.
55. Yanagisawa, H., Fukushima, M., Ando, A., and Nakao, H. 1976. *Tetrahedron Lett.*, 259–262.
56. Yanagisawa, H., Nakao, H., Sadao, I., Nakayama, A. A., Nakazawa, J., Shimizu, B., Kaneko, M., Nagano, M., and Sagawara, S. 1979. *J. Antibiot.*, **32**, 320–329.

5 MODE OF ACTION

FUNCTIONS OF PENICILLIN-BINDING PROTEINS 5 AND 6 OF *ESCHERICHIA COLI*

Hiroshi AMANUMA and Jack L. STROMINGER

*The Biological Laboratories, Harvard University**

In order to elucidate the molecular mechanism by which β-lactam antibiotics exert their lethal effects toward sensitive bacterial cells, much effort has recently been directed to the study of penicillin-binding proteins (PBPs) (*16*). Because of the inherent nature of PBPs, namely the ability to bind β-lactam antibiotics specifically and covalently, these proteins are amenable to extensive biochemical characterization. After binding with radioactively labeled β-lactam antibiotics (usually [^{14}C]-PCG) PBPs can be conveniently detected and identified by SDS-polyacrylamide gel electrophoresis and subsequent fluorography (*2, 14*). Since the covalent linkage between native PBPs and β-lactams is usually reversible in the presence of a nucleophile, such as neutral hydroxylamine (*7, 8*), PBPs can be purified rapidly and efficiently by covalent affinity chromatography utilizing a β-lactam as an affinity ligand (*3*). Using this method a number of PBPs are easily purified to protein homogeneity in mg amounts (*1, 3, 21*).

Each bacterial species so far examined has a distinct number of PBPs in its cytoplasmic membranes. The existence of multiple PBPs in each bacterial species suggests the complexity of the β-lactam antibiotic-sensitive enzyme system which is involved in forming and regulating the crosslinkage of bacterial cell-wall peptidoglycan. Currently the main objectives in the study of PBPs are to demonstrate a biochemical reaction(s) catalyzed by each PBP, to examine a precise mode of interaction of β-lactam antibiotics with PBPs, and to elucidate how each PBP is involved in the metabolism of peptidoglycan *in vivo*.

Some of our recent findings that are related to these problems are briefly described below. For more extensive description on the subject, several review articles are available (*4, 18, 19*).

* Cambridge, Massachusetts 02138, U.S.A.

PURIFICATION AND ENZYME ACTIVITIES OF PBPs 5 AND 6 OF *ESCHERICHIA COLI*

At least seven PBPs are detected in the membranes of *E. coli* K12 (*13*). PBPs of this organism have been by far the most extensively studied. Each of the lower molecular weight PBPs, namely PBP 4 (MW 49,000), PBP 5 (MW 42,000), and PBP 6 (MW 40,000), was shown to catalyze penicillin-sensitive D-alanine carboxypeptidase (CPase) activity *in vitro* toward various natural and synthetic substrates.

Using conventional column chromatography Tamura *et al.* (*17*) purified two protein fractions each showing CPase activity (CPase IA and CPase IB-C). The purified CPase IB-C was found to contain one polypeptide on SDS-polyacrylamide gel electrophoresis. This CPase also catalyzed a penicillin-sensitive endopeptidase activity which hydrolyzes crosslinked bis(disaccharide-tetrapeptide) to form disaccharide-tetrapeptide monomers. Subsequent isolation by two laboratories (*6, 10*) of mutants (*dacB*) which lack the CPase IB-C activity showed that these mutants also have a deletion in PBP 4, indicating that PBP 4 is identical with CPase IB-C. The purified preparation of CPase IA, which catalyzed model transpeptidase activity in addition to CPase, was composed of two polypeptides. Based on the observed properties, such as molecular weight and interactions with penicillin G, these two polypeptides were later identified as PBP 5 and PBP 6 (*15*).

Each of PBPs 5 and 6 has recently been purified to protein homogeneity from *E. coli* strain PA3092 (Fig. 1) (*1*). Purification procedures included three crucial steps, namely selective solubilization of certain PBPs from the membranes, covalent affinity chromatography, and column chromatography on carboxymethyl (CM)-cellulose. Treatment of the membranes with Triton X-100 at relatively low ionic strength (50 mM KP_1 (pH 7.2)) extracted only PBP 1A, 5, and 6, leaving other PBPs in the pellet. The latter PBPs required the presence of 0.5 M NaCl in addition to Triton X-100 for solubilization. Several CPases from different bacteria have been purified very efficiently by covalent affinity chromatography (*3, 5, 21*). These CPases, usually the lowest molecular weight PBP in each bacterium, bind penicillins but do not bind cephalosporins. The higher molecular weight PBPs bind both penicillins and cephalosporins. Thus the affinity chromatography of a crude detergent extract pretreated with an appropriate cephalosporin (such as cephalothin (CET)) on a resin containing 6-aminopenicillanic acid (6APA) as a ligand yields a pure CPase. While a similar method may be useful for purification of a mixture of PBPs 5 and 6 of *E. coli*, it cannot be used for the separation of PBPs 5 and 6 from each other, since PBPs 5 and 6 have very similar properties in their interactions with β-lactam antibiotics (*12*). Instead, it was found that the binding of PBP 5 to a 6APA-resin requires a long spacer group which links 6APA with a matrix (Sepharose), while that of PBP 6 does not. Thus, the Triton extract was first treated with 6APA-CM-Sepharose CL-6B which trapped almost all the PBPs 1A and 6 and a trace amount of PBP 5. The untrapped fraction from this resin, containing PBP 5 as the sole PBP, was then incu-

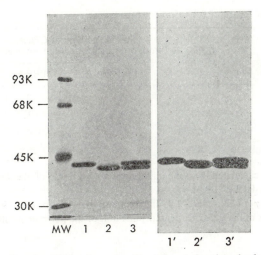

FIG. 1.   SDS-polyacrylamide slab gel showing the homogeneity of the purified PBPs
5 and 6 (1).
Purified PBPs 5 and 6, after binding with [¹⁴C]PCG, were subjected to SDS-gel electrophoresis (13). Coomassie brilliant blue-stained protein profile (lanes 1–3) and fluorography of the same gel (lanes 1′–3′). Lane 1, PBP 5 (1.8 μg); lane 2, PBP 6 (2.1 μg);
lane 3, PBP 5 (1.8 μg) and PBP 6 (2.1 μg); MW, molecular weight markers.

bated with 6APA-succinylamino(2-hydroxy)propyl (SAP)-Sepharose 4B, which bound
PBP 5 effectively. The use of the hydrophilic spacer, SAP, significantly reduced the
nonspecific binding of contaminant proteins to the affinity resin. The hydroxylamine
eluate from 6APA-SAP-Sepharose contained almost pure PBP 5. A trace amount
of contaminant proteins could be removed by a column of DEAE-cellulose. The
hydroxylamine eluate from 6APA-CM-Sepharose contained PBPs 1A and 5 in addition to PBP 6. PBP 1A was removed by a column of DEAE-cellulose from which
PBPs 6 and 5 were recovered in the flowthrough. PBP 6 was separated from PBP 5
by a column of CM-cellulose using an elution with a shallow linear gradient of Na
acetate buffer (pH 5.2). From 170 g wet weight of cells, 1.0 mg of PBP 5 and 0.37
mg of PBP 6 were obtained, reflecting the relative ratio of these proteins in the membranes (12).
    The fact that PBP 5 is separable from PBP 6 by penicillin affinity chromatog-
raphy and by CM-cellulose chromatography suggests that these two PBPs do not
form a specific protein-protein complex in mild detergent solution. Their similarity
as polypeptides would account for the previous co-purification of these PBPs as
CPase IA after several column chromatographic steps (17). Peptide mapping of the
two PBPs by one-dimensional SDS-polyacrylamide gel electrophoresis after partial
digestion with proteases and cyanogen bromide, however, established that these two
PBPs are distinct polypeptides (1).

TABLE I. Specific Activities of CPase of PBPs 5 and 6 (1)

Substrate	Conc. (μM)	Specific activity of CPase (pmol product formed/min/μg protein)	
		PBP 5	PBP 6
UDP-MurNAc-pentapeptide[a]	24	95	22
Diacetyl-L-Lys-D-Ala-D-Ala	14	4. 4	1. 7
Diacetyl-L-Lys-D-Ala-D-lactate	22	92	156
Linear, uncross linked peptidoglkcan	19[b]	72	26

Specific activities of CPase were calculated from the initial rates of hydrolysis of the various substrates at 37°C in 50 mM Tris-HCl (pH 8.6).
[a] UDP-N-acetylmuramyl-L-Ala-γ-D-Glu-meso-2,6-diaminopimelyl-D-Ala-D-Ala. [b] The value indicates the concentration of disaccharide-pentapeptide unit of the polymer substrate.

Several enzyme activities were examined using purified PBPs 5 and 6 (1). Both PBPs were found to catalyze a CPase activity independently toward various natural and synthetic substrates including linear, uncrosslinked peptidoglycan (20) which was prepared from the culture medium of *Bacillus subtilis* cells grown in the presence of a sublethal concentration of PCG. For most substrates PBP 5 showed 3-to 4-fold higher specific activities than PBP 6 (Table I). Both PBPs also catalyzed a model transpeptidase activity using diacetyl-L-Lys-D-Ala-D-Ala-or diacetyl-L-Lys-D-Ala-D-lactate as a donor and glycine as an acceptor. No evidence, however, was obtained which indicated the formation of crosslinkage between adjacent peptide side chains when these PBPs were incubated with linear, uncrosslinked peptidoglycan. CPase activities of the two PBPs had broad pH optima (pH 8.5–10) and were similarly inhibited by MgCl$_2$. Almost stoichiometric binding of [^{14}C]PCG was attained with each PBP at saturation, and the bound [^{14}C]PCG was spontaneously released from the PBPs as reported previously (12).

More recently the same method was employed for the purification of PBPs 5 and 6 from a strain containing the *dacA* mutation (*E. coli* JE 11191) (H. Amanuma and J. L. Strominger, manuscript in preparation). Matsuhashi *et al.* (9) previously isolated a mutant (*dacA*) which lacked the activity of CPase IA when assayed using a crude detergent extract of the membranes. This mutant contained both PBPs 5 and 6 which are active in binding PCG. Subsequently the *dacA* mutation was genetically correlated with the loss of PCG-releasing activity of PBP 5 (11). With regard to the interactions with PCG PBP 6 of this mutant seemed to be normal. PBP 6 was purified to protein homogeneity. It showed the same degree of CPase activity as wild-type PBP 6. The purified PBP 5 bound an almost stoichiometric amount of PCG but did not release it spontaneously. Hydroxylamine, on the other hand, could cause the release of bound PCG. No CPase activities were detected with the purified PBP 5 using various substrates. Thus it is clear that the *dacA* mutant cells still contain an intact PBP 6. The failure to detect any CPase IA activity in *dacA* cells using crude detergent extract might have been due to the fact (*1*) that the CPase activity catalyzed by PBP 6 is responsible for 7–11% of the total CPase IA activity in wild type cells. Neither the *dacB* or *dacA* mutation seemed to cause any growth defect under various conditions (*6, 9, 10*). Moreover, a double mutant containing both *dacA* and *dacB* was reported to grow normally (*9*). So far no conclusive evidence has been obtained on whether the CPase activity in any bacterium is indispensable for cell growth. These CPases might function in regulating the degree of crosslinkage of the peptidoglycan, as suggested by the finding that PBPs 5 and 6 catalyze the CPase activity toward linear, uncrosslinked peptidoglycan, and might constitute a lethal target for β-lactam antibiotics. Isolation of a mutant having a defective PBP 6 would resolve this problem.

Acknowledgments
We are most grateful to Dr. T. A. O'Brien for useful comments on the manuscript. The research done by the authors was supported by a Research Grant from the National Institutes of Health (AI-09152).

REFERENCES

1. Amanuma, H. and Strominger, J. L. 1980. *J. Biol. Chem.*, **255**, 11173–11180.
2. Blumberg, P. M. and Strominger, J. L. 1972. *J. Biol. Chem.*, **247**, 8107–8113.
3. Blumberg, P. M. and Strominger, J. L. 1972. *Proc. Natl. Acad. Sci. U.S.A.*, **69**, 3751–3755.
4. Blumberg, P. M. and Strominger, J. L. 1974. *Bacteriol. Rev.*, **38**, 291–335.
5. Chase, H. A., Shepherd, S. T., and Reynolds, P. E. 1977. *FEBS Lett.*, **76**, 199–203.
6. Iwaya, M. and Strominger, J. L. 1977. *Proc. Natl. Acad. Sci. U.S.A.*, **74**, 2980–2984.
7. Kozarich, J. W., Nishino, T., Willoughby, E., and Strominger, J. L. 1977. *J. Biol. Chem.*, **252**, 7525–7529.
8. Lawrence, P. J. and Strominger, J. L. 1970. *J. Biol. Chem.*, **245**, 3660–3666.
9. Matsuhashi, M., Maruyama, I. N., Takagaki, Y., Tamaki, S., Nishimura, Y., and Hirota, Y. 1978. *Proc. Natl. Acad. Sci. U.S.A.*, **75**, 2631–2635.
10. Matsuhashi, M., Takagaki, Y., Maruyama, I. N., Tamaki, S., Nishimura, Y., Suzuki, H., Ogino, U., and Hirota, Y. 1977. *Proc. Natl. Acad. Sci. U.S.A.*, **74**, 2976–2979.
11. Matsuhashi, M., Tamaki, S., Curtis, S. J., and Strominger, J. L. 1979. *J. Bacteriol.*, **137**, 644–647.
12. Spratt, B. G. 1977. *Eur. J. Biochem.*, **72**, 341–352.
13. Spratt, B. G., Jobanputra, V., and Schwarz, U. 1977. *FEBS Lett.*, **79**, 374–378.
14. Spratt, B. G. and Pardee, A. B. 1975. *Nature*, **254**, 516–517.
15. Spratt, B. G. and Strominger, J. L. 1976. *J. Bacteriol.*, **127**, 660–663.

16. Suginaka, H., Blumberg, P. M., and Strominger, J. L. 1972. *J. Biol. Chem.*, **247**, 5279–5288.
17. Tamura, T., Imae, Y., and Strominger, J. L. 1976. *J. Biol. Chem.*, **251**, 414–423.
18. Waxman, D. J. and Strominger, J. L. 1981. *In* "β-Lactam Antibiotics: Chemistry and Biology," ed. by M. Gorman and R. B. Morin, Academic Press, New York, Vol. I, in press.
19. Waxman, D. J., Yocum, R. R., and Strominger, J. L. 1980. *Phil. Trans. Roy. Soc. Lond. B*, **289**, 257–271.
20. Waxman, D. J., Yu, W., and Strominger, J. L. 1980. *J. Biol. Chem.*, **255**, 11577–11587.
21. Yocum, R. R., Rasmussen, J. R., and Strominger, J. L. 1980. *J. Biol. Chem.*, **255**, 3977–3986.

MECHANISTIC PROPERTIES AND FUNCTIONING
OF DD-CARBOXYPEPTIDASES

J. M. Ghuysen,[*1] J. M. Frère,[*1] M. Leyh-Bouille,[*1] J. Coyette,[*1] C. Duez,[*1] B. Joris,[*1] J. Dusart,[*1] M. Nguysen-Distèche,[*1] O. Dideberg,[*2] P. Charlier,[*2] J. R. Knox,[*3] J. A. Kelly,[*3] P. C. Moews,[*3] and M. L. DeLucia[*3]

*Service de Microbiologie, Faculté de Médecine, Institut de Chimie[*1] and Service de Christallographie, Faculté des Sciences, Institut de Physique[*2], Université de Liege, and Biological Sciences Group, University of Connecticut[*3]*

The bacterial target of β-lactam antibiotics consists of a set of multiple receptors which are localized within the plasma membrane. Fluorography of polyacrylamide gel electrophoreses in SDS of membranes radioactively labeled by reaction with [^{14}C]benzylpenicillin permits detection of the receptors, or at least some of them, as penicillin binding proteins (52). Their apparent molecular weights range between 25 and 140 Kdaltons. Some of these proteins have been characterized as penicillin-sensitive enzymes; they are DD-carboxypeptidases, transpeptidases, and endopeptidases. The affinities of the β-lactam antibiotics for their receptors vary widely depending upon the protein or the enzyme under consideration, the organism, and the nature of the β-lactam compound. Wide variations also occur with respect to the number of copies (from 20 to several thousands) of penicillin-binding proteins present in one given bacterial cell.

Obtaining DD-carboxypeptidases in a truly water-soluble form and devising peptides with substrate activities for these isolated enzymes are all the more important for a detailed understanding of the functioning of these penicillin receptors.

Assays have been developed that employ synthetic and/or natural peptides functioning directly as donors and, for transpeptidation reactions, as amino acceptors of the DD-carboxypeptidases (33). In addition, truly water-soluble DD-carboxypeptidases can be obtained in a number of ways. For example, the 43-Kdalton DD-carboxypeptidase 4 of various gram-negative bacteria is solubilized by treating the cells with a Ribi fractionator or by submitting the isolated membranes to hypertonic conditions (53). Conversion of the cells of various *Streptomyces* strains into protoplasts is accompanied by the release of a water-soluble 40-Kdalton DD-car-

[*1,*2] B-4000 Start Tilman, Liège, Belgium.
[*3] Storrs, Connecticut 06268, U.S.A.

boxypeptidase (43). Removal by trypsin action of a 2–3-Kdalton fragment from the C-terminal of membrane-bound DD-carboxypeptidases of *Bacilli* yields slightly shortened and water-soluble enzymes (56). Similarly, the membrane-bound, 43-K dalton DD-carboxypeptidase of *S. faecalis* is converted under trypsin action into a water-soluble 30-Kdalton protein (6). Although one third of the original molecule is eliminated, this 30-Kdalton protein still functions perfectly as a DD-carboxypeptidase and penicillin-binding protein. During incubation of the isolated membranes of *S. faecalis* at 37°C and at alkaline pH, the 80-Kdalton penicillin-binding protein (of unknown enzyme activity) undergoes rapid and quantitative conversion (probably as a result of some endogenous proteolytic activity) into a water-soluble 73-Kdalton penicillin binding protein (6). Finally, various strains of *Actinomycetes* have the property, apparently unique, to excrete DD-carboxypeptidases in the external medium during growth. The release mechanism is under study. These organisms have been widely used as sources of water-soluble DD-carboxypeptidases. The R61 enzyme (from *Streptomyces* R61) (24), the G enzyme (from *S. albus* G) (14), and the R39 enzyme (from *Actinomadura* R39) (30) have been purified to protein homogeneity. Both the R61 (41) and G enzymes (12) have been crystallized.

In this paper, the current state of our knowledge of the mechanistic properties and functioning of the enzyme active centers of the DD-carboxypeptidases is presented.

THE REACTIONS CATALYZED

The DD-carboxypeptidases are involved in the last stages of wall peptidoglycan synthesis. Like the proteases, they catalyze the opening of amide bonds and transfer the carbonyl carbon to an exogenous nucleophile (HY):

$$\begin{array}{cc} O & O \\ \| & \| \\ -C-N< + HY \rightarrow -C-Y + HN< . \end{array}$$

The DD-carboxypeptidases are specifically designed to operate on the amide bond of the D-Ala-D-Ala dipeptide of L-R-D-Ala-D-Ala terminated peptides (where R is most often a diamino acid residue). In addition, β-lactam antibiotics are also used in a manner analogous to the natural carbonyl donors. The endocyclic amide bond is exposed on the α face of the β-lactam antibiotics in a position roughly equivalent to that of the amide bond of D-Ala-D-Ala (Fig. 1).

Depending on the nucleophile that serves as acceptor of the L-R-D-alanyl moiety, the enzymes function as hydrolases (HY=H$_2$O) or transpeptidases (HY=a suitable amino compound). Hydrolysis and transpeptidation may occur concomitantly; they compete with each other and the channelling of the enzyme activity in either pathway depends on the microenvironmental conditions (25, 38).

The enzyme requirements for a D-amino acid residue at the C-terminal position of the peptide substrates are not strictly restricted to D-alanine, which can be replaced at this position by other D-amino acids or Gly, although most often at the expense

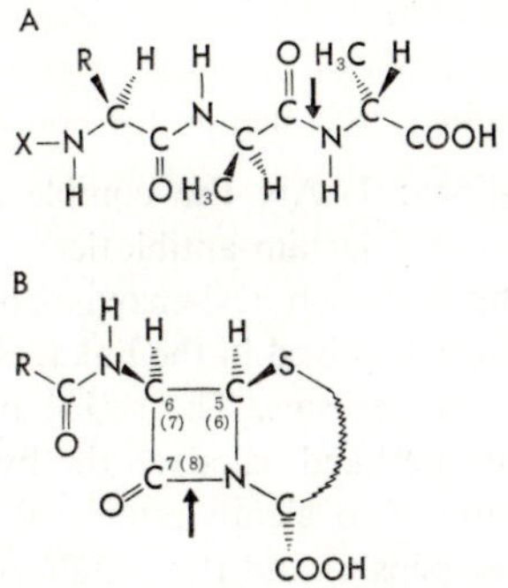

FIG. 1.   Amide bonds (arrows) attacked by the DD-carboxypeptidases.
A: L-R-D-Ala-D-Ala terminated peptides. The N-terminal amino group is substituted
by X.   B: β-lactam antibiotics. The carbon atoms in the β-lactam ring are num-
bered 5, 6, 7 in the penicillins and (6), (7), (8) in the $\varDelta^3$-cephalosporins.

of substrate activity. The DD-carboxypeptidases vary widely in this respect. Some of
them have a high propensity to hydrolyze D-Ala-D-X linkages where the D-center of
the C-terminal X residue is substituted by very bulky groups (44), as for example,
the D-Ala-(D)-*meso*-diaminopimelic interpeptide linkages which in the peptidoglycans
of many gram-negative bacteria occur in the α-position to a free carboxyl group.
Such enzymes may function as powerful endopeptidases.

The general equation of the reaction for both L-R-D-Ala-D-Ala terminated
peptides and β-lactam antibiotics is:

$$E+C \underset{}{\overset{K}{\rightleftharpoons}} E.C \overset{k_3}{\longrightarrow} E\text{-}C^* \underset{(+HY)}{\overset{k_4}{\longrightarrow}} E+Ps$$

where E=enzyme; C=carbonyl donor; E. C=first stoichiometric complex; E-C*=
modified complex; Ps=reaction products; K=dissociation constant of complex
E.C; and k_3 and k_4=first-order rate constants. The interaction between enzyme,
peptide, and β-lactam drug is a competition between substrates (22, 23). However,
while k_4 is high with the L-R-D-Ala-D-Ala terminated peptides (high turnover numbers), it is very low with the β-lactam antibiotics. β-Lactam drugs are suicide substrates, which explains their potency as enzyme inactivators. Although somewhat
arbitrarily, a good β-lactam inactivator of a given enzyme should have a k_3/K value
of 1,000 M^{-1} sec^{-1} or more, and a k_4 value of 1×10^{-4} sec^{-1} or less. Under these conditions, at a β-lactam drug concentration smaller than the dissociation constant K,
99% of the enzyme is inactivated in the steady state and the time required for the
reaction to reach 95% of the steady state is about 5 min (36).

MECHANISTIC PROPERTIES

Central to the problem are the following questions: 1) Are the complexes E-C* formed with L-R-D-Ala-D-Ala terminated peptides or β-lactam antibiotics covalently bound to acyl-enzyme intermediates? 2) Assuming that such acyl-enzyme complexes are formed, what are the enzyme amino acid residues involved in the linkages?

Proteases operate by at least four different mechanisms. The serine proteases (trypsin) and the thiol proteases (papain), on the one hand, catalyze the hydrolysis of sensitive amide bonds *via* the transitory formation of covalently ester or thiolester-linked acyl-enzyme complexes, The acid proteases (pepsin) and the metalloproteases (carboxypeptidase A), on the other hand, are thought not to form acyl-enzyme complexes. Recent progress has established that the DD-carboxypeptidases also fall into several classes depending upon their distinctive mechanistic properties.

1. The Serine R61 DD-Carboxypeptidase

The water-soluble, 38-K dalton R61 enzyme has been crystallized (Fig. 2) (*41*). X-ray diffraction photographs of well-formed octahedral crystals show orthorhombic 222 Laue symmetry. The unit cell dimensions are: $a=51.1$ Å, $b=67.4$ Å, and $c=102.9$ Å. The space group is $P2_12_12_1$. With four molecules of molecular weight 38,000,

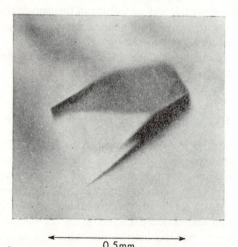

◄————————————► 0.5mm

FIG. 2.   Orthorhombic crystal of the R61 serine DD-carboxypeptidase.
The enzyme was crystallized from polyethylene glycol (MW 6,000–7,500) solution at pH 7.6. Well-formed octahedral crystals developed from a solution containing 14 g of polyethylene glycol per 100 ml of 0.05 M imidazole-HCl buffer. The final protein concentration was 13.3 mg/ml. After centrifugation, the protein solution was slowly concentrated over a reservoir of 28% polyethylene glycol solution by vapor diffusion at 10°C.

Origin   y

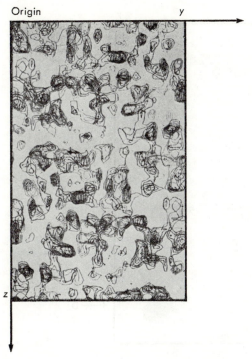

z

FIG. 3. Fourier map of the native R61 enzyme at 5-Å resolution phased by uranyl derivative.
The x-axis is perpendicular to the plane of the figure. One-sixth of the sections of the x-axis is included in the figure.

the $Å^3$/dalton ratio for the cell is 2.33. Data have been collected to 5-Å resolution for both the native crystal and a very isomorphous uranyl derivative ($K_3UO_2F_5$). Figure 3 shows a portion of the Fourier map of the native enzyme, phased by the uranyl derivative (figure of merit, 0.70). The radius of gyration of the native enzyme, as measured by small angle X-ray scattering, is 20.8 ± 0.5 Å (in 10 mM phosphate buffer, pH 7.8, and for a protein concentration of 16 mg/ml). Assuming that the molecule is spherical, this value corresponds to a molecular diameter of 52 Å, a value close to that for the crystallographic a unit cell dimension.

The characterization of the R61 enzyme as a serine DD-carboxypeptidase has been established by various procedures carried out on both β-lactam antibiotics and L-R-D-Ala-D-Ala-terminated peptides. Because of the very low k_4 value of the reaction, the complexes E-C* formed with various β-lactam antibiotics are stable enough to be easily isolated (29). NMR studies of complex E-C* formed with benzylpenicillin showed that the penicilloyl moiety is covalently bound in the denatured complex, with the penicilloyl group able to epimerize while still attached to the protein (9).

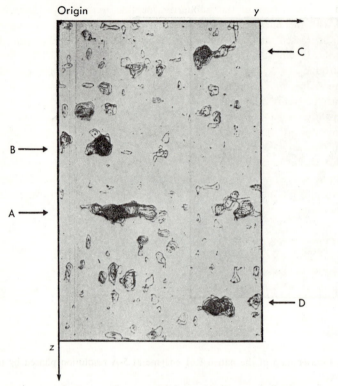

Fig. 4.   Native R61 enzyme—*ortho*-iodo-phenyl penicillin difference map.
The *x*-axis is perpendicular to the plane of the figure. One-third of the sections of the *x*-axis is included in the figure. Peaks A and B: see text. The two peaks C and D on the right of the figure are symmetry equivalents of the two peaks on the left. This second set of peaks is centered on an *x*-level just above those sections included in the photograph.

Degradation of complex E-C* formed with [^{14}C]benzylpenicillin generated a tripeptide, Val-Gly-Ser, with the radioactive penicilloyl group ester-linked to the serine residue (*18*). The β-lactam *ortho*-iodo-phenylpenicillin was successfully diffused into a native crystal, and the difference Fourier map at 5-Å resolution was calculated (*10*). In Fig. 4, the site of interaction is well visualized as the 22-Å segment of difference density elongated in the *y* direction of the map (peak A). Also observed in Fig. 4 is a peak at similar *x* and *y* coordinates but at a lower *z* coordinate. This peak B is probably associated with a conformational change induced in the native structure upon interaction with this penicillin.

The isolation and characterization of complex E-C* from L-R-D-Ala-D-Ala-terminated peptides was made possible by using as a substrate the depsipeptide Ac$_2$-

L-Lys-D-Ala-D-lactate instead of the standard tripeptide Ac$_2$-L-Lys-D-Ala-D-Ala. As first observed with the *Bacilli* DD-carboxypeptidases, the k_3 term of the reaction is then markedly increased and becomes higher than the k_4 term so that complex E-C* accumulates (51). On this basis, the reaction with the R61 enzyme was shown by Yocum and Strominger (59) to proceed through an acyl-enzyme complex. In addition, the Ac$_2$-L-Lys-D-alanyl and penicilloyl moieties were shown to be covalently bound to the same enzyme serine residue (59).

The effects of serine-containing active site directed reagents were studied. Phenylmethanesulfonyl fluoride had no effect on the enzyme activity nor on its ability to bind penicillin (18), but methanesulfonyl fluoride and diisopropylphosphofluoridate inhibited both the enzyme activity on substrate analogs and benzylpenicillin binding with second order rate constants of 0.5 and 1.2 M^{-1} sec^{-1} (32). The inactivation rate with diisopropylphosphofluoridate, however, is considerably smaller than that observed with the serine proteases, suggesting inefficient binding.

2. Serine DD-Carboxypeptidases Other than the R61 Enzyme

With the membrane-bound 40-K dalton DD-carboxypeptidases of *B. subtilis* and *B. stearothermophilus* (which can be converted into water-soluble forms by trypsin action), it has been shown that the Ac$_2$-L-Lys-D-alanyl (from Ac$_2$-L-Lys-D-Ala-D-lactate) and penicilloyl moieties are covalently linked to the same enzyme serine residue (60). The sequences of the NH$_2$-terminal 40 amino acid residues of the two *Bacilli* enzymes are known, and in both cases the active serine occurs at the 36-position (57). By aligning these sequences with those of the serine β-lactamases at the active serine, DD-carboxypeptidases and β-lactamases might exhibit some degree of homology, at least in this region of the molecules.

The water-soluble 57-Kdalton R39 enzyme is another serine DD-carboxypeptidase. When covalently bound to this enzyme, cephaloglycine, cephalexin, and cephalosporin C have their ε_{260} decreased to the same extent as that obtained after β-lactamase action (31) and nitrocefin has a $\varepsilon_{482}/\varepsilon_{386}$ ratio of 2.40, which is also that obtained after β-lactamase action. Moreover, degradation of complex E-C* formed with [^{14}C]benzylpenicillin yielded a heptapeptide Leu-Pro-Ala-Ser-Asn-Gly-Val with the radioactive penicilloyl moiety ester-linked to the serine residue (15).

3. The Metallo G DD-Carboxypeptidase

The water-soluble 18-Kdalton G DD-carboxypeptidase effectively hydrolyzes R-D-Ala-D-Ala terminated peptides with a turnover number one order of magnitude lower than those of the R61 or R39 serine DD-carboxypeptidases (14, 44). However, the G enzyme differs drastically from the latter enzymes in several respects: i) the G enzyme utilizes only H$_2$O as a nucleophile and is unable to catalyze transpeptidation reactions, suggesting that it lacks a structured acceptor site for amino compounds (50); ii) it exhibits high endopeptidase activities (44); and iii) it has a low propensity to react with β-lactam antibiotics, especially with the penicillins. The k_3/K values which govern the formation of complexes E-C* are very low: 9×10^{-3} M^{-1} sec^{-1} for benzylpenicillin and 6×10^{-2} M^{-1} sec^{-1} for cephalosporin C (*19*). For comparison, the corresponding values for the same antibiotics are 14,000 and 1,150 M^{-1} sec^{-1} with the R61 enzyme (*22*) and >90,000 and 67,000 M^{-1} sec^{-1} with the R39 enzyme (*31*). Because of these very low k_3/K values, detection of the G enzyme as a penicillin binding protein requires high [^{14}C]benzylpenicillin concentrations and prolonged periods of incubation. Although low, these k_3/K values are nevertheless 10- to 100-fold higher than those observed with proteins such as lysozyme or insulin (*3*) which are completely devoid of DD-carboxypeptidase activity.

As shown by proton-induced X-ray emission studies, the native G enzyme possesses one Zn^{2+} ion per molecule (*13*). The affinity of the Zn^{2+} ion for the apoprotein expressed by an association constant of about 1×10^{13} M^{-1}, is of the same order of magnitude as for EDTA. The Zn^{2+} cofactor, or its Co^{2+} substitute, is required for activity on Ac$_2$-L-Lys-D-Ala-D-Ala and, apparently, for penicillin binding (high concentrations of EDTA cause a 10-fold decrease in the k_3/K value) (*13*). The Zn^{2+} (Co^{2+}) ligands have not been characterized and the nature of the complexes E-C* formed with the G enzyme is unknown. With the Zn^{2+} β-lactamase II of *B. cereus*, the reaction that this enzyme catalyzes on its substrate, penicillin, probably proceeds through a random mechanism in which the ternary complex enzyme-metal-penicillin may be reached by alternative pathways (*39*). The Zn^{2+} (Co^{2+}) ligands in this β-lactamase II are three histidine residues and the solitary cysteine residue (*39*).

The G enzyme has been crystallized (*12*) (Fig. 5). Precession X-ray photographs of well-formed prismatic crystals show that the crystals belong to the P2$_1$ space group, with unit cell dimensions $a=51.1$ Å, $b=49.7$ Å, $c=38.7$ Å, $\beta=100.6$ Å, and

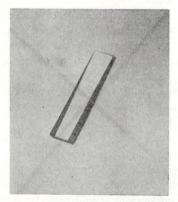

FIG. 5. Crystal of the Zn^{2+} G DD-carboxypeptidase.
The enzyme was crystallized using the vapor diffusion method. Droplets (10 μl) of the enzyme preparation (2% protein, final concentration) in 50 mM Tris-HCl, 5 mM MgCl$_2$, 10 mM NaN$_3$, 6% (w/v) polyethylene glycol 6000 were equilibrated against 12% (w/v) polyethylene glycol solution. The crystals grew in a few weeks, with a prismatic shape, to a maximum size of $1.4 \times 0.6 \times 0.6$ mm^3.

A   B

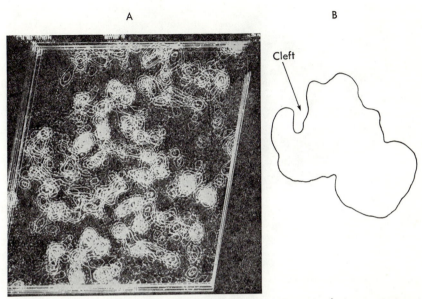

FIG. 6. A: Portion of Fourier map of the native G enzyme at 4.5-Å resolution phased by three heavy atom derivatives. The map is viewed down to the *y*-axis. B: Schematic representation of the molecular envelope as devised from A.

one molecule in the asymmetric unit. Data have been collected to 4.5-Å resolution for the native crystal and three heavy atom derivatives, K_2PtCl_4, $NaUO_2(CH_3COO)_3$, and $K_2Pt(C_2O_4)_2$, respectively (11) (Figs. 6 and 7). The Fourier map of the native enzyme phased by these three derivatives (figure of merit, 0.86) reveals the presence of two enzyme molecules per unit cell, surrounded by a very low electron density region. Each enzyme molecule can be inscribed in a 48 Å × 34 Å × 28 Å ellipsoid, and consists of two globular domains connected by three strands of electron density. The largest domain has a deep cleft (20 Å × 6 Å × 6 Å) in the vicinity of which the map shows a prominent peak, presumed to be the Zn^{2+} ion cofactor.

Crystallographic studies have also permitted the visualization of the enzyme active center (11). The dipeptide Ac-D-Ala-D-Glu (a competitive inhibitor of the hydrolysis of Ac$_2$-L-Lys-D-Ala-D-Ala) and the β-lactam *para*-iodo-7-β-phenylacetyl-aminocephalosporanic acid were successfully diffused in native crystals and the difference Fourier maps calculated at 4.5 Å. The difference Fourier synthesis for the enzyme-dipeptide inhibitor complex gave one peak which was three times higher than any other feature in the map. The site of interaction is well visualized as a 12-Å segment of difference density elongated in the *y* direction of the map, inside the cavity and close to the Zn^{2+} ion site. Although the difference Fourier synthesis for the enzyme-β-lactam complex was much more noisy, the highest peak found

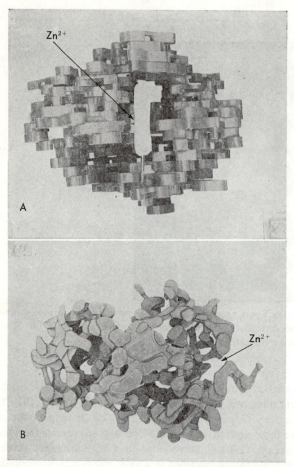

FIG. 7.   A: Model of the G enzyme molecule looking into the cleft of the large domain. Arrow marks the Zn^{2+} ion site.   B: Model of the G enzyme molecule viewed along the y-axis and showing the two domains. Arrow marks the Zn^{2+} ion site. The difference density observed with the peptide inhibitor is represented in white, inside the cleft.

in the map was also located in the same cavity. These data suggest that the enzyme active center, where binding of the dipeptide and the *para*-iodo-cephalosporin inhibitors occurs, is situated in the vicinity of the Zn^{2+} ion site. In agreement with this conclusion, the inhibition of the enzyme activity on Ac_2-L-Lys-D-Ala-D-Ala by 7-aminocephalosporanic acid was found to be competitive, under conditions where inhibition was due exclusively to the formation of the first complex E. C between enzyme and the β-lactam compound (40). Surprisingly, under similar conditions, cephalosporin C behaved as a noncompetitive inhibitor (*19*). The reason why the two β-lactam compounds behave differently is not understood.

4. Other Possible Classes of DD-Carboxypeptidases

The *S. faecalis* membrane-bound 43-Kdalton DD-carboxypeptidase and its water-soluble 30-Kdalton derivative differ from the aforedescribed DD-carboxypeptidases in that their enzyme activities and penicillin-binding abilities are inhibited by low dose levels of *para*-chloromercuribenzoate, and dinitro 5,5′-dithiobis-(2-nitroben-zoate) (*6*), suggesting that this enzyme might be a thiol DD-carboxypeptidase. Further experiments, however, are required to confirm this possibility since the effects of chemical reagents of this type and others may be caused by reaction with some satellite amino acid residues which operate in conjunction with, for example, the serine residue or the Zn^{2+} cofactor and its ligands, in the active centers of the corresponding enzymes.

Low concentrations of *para*-chloromercuribenzoate inhibit the enzyme activity of the *E. coli* DD-carboxypeptidase 1A but not its penicillin-binding ability (*8*). The interpretation has been that one enzyme SH group, not involved in the formation of the presumed acyl-enzyme complexes, is essential for the deacylation processes (k_4), which are therefore prevented from occurring in the presence of the thiol reagent. With the serine R61 enzyme, the use of *ortho*-methylisourea or 2,4-dinitrobenzene suggests that one ε-amino group of lysine is probably involved in both enzyme activity and penicillin binding (*2*). Methylglyoxal, 2,3-butanedione, and phenyl-glyoxal are also inhibitors of the R61 enzyme activity on the peptide substrates, suggesting the involvement of an arginine residue (*32*). The same α-dicarbonyls inhibit benzylpenicillin binding but to a much lesser degree, depending on the size of the α-dicarbonyl side chain (*32*). Characterization of these satellite amino acid residues is a topic for future research.

FUNCTIONING

One approach to an understanding of the functioning of the enzyme active centers has been to study the effects that each residue of the tripeptide Ac_2-L-Lys-D-Ala-D-Ala or each portion of the β-lactam antibiotic molecules exerts on the various kinetic parameters of the corresponding reactions. Since the carbonyl carbon that is transferred to the exogenous nucleophile belongs to the amide bond of D-Ala-D-Ala or the β-lactam ring, the fused bicyclic ring and the 6(7)-β-substituent in the penicillins or Δ^3-cephalosporins are regarded as the counterparts of the D-Ala-D-Ala sequence and the preceding L-residue in the tripeptide substrate, respectively (Fig. 1).

With the β-lactam compounds and because of the high stability of the corresponding acyl-enzyme complexes, the k_4 term, k_3/K ratio, and, in some cases, the K and k_3 terms of the reaction can be determined directly (*17, 22, 23, 26, 29, 31*). With the peptide substrates and because of the very low stability of the corresponding acyl-enzyme complexes, the terms of the reaction that could be measured were K_m

and V_{max} (*42, 44, 45*). As a first approximation, K_m and V_{max} were considered as equivalent to K and k_3. Note that with Ac_2-L-Lys-D-Ala-D-Ala, $k_4 > k_3$ and therefore $V_{max} = k_3[E_0]$. If, in addition, $k_2 \gg k_3$ ($E + C \underset{k_2}{\overset{k_1}{\rightleftharpoons}} E.C$; with $k_2/k_1 = K$), then $K_m = K$.

1. The Serine DD-Carboxypeptidases

The R61 and R39 enzymes have been studied extensively and the results have been reviewed in detail elsewhere (*17, 33–36*). The main conclusions are presented here. From the data so far available, the same conclusions probably apply to the serine DD-carboxypeptidases of *Bacilli* (*55*) as well as to the presumed thiol DD-carboxypeptidase of *S. faecalis* (*4–7*).

1) Initial binding (K)

Three distinct features characterize the first step of the reaction. i) Neither the L-residue of the peptide nor the 6(7)-β-substituent of the β-lactam is involved, at least substantially, in initial binding. On the contrary, that part of the relevant molecules which is mainly responsible for binding to the enzyme binding site n°1 is the C-terminal D-Ala-D-Ala sequence or the equivalent portion of the bicyclic fused ring system. ii) There is a strict requirement for the occurrence of a D-Ala residue at the penultimate position or an intact β-lactam ring. Conversely, the enzymes have a less strict requirement for a D-Ala at the C-terminal position, and, similarly, the β-lactam ring may be fused to various cyclic compounds (thiazolidine in the penicillins, dihydrothiazine in the Δ^3-cephalosporins, *etc.*). iii) Whether the peptides have high or poor substrate activities, or are nonsubstrate inhibitors (*48*), and whether the β-lactam compounds have high or poor inactivating properties, the K term of the reaction is always rather high (0.1–10 mM). One may thus conclude that initial binding is not very selective nor very efficient.

2) Enzyme acylation (k₃)

The second step of the reaction consists of a series of connected events. Once the peptide or the antibiotic is bound to the enzyme, a suitable lateral chain on the L-residue or a suitable 6(7)-β-substituent on the β-lactam ring interacts with some specific enzyme groupings (binding sites n°2), inducing conformational changes in the protein. As a result, the enzyme center thus made catalytically active is then able to considerably increase the electrophilic character of the carbonyl carbon of the penultimate D-Ala or the β-lactam ring, so that, eventually, enzyme acylation is achieved. Induced conformational changes are suggested by X-ray crystallographic studies of the complex formed between the R61 enzyme and *para*-iodo-phenyl-penicillin (see above). They are also reflected by the fluorescence quenching and alterations in the CD spectrum observed as a result of penicilloylation of this enzyme (*47*).

The interaction between a suitable side chain at the positions under consideration and the enzyme binding sites n°2 is remarkable in several respects as follow:

i) The interaction may be extremely effective. Thus, with the R61 enzyme, the k_3 value is about 200 sec^{-1} for benzylpenicillin, 1 sec^{-1} for ampicillin, and 2×10^{-4}

sec^{-1} for the 6-(β)unsubstituted aminopenicillanic acid. Similarly, the turnover number on Ac$_2$-L-Lys-D-Ala-D-Ala is 3,300; it is decreased by 15% with Ac$_2$-L-A$_2$bu-D-Ala-D-Ala and by 99% for Ac-D-Ala-D-Ala, which in fact, becomes an inhibitor of the enzyme activity on Ac$_2$-L-Lys-D-Ala-D-Ala. Similar observations have been made with the R39 enzyme.

ii) The interaction may be extremely specific. Thus, although a long side chain at the L-position in the peptide is a general requirement for substrate activity, the occurrence of charged groups at this terminal position may exert very specific effects. Succinylation instead of acetylation of the ε-amino group of L-lysine, lack of substitution of this amino group, or replacement by other charged groups may, depending on the enzyme, increase, decrease, or suppress substrate activity. Similarly, the effects of a given side chain on the 6(7)-β-position of the β-lactam antibiotics, in particular its degree of steric hindrance and rigidity, the occurrence of charged groups, etc., vary widely depending on the enzymes.

iii) Effective side chains on the L-residue of the peptide or at the 6(7)-β-position in the antibiotic molecule are (apparently) completely unrelated, suggesting the occurrence, in a given enzyme, of two binding sites n°2, for the bound peptide and the bound β-lactam compound, respectively.

iv) In its ground state conformation, the amide nitrogen of the β-lactam ring of penicillins and Δ^3-cephalosporins, on the one hand, is pyramidal, and must be so for the reaction to occur effectively. Δ^2-Cephalosporins, in which the nonplanarity of the β-lactam nitrogen is less pronounced, and monocyclic β-lactam compounds are weak acylating agents and poor enzyme inactivators. The amide nitrogen of D-Ala-D-Ala, on the other hand, is planar and, in spite of this lack of reactivity, hydrolysis of sensitive peptides may occur at very high rates. Thus, there are considerable differences in the heights of the barrier to reaction with the enzyme that are overcome as a result of the interaction of the lateral side chain of the bound peptide or the 6(7)-β-substituent of the bound β-lactam molecule, with the relevant enzyme binding sites n°2. Some of the recently discovered Δ^2-penems and 1-carba-Δ^2-penems, with no or very simple side chains, exhibit antibacterial activities. The nonplanarity of their β-lactam nitrogen is considerably more pronounced than in penicillins and Δ^3-cephalosporins (58) so that binding of the nucleus itself to at least some enzyme receptors may be sufficient to cause rapid opening of the β-lactam ring and acylation of the enzyme active centers.

3) Deacylation (k_4) of L-R-D-alanyl-enzyme complexes

Enzyme deacylation is the process through which the serine ester linkage formed during enzyme acylation is, in turn, broken down with concomitant transfer of the acyl moiety to an exogenous nucleophile. With the peptide substrates, deacylation is a rapid process and water can serve as a nonspecific acceptor (DD-carboxypeptidase activity). The serine enzymes, however (at least the R61 and R39 enzymes), also possess structured amino acceptor sites which confer on them very specific transpeptidase activities (28, 37, 38, 49, 61). Thus by using peptide monomers such as

$$\text{Ac-L-Lys-D-Ala-D-Ala or L-Ala-D-Glu-}\underset{\text{D}}{\overset{\text{L}}{\underset{|}{\overline{\text{A}_2\text{pm}}}}}\text{-D-Ala-D-Ala}$$
$$\text{Gly}\rule[-0.3em]{0pt}{0pt}\rfloor$$

where the N-terminal glycine or the N-terminal group of the D center of meso-di-aminopimelic acid, fits the acceptor sites of the R61 and R39 enzymes, respectively, peptide dimers can be synthesized *in vitro* that are identical or very similar to those synthesized *in vivo* during wall peptidoglycan synthesis in the corresponding bacteria. Steady-state kinetic studies suggest that transpeptidation follows an ordered pathway in which binding of the amino nucleophile to the enzyme occurs before binding of the carbonyl carbon donor (25). In aqueous media and with simple amino compounds such as D-Ala or Gly, hydrolysis and transpeptidation interfere with each other on a simple competitive basis. With complex amino nucleophiles related to wall pep-tidoglycan synthesis, the phenomenon is more complicated (25, 38). In the presence of increasing concentrations of such amino compounds, not only is hydrolysis pro-gressively inhibited but transpeptidation, after rising to a maximum, is in turn pro-gressively inhibited so that, eventually, the enzyme may be frozen in a nonopera-tional state. Hence, these amino nucleophiles not only serve as acceptors of the L-R-D-Ala-D-Ala moiety but may also act as modulators of enzyme activity. Crys-tallographic studies should contribute, in the near future, to a better understanding of these phenomena.

4) Deacylation (k_4) of penicilloyl (cephalosporoyl)-enzyme complexes

With the β-lactam antibiotics, enzyme deacylation is a low or very low process with k_4 values ranging, for instance, from 2.8×10^{-4} sec^{-1} for the interaction between the R61 enzyme and phenoxymethylpenicillin, and 3×10^{-7} sec^{-1} for the interaction between the R39 enzyme and cephalosporin C. The stability of the corresponding acyl-enzyme complexes has been attributed to a specific interaction between the monocyclic thiazolidine (dihydrothiazine) ring and a specific enzyme binding site n°3, conferring on the acyl-enzyme complex a conformation that is not suitable for attack by an exogenous nucleophile (34–36). This interpretation rests upon the ob-servation that with the penicilloyl-R61 enzyme complex, once the stabilization effect has been eliminated by C-5–C-6 cleavage of the penicilloyl moiety and protonation at C-6 (Fig. 1), the serine ester-linked N-acylglycyl fragment thus produced is then susceptible to immediate nucleophilic attack (by water or a suitable amino nucle-ophile) (20, 21, 27, 46). Fragmentation is the rate limiting step of the deacylation process. The mechanism is not yet understood. It might proceed *via* an oxazolinone-thiazolidine derivative (54). It is known that the thiazolidine part of the penicilloyl moiety is converted into as yet an unidentified compound Z which is further proc-essed to give rise to N-formyl-D-penicillamine (1).

Enzyme deacylation may also (slowly) proceed by elimination, without fragmen-tation, of the bound metabolite. Thus the product of the reaction between the R61 enzyme and nitrocefin is the corresponding cephalosporoic acid (unpublished results). This latter pathway may also occur with other Δ^3-cephalosporins but the charac-terization of the product(s) thus formed is a difficult problem, since it is known that hydrolysis of the β-lactam amide bond in the Δ^3-cephalosporins (by β-lactamase action) is usually accompanied by a series of further changes in the molecules.

From the foregoing, it appears that the thiazolidine (dihydrothiazine) part of the β-lactam molecule fulfils antagonistic functions. By distorting the β-lactam ring, it forces the β-lactam nitrogen to adopt a pyramidal character, a feature which is essential for enzyme action. By interreacting with the enzyme binding site n°3, the same thiazolidine (dihydrothiazine) forces the reaction to stop at the abortive level of the acyl-enzyme intermediate.

2. The Metallo G Enzyme

Although mechanistically different from the serine R61 and R39 DD-carboxypeptidases, the Zn^{2+} G enzyme is a DD-carboxypeptidase of comparable efficiency and with similar substrate requirements for L-R-D-Ala-D-Ala-terminated peptides. Moreover, and in complete analogy with the serine enzymes, the conformation of the Zn^{2+}-containing active center in the G enzyme is modulated by the structure of the side chain at the L position of the peptide substrates (44). In marked contrast, the G enzyme has an extremely low propensity to react with β-lactam antibiotics (see above), not that binding (K) is less efficient, at least with Δ^3-cephalosporins, but because, irrespective of the structure of the 6(7)-β-substituent, the k_3 term of the reaction is always extremely low ($\geq 1 \times 10^{-3} sec^{-1}$) (19). Phenotypically, the G enzyme, which has an effective binding site n°2 for bound peptides, lacks the binding site n°2 for bound β-lactam compounds. Fianlly, breakdown of complex E-C* (whatever its structure) formed with benzylpenicillin (at high concentrations and after prolonged incubation) releases benzylpenicilloate ($k_4 = 0.6 \times 10^{-4} sec^{-1}$) (16). The G enzyme behaves as a penicillinase of very low efficiency.

Acknowledgments

The work at the University of Liège has been supported in part by the National Institutes of Health, U.S.A. (contract n°2 R01 AI13364-04), the Fonds de la Recherche Scientifique Médicale, Brussels (contract n°3.4501.79), the Fonds National de la Recherche Scientifique, Brussels (contract n°S2/5-FG-E20), and the Actions Concertées (convention n°79/84-I1). P. Charlier is a fellow of the Institut pour l'Encouragement de la Recherche Scientifique dans l'Industrie at l'Agriculture (IRSIA), Brussels, Belgium; O. Dideberg thanks the European Molecular Biology Organization for support; and J. A. Kelly has been working at the University of Liège under a one-year research fellowship from the United States Public Health Service, National Institute of Allergy and Infectious Diseases (grant 1 F32 AI05735-01).

The work at the University of Connecticut has been supported by the United States Public Health Service, National Institute of Allergy and Infectious Diseases (grant AI-10925 to J.R.K.).

REFERENCES

1. Adriaens, P., Meesschaert, B., Frère, J. M., Vanderhaeghe, H., Degelaen, J., Ghuysen, J. M., and Eyssen, H. 1978. *J. Biol. Chem.*, **33**, 3660–3665.
2. Charlier, P. 1978. M. S. Thesis, University of Liège.
3. Corran, P. H. and Waley, S. G. 1975. *Biochem. J.*, **149**, 357–364.
4. Coyette, J., Ghuysen, J. M., Binot, F., Adriaens, P., Meesschaert, B., and Vanderhaeghe, H. 1977. *Eur. J. Biochem.*, **75**, 231–239.
5. Coyette, J., Ghuysen, J. M., and Fontana, R. 1978. *Eur. J. Biochem.*, **88**, 297–305.
6. Coyette, J., Ghuysen, J.M., and Fontana, R. 1980. *Eur. J. Biochem.*, **110**, 445–456.
7. Coyette, J., Perkins, H. R., Polacheck, I., Shockman, G. D., and Ghuysen, J. M. 1974. *Eur. J. Biochem.*, **44**, 459–468.
8. Curtis, S. J. and Strominger, J. L. 1978. *J. Biol. Chem.*, **253**, 2584–2588.
9. Degelaen, J., Feeney, J., Roberts, G. C. K., Burgen, A. S. V., Frère, J. M., and Ghuysen, J. M. 1979. *FEBS Lett.*, **98**, 53–56.
10. DeLucia, M. L., Kelly, J. A., Mangion, M. M., Moews, P. C., and Knox, J. R. 1980. *Phil. Trans. Roy. Soc. Lond. B.*, **289**, 374–376.
11. Dideberg, O., Charlier, P., Dupont, L., Vermeirem, M., Frère, J. M., and Ghuysen, J. M. 1980. *FEBS Lett.*, **117**, 212–214.
12. Dideberg, O., Frère, J. M., and Ghuysen, J. M. 1979. *J. Mol. Biol.*, **129**, 677–679.
13. Dideberg, O., Joris, B., Frère, J. M., Ghuysen, J. M., Weber, G., Robaye, R., Delbrouck, J. M., and Roelandts, I. 1980. *FEBS Lett.*, **117**, 215–218.
14. Duez, C., Frère, J. M., Geurts, F., Ghuysen, J. M., Dierickx, L., and Delcambe, L. 1978. *Biochem. J.*, **175**, 793–800.
15. Duez, C., Joris, B., Frère, J. M., Ghuysen, J. M., and Van Beeumen, J. 1981. *Biochem. J.*, **193**, 83–86.
16. Duez, C., Frère, J. M., Klein, D., Noël, M., Ghuysen, J. M., Delcambe, L., and Dierickx, L. 1981. *Biochem. J.*, **193**, 75–82.
17. Frère, J. M., Duez, C., Dusart, J., Coyette, J., Leyn-Bouille, M., Ghuysen, J. M., Dideberg, O., and Knox, J. R. 1980. *In* "Enzyme Inhibitors as Drugs," ed. by M. Sandler, MacMillan Press, London, pp. 183–207.
18. Frère, J. M., Duez, C., Ghuysen, J. M., and Vandekerckhove, J. 1976. *FEBS Lett.*, **70**, 257–260.
19. Frère, J. M., Geurts, F., and Ghuysen, J. M. 1978. *Biochem. J.*, **175**, 801–805.
20. Frère, J. M., Ghuysen, J. M., Degelaen, J., Loffet, A., and Perkins, H. R. 1975. *Nature*, **258**, 168–170.
21. Frère, J. M., Ghuysen, J. M., and De Graeve, J. 1978. *FEBS Lett.*, **88**, 147–150.

22. Frère, J. M., Ghuysen, J. M., and Iwatsubo, M. 1975. *Eur. J. Biochem.*, **57**, 343–351.
23. Frère, J. M., Ghuysen, J. M., and Perkins, H. R. 1975. *Eur. J. Biochem.*, **57**, 353–359.
24. Frère, J. M., Ghuysen, J. M., Perkins, H. R., and Nieto, M. 1973. *Biochem. J.*, **135**, 463–468.
25. Frère, J. M., Ghuysen, J. M., Perkins, H. R., and Nieto, M. 1973. *Biochem. J.*, **135**, 483–492.
26. Frère, J. M., Ghuysen, J. M., Reynolds, P. E., Moreno, R., and Perkins, H. R. 1974. *Biochem. J.*, **143**, 241–249.
27. Frère, J. M., Ghuysen, J. M., Vanderhaeghe, H., Adriaens, P., and Degelaen, J. 1976. *Nature*, **260**, 451–454.
28. Frère, J. M., Ghuysen, J. M., Zeiger, A. R., and Perkins, H. R. 1976. *FEBS Lett.*, **63**, 112–116.
29. Frère, J. M., Leyh-Bouille, M., Ghuysen, J. M., and Perkins, H. R. 1974. *Eur. J. Biochem.*, **50**, 203–214.
30. Frère, J. M., Moreno, R., Ghuysen, J. M., Perkins, H. R., Dierickx, L., and Delcambe, L. 1974. *Biochem. J.*, **143**, 233–240.
31. Fuad, N., Frère, J. M., Ghuysen, J. M., Duez, C., and Iwatsubo, M. 1976. *Biochem. J.*, **155**, 623–629.
32. Georgopapadakou, N. H., Lui, F. Y., Ryono, D. E., Neubeck, R., Sabo, E. F., and Ondetti, M.A. 1981. *Eur. J. Biochem.*, in press.
33. Ghuysen, J. M. 1977. The Bacterial DD-Carboxypeptidase-Transpeptidase Enzyme System. A New Insight into the Mode of Action of Penicillin. E. R. Squibb Lectures on Chemistry of Microbial Products. Series Editor: W. E. Brown, Univ. Tokyo Press, Tokyo, 162 pp.
34. Ghuysen, J. M. 1980. *In* "Topics in Antibiotic Chemistry," ed. by P. G. Sammes, Ellis Horwood, Chichester, West Sussex, Vol. 5, pp. 9–17.
35. Ghuysen, J. M., Frère, J. M., Leyh-Bouille, M., Coyette, J., Dusart, J., and Nguyen-Distèche, M. 1979. *Annu. Rev. Biochem.*, **48**, 73–101.
36. Ghuysen, J. M., Frère, J. M., Leyh-Bouille, M., Perkins, H. R., and Nieto, M. 1980. *Phil. Trans. Roy. Soc. Lond. B*, **289**, 285–301.
37. Ghuysen, J. M., Leyh-Bouille, M., Campbell, J. N., Moreno, R., Frère, J. M., Duez, C., Nieto, M., and Perkins, H. R. 1973. *Biochemistry*, **12**, 1243–1251.
38. Ghuysen, J. M., Reynolds, P. E., Perkins, H. R., Frère, J. M., and Moreno, R. 1974. *Biochemistry*, **13**, 2539–2547.
39. Hill, H. A. O., Sammes, P. G., and Waley, S. G. 1980. *Phil. Trans. Roy. Soc. Lond. B*, **289**, 333–344.
40. Kelly, J. A., Frère, J. M., Klein, D., and Ghuysen, J. M. Manuscript in preparation.
41. Knox, J. R., DeLucia, M. L., Murthy, N. S., Kelly, J. A., Moews, P. C., Frère, J. M., and Ghuysen, J. M. 1979. *J. Mol. Biol.*, **127**, 217–218.

42. Leyh-Bouille, M., Coyette, J., Ghuysen, J. M., Idczak, J., Perkins, H. R., and Nieto, M. 1971. *Biochemistry*, **10**, 2163–2170.
43. Leyh-Bouille, M., Dusart, J., Nguyen-Distèche, M., Ghuysen, J. M., Reynolds, P. E., and Perkins, H. R. 1977. *Eur. J. Biochem.*, **81**, 19–28.
44. Leyh-Bouille, M., Ghuysen, J. M., Bonaly, R., Nieto, M., Perkins, H. R., Schleifer, K. H., and Kandler, O. 1970. *Biochemistry*, **9**, 2961–2971.
45. Leyh-Bouille, M., Nakel, M., Frère, J. M., Johnson, K., Ghuysen, J. M., Nieto, M., and Perkins, H. R. 1972. *Biochemistry*, **11**, 1290–1298.
46. Marquet, A., Frère, J. M., Ghuysen, J. M., and Loffet, A. 1979. *Biochem. J.*, **177**, 909–916.
47. Nieto, M., Perkins, H. R., Frère, J. M., and Ghuysen, J. M. 1973. *Biochem. J.*, **135**, 493–505.
48. Nieto, M., Perkins, H. R., Leyh-Bouille, M., Frère, J. M., and Ghuysen, J. M. 1973. *Biochem. J.*, **131**, 163–171.
49. Perkins, H. R., Nieto, M., Frère, J. M., Leyh-Bouille, M., and Ghuysen, J. M. 1973. *Biochem. J.*, **131**, 707–718.
50. Pollock, J. J., Ghuysen, J. M., Linder, R., Salton, M. R. J., Perkins, H. R., Nieto, M., Leyh-Bouille, M., Frère, J. M., and Johnson, K. 1972. *Proc. Natl. Acad. Sci. U.S.A.*, **69**, 662–666.
51. Rasmussen, J. R. and Strominger, J. L. 1978. *Proc. Natl. Acad. Sci. U.S.A.*, **75**, 84–88.
52. Spratt, B. G. 1980. *Phil. Trans. Roy. Soc. Lond. B*, **289**, 273–283.
53. Tamura, T., Imae, Y., and Strominger, J. L. 1976. *J. Biol. Chem.*, **251**, 414–423.
54. Thomas, R. 1979. *J. Chem. Soc. Chem. Commun.*, 1176–1177.
55. Umbreit, J. N. and Strominger, J. L. 1973. *J. Biol. Chem.*, **248**, 6767–6771.
56. Waxman, D. J. and Strominger, J. L. 1979. *J. Biol. Chem.*, **254**, 4863–4875.
57. Waxman, D. J., Yocum, R. R., and Strominger, J. L. 1980. *Phil. Trans. Roy. Soc. Lond. B*, **289**, 257–271.
58. Woodward, R. B. 1980. *Phil. Trans. Roy. Soc. Lond. B*, **289**, 239–250.
59. Yocum, R. R. and Strominger, J. L. Manuscript in preparation.
60. Yocum, R. R., Waxman, D. J., Rasmussen, J. R., and Strominger, J. L. 1979. *Proc. Natl. Acad. Sci. U.S.A.*, **76**, 2730–2734.
61. Zeiger, A. R., Frère, J. M., Ghuysen, J. M., and Perkins, H. R. 1975. *FEBS Lett.*, **52**, 221–225.

PENICILLIN-BINDING PROTEINS: THEIR NATURE AND FUNCTIONS IN THE CELLULAR DUPLICATION AND MECHANISM OF ACTION OF β-LACTAM ANTIBIOTICS IN *ESCHERICHIA COLI*

Michio Matsuhashi, Jun-ichi Nakagawa, Fumitoshi Ishino, Sadayo Nakajima-Iijima, Shigeo Tomioka, Masaki Doi, and Shigeo Tamaki

*Institute of Applied Microbiology, University of Tokyo**

It is now widely accepted that certain penicillin-binding proteins (PBPs) play essential roles in the proliferation of bacterial cells. These PBPs seem to be differentiated in order to function in different steps of the cell cycle, namely, cell elongation, septum formation, and determination of morphology (*42*). In *Escherichia coli*, seven major PBPs have been separated by sodium dodecylsulfate (SDS)/polyacrylamide gel electrophoresis (*42, 43, 50, 54*). Of these, the higher molecular weight PBPs (1A, 1Bs, 2, and 3) have been supposed to play more important roles than the lower molecular weight ones (PBP-4, 5, and 6) (*19, 20, 21*). PBP-1A and 1Bs are thought to function in cell elongation (*42, 47*), PBP-2 in formation of the rod-shape of cells (*42, 46*), and PBP-3 in septum formation (*42, 44*). Until recently their function was supposed to be to crosslink peptidoglycan (*3, 12, 13, 54*), a constituent of the bag-shaped cell wall basal structure, because penicillin and other β-lactam antibiotics inhibit these crosslinking reactions (*12, 13*) to prevent formation of the network of peptidoglycan (*3, 57, 61*) in the cell wall and septum.

These ideas have been modified by our recent findings. In 1979 we purified PBP-1Bs from *E. coli* as proteins forming triplet bands on gel, free from contaminating proteins (*27, 28*). The purified preparation showed two enzyme activities (*19a, 28*) that catalyze successive reactions to form crosslinked peptidoglycan from its lipid-linked precursor; namely, peptidoglycan transglycosylase activity for the formation of glycan chains (*1a, 12, 13*) and penicillin-sensitive transpeptidase activity for the formation of cross-bridges (*12, 13*). Probably these two activities reside on the same protein molecule, and so the *de novo* synthesis of the peptidoglycan network can be performed efficiently by the action of a single bifunctional enzyme protein at the growing point of the cell. Subsequently bifunctional enzyme activities for the synthesis of peptidoglycan were also demonstrated in PBP-1A (*9, 18c*) and PBP-3 (ref. *8* and Ishino and

* Yayoi 1-1-1, Bunkyo-ku, Tokyo 113, Japan.

Matsuhashi, manuscript submitted for publication) in *E. coli*. Enzyme activities due to PBP-2 is under the investigation. New observations indicating the enzyme activity and function of *E. coli* PBPs will be mainly described in this article.

PENICILLIN-BINDING PROTEINS 1Bs AND 1A IN *E. COLI*

1. Occurrence and Behavior

Under the conditions of the SDS/acrylamide slab gel electrophoresis originally used by Spratt and Pardee (*48*), PBP-1A and PBP-1Bs showed very similar mobilities. After modifying the conditions (*47, 50, 54*) they were separated into two groups of bands, a slower moving single band of PBP-1A and faster moving triplet bands of PBP-1Bs. The amounts of the three components of PBP-1Bs varied according to the physiological conditions of cells. In some cases the component with the slowest mobility was found in the largest amount among the three components, but in most other cases the second one was found more abundantly.

These three components of PBP-1Bs had very similar biochemical properties: thermoresistance at 60°C (*27*) and resistance to treatment with 1% sodium dodecyl-N-sarcosinate (Sarkosyl, Ciba Geighy) (*27*). PBP-1A and all other PBPs are nearly inactivated by these treatments (*27*). The three components of PBP-1Bs showed affinities toward the β-lactam antibiotics so far tested indistinguishable from each other in specificity and magnitude. Moreover, PBP-1Bs eluted from the membrane were split by the action of trypsin to form duplex (or triplex) fragments with molecular weights of about 50,000 which still retained the activity to bind penicillin G and smaller peptides (*26a*) (Fig. 1).

These results may suggest that the three components of PBP-1Bs have chemical structures similar to each other. This was also suggested by genetical observations as described in the next section. However more precise characterization has to be done by amino acid sequence analysis of the trypsin fragments. Nothing is yet known about the amino acids in the active center of the proteins to which penicillin G binds.

2. Mutations in PBP-1Bs and PBP-1A

A mutation in the *mrc* (*m*urein cluster *c*) gene located at 3.2 min (*22, 50, 54*) on the *E. coli* chromosome map (*2*) caused disappearance of all the three components of PBP-1Bs (*22, 50, 54*). The *mrc* mutant strain JST975 was supersensitive to most β-lactam antibiotics and was thermosensitive, being lysed at 42°C (*22, 54*). These β-lactam supersensitivities and thermosensitivity of growth were partially recovered by a suppressive mutation (*54*) in the *mre* (*m*urein cluster *e*) *A* gene, which was recently mapped at 70.7 min on the *E. coli* chromosome map (about 14% co-transduction linkage with *aroE* by phage P1) (ref. *29* and manuscript in preparation). The most plausible gene order may be *mreA-aroE-strA*. The *mreA* mutation caused production of an excessively large amount of PBP-1A and 2 and was recessive as judged by the formation of wild-type meroheterodiploids.

The *mrc*-975 mutation also caused the complete loss of enzymatic activity of the

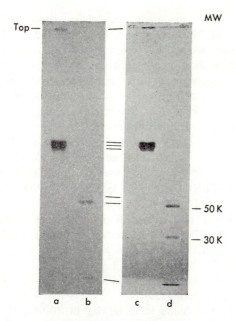

FIG. 1.   Purified PBP-1Bs obtained from the membrane of *E. coli* strain pLC19-19 (*4*) and peptides obtained by digestion of purified PBP-1Bs with trypsin shown by SDS/acrylamide slab gel electrophoresis.

Procedures of purification of PBP-1Bs and conditions for electrophoresis were as described previously (*26a*). A suspension of purified PBP-1Bs (23 μg in 30 μl 0.05 M Tris HCl buffer, pH 7.6, containing 0.1 mM $MgCl_2$ and 1 mM 2-mercaptoethanol) was solubilized by addition of 2 μl of 15% Sarkosyl and then digested with trypsin (Worthington, final 10 μg per ml) for 1.5 min at 30°C. Digestion was complete under these conditions. After addition of 0.7 μg trypsin inhibitor (Miles Laboratories), [^{14}C]penicillin G-protein complexes (left) and untreated proteins (right) were detected as follows. Sarkosyl, trypsin, and trypsin inhibitor were omitted from the control experiments (lanes a and c). Left: [^{14}C]penicillin G (60 Ci per mol, 2.4 nmol) was added to 30 μl aliquots of samples and the binding reaction was carried out. A fluorogram is shown. Right: aliquots of 30 μl samples were mixed with 20 μl of a solution of 0.15 M Tris HCl buffer, pH 6.8, 2.2% SDS, 22% glycerol and 3.5 M 2-mercaptoethanol. The mixtures were boiled for 2 min and then subjected to electrophoresis. a and c, purified PBP-1Bs; b and d trypsin digest of purified PBP-1Bs. The low penicillin-binding activity of 50 K fragments (lane b) is owing to the presence of Sarkosyl in the binding reaction.

membrane fraction to form peptidoglycan from their lipid-linked precursor by the assay method previously reported (*12, 13, 54*). The sequence of enzymatic reactions forming crosslinked peptidoglycan from their lipid-linked precursor, namely, reactions due to peptidoglycan transglycosylase which elongates glycosidic chains and penicillin-sensitive transpeptidase which constructs crossbridges between glycan chains, was found originally by Izaki, Matsuhashi, and Strominger (12, 13) in the *E. coli* membrane. Recently, however, we realized that both activities of the trans-glycosylase and transpeptidase are residing on the purified PBP-1Bs (19b, 27, 28). Moreover, more recently Ishino et al. succeeded in demonstrating similar dual enzyme activities, also in a purified preparation of PBP-1A (9, 18c) and PBP-3 (ref. 8 and Ishino and Matsuhashi, manuscript in preparation). The activities belonging to PBP-1A and 1B(s) seemed to require different conditions for reaction.

Other *mrc* mutations were obtained which caused change in phenotypes different from the *mrc*-975 mutation. An example will be described here. Mutation in strain JST977 caused a simultaneous increase in the electrophoretical mobilities of all the (three) components of PBP-1Bs. Probably the peptide lengths of PBP-1Bs in this mutant are shorter than those of the wild-type PBP-1Bs; alternatively, the mutant PBP-1Bs are different in some additional structures such as the presence or absence of glycosidic residues from wild type PBP-1Bs. The mutant was supersensitive to most β-lactam antibiotics and showed thermosensitive growth at 45°C, and the membrane obtained from this mutant seemed to have a lower activity of formation of peptidoglycan in the assay method of Izaki et al. (12, 13). A similar mutant with modified PBP-1Bs has previously been reported (50).

A mutant strain, HAT293 (14), was found to be lacking in PBP-1A (27, 54). The mutation was located close to *aroB* (74.1 min). It did not cause any discernible phenotypical change in the cell. No increase in the sensitivity of the cells to β-lactam antibiotics tested and no thermosensitivity of growth of the mutant were observed. However, in PBP-1A^{-} mutants (27, 47) there was observed an appreciable increase in the amount of PBP-1Bs, suggesting the compensatory functions of these proteins (50, 54). The PBP-1A^{-} mutation in strain HAT293 was found to be recessive and introduction of a colE1 plasmid (4) carrying a chromosomal part covering the putative structural gene of PBP-1A (56) to the mutant cell caused production in an excessively large amount of PBP-1A. Therefore it is highly probable that the mutation in the mutant strain HAT293 is concerned with the structural gene of PBP-1A which has been proposed previously by Suzuki, Nishimura, and Hirota, who isolated a mutant with thermosensitive PBP-1A (50). The name *mrcA* was given by Bachmann and Low (2) to the gene of PBP-1A at 74.2 min and *mrcB* to that of PBP-1Bs at 3.2 min. However, as the two genes cannot belong to the same cluster of genes, their nomen-clature may have to be reconsidered after extensive studies of their neighboring genes. If the peptide chains of PBP-1A, PBP-1Bs, and PBP-3 are respectively composed of two peptide moieties which are responsible for the activities of transglycosylase and transpeptidase, the structural genes of the proteins should also be composed of two parts of genes coding for the two peptide moieties. Probably they are formed originally by fusion of the two ancestral genes.

3. Purification of PBP-1Bs

The *E. coli* membrane fraction on which PBPs reside carries out the synthesis of crosslinked peptidoglycan from its lipid-linked precursor and the enzyme activities of PBP-1Bs (peptidoglycan transglycosylase and penicillin-sensitive transpeptidase) can be extracted with Sarkosyl and purified by ammonium sulfate precipitation and by column chromatography on ampicillin-Sepharose (28). Membranes were obtained from E. coli strain pLC19-19 (4), which contains colEl-plasmids carrying the chromosomal part covering the structural gene of PBP-1Bs (28, 56). The procedures for preparation of membranes, extraction of PBP-1Bs with 1% Sarkosyl at 20°C, and fractionation with ammonium sulfate were essentially as described previously (28). Enzyme activities for forming lipid-linked intermediates from UDP-linked precursors, i.e., UDP-N-acetylmuramyl-pentapeptide(L-Ala-D-Glu-meso-A₂pm-D-Ala-D'-Ala): undecaprenol-phosphate phospho-N-acetylmuramyl-pentapeptide transferase and UDP-N-acetylglucosamine: undecaprenol-diphospho-N-acetylmuramyl-pentapeptide acetylglucosaminyl transferase, could also be extracted from the membrane with 1% Sarkosyl in the active state but they seemed to be separated from PBP-1Bs during the procedures of fractionation with ammonium sulfate and affinity chromatography on ampicillin-Sepharose (Table I). Purification on an affinity column of ampicillin-Sepharose was carried out by the procedures of Shepherd, Chase, and Reynolds (40) except that all buffer solution contained 1% Sarkosyl. We achieved extensive purification (950-fold with respect to the transglycosylase activity) of the activities

TABLE I.   Fractionation of Enzyme Activities of Peptidoglycan Synthesis from E. coli Membrane (28)

Fraction	Assay 1		Assay 2	
	Peptidoglycan	Lipid-linked precursors	Peptidoglycan	D-Alanine
Membrane	340	143	31	42
1% Sarkosyl extract	376	73	343	113
Ammonium sulfate				
0–45% saturation	24	11	332	122
45–60% saturation	77	497	31	53
60–100% saturation	0	780	0	4
Mixture of 3 fractions	291	245	203	78

Results are expressed as pmol D-alanine per mg protein. Experimental procedures are as described in ref. 28. The compositions of the assay mixtures in a final volume of 30 μl were as follows. Assay 1: 2 μmol Tris-HCl, pH 8.5, 1 μmol MgCl₂, 8.45 nCi labeled UDP-N-acetylmuramyl-L-Ala-D-Glu-meso-A₂pm-D-[¹⁴C]Ala-D-[¹⁴C]Ala (8.8 μCi per μmol D-Ala), 10 nmol UDP-N-acetylglucosamine, 50 nmol 2-mercaptoethanol, 30–300 μg protein; Assay 2: 2 μmol Tris HCl, pH 8.5, 1 μmol MgCl₂, 6.7 nCi undecaprenol-PP-disaccharide pentapeptide labeled with D-[¹⁴C]Ala-D-[¹⁴C]Ala (45 μCi per μmol D-Ala), 50 nmol 2-mercaptoethanol, and enzyme proteins as in Assay 1. Reactions were carried out at 42°C for 60 min. Peptidoglycan formed was crosslinked, as estimated after lysozyme digestion.

of penicillin-binding, transglycosylase and penicillin-sensitive transpeptidase without their separation from each other.

The purified preparation of PBP-1Bs was treated with [^{14}C]penicillin G and subjected to SDS/polyacrylamide slab gel electrophoresis. The pattern of protein on the purified sample was identical to that of the fluorogram of the [^{14}C]penicillin G-protein complexes and no other proteins or radioactive bands were detectable, except for a trace of protein remaining at the top of the gel (see Fig. 1, lanes a and c).

4. PBP-1B(s), a Bifunctional Protein(s) with Activities of Peptidoglycan Transglycosylase and Penicillin-sensitive Transpeptidase

The purified PBP-1Bs catalyzed formation of crosslinked peptidoglycan from its lipid-linked precursor, N-acetylglucosaminyl-N-acetylmuramyl(pentapeptide)-PP-undecaprenol (Table II). The extent of crosslinking varied from 16 to 24% according to the reaction conditions. Release of D-alanine amounted to about one-sixth to one-fourth of the amount incorporated into peptidoglycan, suggesting that the purified PBP-1Bs contained little if any activity of D-alanine carboxypeptidase, which is supposed to remove the terminal D-alanine molecules of the pentapeptide side chains in the peptidoglycan that are not utilized for crosslink formation. The transglycosylase reaction required 10 mM MgCl$_2$ (at pH 8.5) for its maximal activity, was insensitive to 10 mM p-chloromercuribenzoate, but was very sensitive to macarbomycin or moenomycin (ID$_{50}$ values, less than 0.1 μg per ml), and moderately sensitive to enramycin (ID$_{50}$ value, about 5 μg per ml). Release of D-alanine also did not occur in the presence of these antibiotics.

Penicillin G inhibited the crosslinking reaction and the concomitant release of D-alanine, which are supposed to be mainly due to the transpeptidase reaction (18c) (Table II). But under certain conditions, it greatly increased formation of uncrosslinked peptidoglycan. About 150% as much peptidoglycan was formed in the presence of 10 μg per ml penicillin G as in its absence. The stimulation of transglycosylase activity by penicillin G could owe to the uncoupling of the two successive reactions, i.e., glycan chain elongation and crossbridge formation, but it could also be a specific phenomenon for each antibiotic. A similar stimulation of the transglycosylase reaction concomitant with inhibition of the crosslinking reaction was also obtained with N-formimidoyl thienamycin (6) under similar conditions, for example, as shown in Table II (18c). Izaki et al. (12, 13) also obtained evidence suggesting that penicillin G increased formation of peptidoglycan by a crude membrane preparation of E. coli. More precise work is necessary to determine how penicillin G stimulates the reaction of transglycosylase while inhibiting that of transpeptidase.

Incubation of the enzyme with 1 μg per ml of penicillin G or N-formimidoyl thienamycin (6) inhibited about 50% of the formation of crosslinkage but 1,000 μg per ml of cephalexin exerted only slight inhibition of the crosslinkage formation.

We have so far not been able to separate the three bands of PBP-1Bs to test the enzymatic activities of each. Probably they are similar proteins and all, or at least

TABLE II.   Peptidoglycan Formation by Purified PBP-1Bs of *E. coli* and Effect of Inhibitors

Condition		Peptidoglycan formation (pmol)	D-Alanine release (pmol)	Degree of crosslinkage (%)
Experiment 1				
Control		37. 6	10. 7	—
+Penicillin G	800 μg/ml	71. 0	0. 1	—
+Macarbomycin	67 μg/ml	0	0	—
Experiment 2				
Control		18. 7	—	17. 8
+Penicillin G	1 μg/ml	18. 9	—	9. 1
+Penicillin G	10 μg/ml	27. 5	—	1. 5
+Cephalexin	1, 000 μg/ml	21. 7	—	13. 8
+Nocardicin A	300 μg/ml	15. 3	—	9. 1
+Enramycin	15 μg/ml	0	—	—
Experiment 3				
Control		9. 8	—	16. 0
+N-formimidoyl thienamycin	1 μg/ml	13. 1	—	7. 5
	10 μg/ml	16. 5	—	0. 1

The reaction mixture in a final volume of 35 μl contained 2 μmol Tris HCl, pH 8.5, 0.33 μmol MgCl$_2$, 50 nmol 2-mercaptoethanol (Exps. 1 and 2), or Na-phosphate buffer, pH 7.0, 1 μmol MgCl$_2$ (Exp. 3), 7.8 μg (Exp. 1) or 6.4 μg (Exps. 2 and 3) purified PBP-1Bs and N-acetyl-glucosaminyl-N-acetylmuramyl-(-L-Ala-D-Glu-meso-A$_2$pm-D-Ala-D-Ala)-diphospho-unde-caprenol in 5 μl methanol, which was labeled in either D-[^{14}C]Ala-D-[^{14}C]Ala (45 Ci per mol, 148 pmol, in terms of D-alanine) (Exp. 1) or meso-[^{14}C]A$_2$pm (44 Ci per mol, 136 pmol) (Exps. 2 and 3).   The reaction was carried out at 37°C for 15 min and terminated by the addition of 10 μl of isobutyric acid.   In inhibition experiments, penicillin G, cephalexin, N-formimidoyl thienamycin, and enramycin were added to the reaction mixture omitting the lipid-linked precursor and the mixture was preincubated for 10 min at 37°C before starting the reaction by adding the lipid-linked precursor; macarbomycin was added just before starting the reaction. The degree of crosslinkage was calculated after paper chromatography of the lysozyme digests from the ratio (radioactivity) of bis (disaccharide-peptide) to [bis(disaccharide-peptide) +disaccharide-peptide].   A ratio of 1 corresponds to 50% crosslinkage.

one of them, functions as a bifunctional enzyme in peptidoglycan synthesis. Assuming that the active sites of both the transglycosylase and the transpeptidase are on a single peptide chain(s) of PBP-1Bs, a mechanism for formation of crosslinked pep-tidoglycan from the lipid-linked precursor by this bifunctional enzyme may be out-lined as in Fig. 2 (*19a*).

PBP-1Bs are very hydrophobic proteins and are precipitated by centrifugation

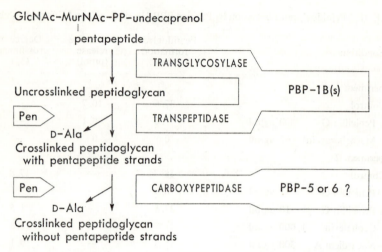

FIG. 2.   A scheme of enzymatic formation of crosslinked peptidoglycan showing bifunctional activity of PBP-1B(s) as peptidoglycan transglycosylase and penicillin-sensitive transpeptidase (*19a*).
PBP-5 or 6 may function as penicillin-sensitive DD-alanine carboxypeptidase to limit the crosslinking reaction.

after removal of Sarkosyl with Bio-Beads (BIO-RAD Laboratories). No enzyme activities were found in the supernatant. Probably, the bifunctional protein is mounted with its hydrophobic moiety on the outside of the cytoplasmic membrane and catalyzes with its transglycosylase moiety formation of glycan chains and with its transpeptidase moiety formation of crossbridges (Fig. 2). PBP-5 or PBP-6 may function as D-alanine carboxypeptidase to remove the terminal D-alanine of residual pentapeptide side chains. (About a year after the publication of our results (*27, 28*), the presence of transglycosylase-transpeptidase activities on PBP-1Bs was confirmed by other investigators (*49, 56*).

5. Purification and Properties of PBP-1A

The bifunctional enzyme activities to synthesize crosslinked peptidoglycan is not unique to PBP-1B(s). We recently demonstrated that a preparation of PBP-1A, the presumptive detour enzyme of PBP-1B(s) (*50, 54*), also catalyzes the formation of peptidoglycan from the lipid-linked precursor (*9, 18c*).

PBP-1A was purified from the cells of *E. coli* producing an excessively large amount of PBP-1A and lacking in PBP-1Bs (*27, 54*) by extraction with 1% Triton X-100, chromatography on a column of DEAE-cellulose, and chromatography on a column of 6-aminopenicillanic acid-Sepharose (*9*). The obtained preparation was free from contaminating proteins as judged by SDS-acrylamide gel electrophoresis and then staining with Coomassie brilliant blue and fluorography (*9*), and carried out synthesis of peptidoglycan from the lipid-linked precursor. The extent of crosslinkage of the peptidoglycan formed was about 8 to 16%. The formation of peptidoglycan (transglycosylase reaction) was completely inhibited in the presence of 0.1 μg per ml of macarbomycin and the crosslinking (transpeptidase reaction) was inhibited 50% or more by 0.1 μg per ml penicillin G, 0.2 μg per ml apalcillin, 10 μg per ml cephalexin, 0.05 μg per ml N-formimidoyl thienamycin, or 10 μg per ml nocardicin A (*6*, *9*, *18a*, *18c*, and unpublished experiments).

More precise work is necessary to determine that the active sites of the two enzymes, transglycosylase and transpeptidase, are located on the single peptide chain of PBP-1A. Because an appreciable difference in reaction conditions for the optimal activities between PBP-1A and PBP-1Bs was observed, these two kinds of proteins may be functioning to compensate for each other in the cells according to the culture conditions. Alternatively, the difference in the optimal reaction conditions could be a reflection of a mechanism regulating the enzyme activities of the two compensative proteins.

PBP-2 AND SPHERICAL MUTATIONS IN *E. COLI*

1. Cluster of Genes, mrdA and mrdB, Responsible for Formation of Rod-shaped Cells
Spratt previously found that mutants with thermosensitive PBP-2 are mecillinam resistant and cannot form a rod-shape at nonpermissive temperatures (*46*). The mutation was located close to the *lip* gene on the *E. coli* chromosome. Tamaki, Matsuzawa, and Matsuhashi (*51*) isolated another type of spherical, conditionally mecillinam-resistant mutants which have normal PBP-2 at both permissive and nonpermissive temperatures. Both mutations were recessive and located very close to each other. Complementation as detected in $+-/-+$ meroheterodiploids having the wild-type phenotype provided strong evidence that the two mutations are in different complementation groups. The mutation responsible for formation of thermosensitive PBP-2 was referred to as *mrd* (*murein cluster d*) *A* and another spherical mutation was referred to as *mrdB* (*51*). Transduction with phage P1 suggested that the most plausible gene order is *lip-mrdB-mrdA-leuS*. Previously Matsuzawa *et al.* (*24*) isolated a spherical mutant of *E. coli* and referred to the mutation as *rodA*, located close to *lip*. The *rodA* mutant had apparently normal PBP-2 and by complementation tests with *mrdA* and *mrdB* mutations the *rodA* gene seemed to be identical to the *mrdB* gene.

The *mrdA* mutants at 42°C had no PBP-2 and were very resistant to mecillinam but supersensitive to many β-lactam antibiotics such as ampicillin, cephalexin, cefoxitin, or nocardicin A at this temperature (*52*). At 30°C both PBP-2 and sensitivity to antibiotics were wild type. Contrary to *mrdA* mutants, *mrdB* mutants were spherical and supersensitive to mecillinam at 30°C, whereas at 42°C they showed phenotypes similar to *mrdA* mutants (*52*). The two genes *mrdA* and *mrdB* are supposed to be related to some step in the formation of the rod-shape of *E. coli*. Probably they are required for an initial step of elongation of the cell wall peptidoglycan sacculus of *E. coli* to ensure the formation of the correct rod-shape of the cell (*42*).

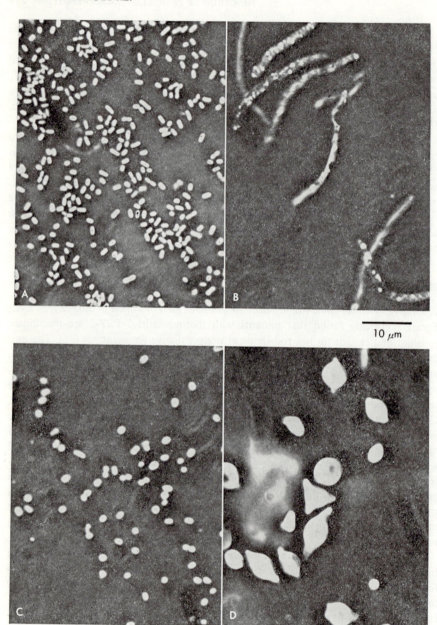

10 μm

10 μm

It is unknown if the loss of PBP-2 is lethal for the cells. The growth of some mutants producing very thermosensitive PBP-2 has been reported to be thermosensitive (*42, 46*). The growth of *mrdA* and *mrdB* mutants (*51*) was not thermosensitive. If the mutation in PBP-2 was combined in a cell with double mutation *mrc*-975-*mreA* (PBP-1A[overproduction] PBP-1Bs⁻ PBP-2⁻), the cell became thermosensitive. Combination of PBP-2⁻ mutation with a single *mreA* mutation caused isolation of a thermosensitive strain which formed elongated cells at 42°C in a low salt medium (Fig. 3A and B), and a thermoresistant strain, which at 42°C in a low salt medium formed very swollen cells with diameters 3 to 5 times larger than normal and with normal-sized caps at both ends (Fig. 3C and D). In high salt media the latter strain formed spherical cells at both temperatures (0.5% NaCl added).

These results may suggest that cells with impaired PBP-2 can abnormally elongate under certain circumstances, probably for instance, when PBP-1A is present in an excessively large amount and cells were cultured in a low salt medium.

Different names have been given to the structural gene of PBP-2: *pbpA* (*44*) and *rodA* (*50*). The latter nomenclature is surely misleading, because the *rodA* gene originally reported (*24*) is distinctly different from the gene of PBP-2. A new nomenclature, *mrdA*, was proposed for the structural gene of PBP-2 (*51*), because it seems to be involved in a cluster of genes related to the formation of the cell wall peptidoglycan sacculus which is located between *lip* and *leuS* on the *E. coli* chromosome, and which we referred to as the *mrd* cluster. The structural gene for PBP-5, which was referred to as *dacA* previously (*19, 21*), is also involved in the *mrd* cluster. Spratt, Boyd, and Stoker (*46a*) recently demonstrated by a fine mapping experiment using transducing phage λ that *dacA* is located between *rodA* (*mrdB*) and *lip* and therefore the gene order of the cluster will be *lip-dacA-rodA*(*mrdB*)*-pbpA*(*mrdA*)*-leuS*. According to our new nomenclature, *dacA* may be referred to as *mrdC*.

2. Genes mreB and mreC, Also Responsible for Formation of Rod-shape and Mecillinam Sensitivity

Normark (*36*) previously isolated a spherical mutant that was very resistant to mecillinam at 37°C. After transduction experiments, however, the original mutation was separated into two independent mutations, *i.e.*, the *envB* mutation, which seemed to be responsible for the formation of a spherical shape and high sensitivity to several β-lactam antibiotics including mecillinam, and the *sloB* mutation, which seemed to

←Fig. 3. Cell shape of *E. coli* double mutants, *mrdA-mreA* (PBP-1A[overproduction] PPB-2⁻).

Cells were grown on the agar plates of a rich low-salt medium (1% polypepton, Daigo Eiyo Chemical Co., Osaka, Japan, 0.5% Difco yeast extract, 0.1% glucose, 1.5% agar, Wako Pure Chemical Ind. Co., Osaka, Japan, 20 μg of thymine per ml, adjusted to pH 7.0). Dark-field phase contrast micrographs are shown. A and B: thermosensitive strain SREM24CD4-4 (derived from strain JST975 (*54*)). C and D: thermoresistant strain SREM24CD4-2 (derived from strain JST975 (*54*)). Incubation temperatures, 30°C (A and C); 42°C (B and D).

be responsible for the resistance to mecillinam (60). The *envB* mutation was mapped at about 70.3 min and the *sloB* mutation at about 72.8 min (2, 60). Similar mutations have been isolated in other laboratories (10, 23). We found a similar pair of mutations located close to *aroE* (71.7 min). The two mutations were tentatively referred to as *mreB* and *mreC*. The *mreB mreC* double mutants originally isolated were spherical and at 30°C supersensitive to mecillinam, but at 42°C they were resistant to this antibiotic. After P1-transduction (donor : *mreB*; recipient : *aroE*; selection : *Aro⁺*), wild type and spherical transductants (*mreB*-type) were obtained. The *mreB*-type transductants were at both temperatures spherical and supersensitive to mecillinam. The *mreB* mutation seemed therefore to be identical to or related to the *envB* mutation of Normark (36). Contrary to *mreB* mutants, the *mreC*-type transductants were rod-shaped and resistant to mecillinam at both temperatures. The *mreB*-type transductants were supersensitive to β-lactam antibiotics such as ampicillin, cephalexin, or cefoxitin at both temperatures, but *mreC*-type transductants were sensitive to these antibiotics. Both *mreB* and *mreC* mutations were recessive and seemed to belong to different complementation groups. A λ phage carrying the chromosomal part involving the *mreA*, *B*, and *C* genes was isolated (S. Nakajima-Iijima, 1981 Dissertation). From these results it seems that the *mreC* and *sloB* mutations are different.

A precise genetical analysis of *mreB* and *mreC* mutations are under investigation. Both *mreB* and *mreC* mutations are supposed to be involved in the process of formation of the rod-shaped cell wall peptidoglycan sacculus. Probably some of the spherical mutants are related to the peptidoglycan nicking (hydrolyzing) enzyme activity which is supposed to play an important role in combination with a peptidoglycan-synthetic enzyme in the formation of the rod-shaped sacculus (see later section, p. 211). Supersensitivity to β-lactam antibiotics of all the spherical mutant cells ever examined suggests that a step in the duplication of the spherical peptidoglycan sacculus is very sensitive to several β-lactam antibiotics, or the spherical peptidoglycan sacculus is more fragile and sensitive to mechanical, osmotic, or enzymatic damage than rodshaped, normal *E. coli* peptidoglycan saccul.

PBP-3 IN *E. COLI*, SEPTUM-SYNTHETASE PEPTIDOGLYCAN

Matsuzawa *et al.* (25) and Miyakawa *et al.* (26) first demonstrated that several genes related to the synthesis of peptidoglycan sacculi are located between *leuA* (1.6 min) and *azi* (2.5 min) on the *E. coli* chromosome (2) forming a cluster of genes. This cluster of genes was referred to as *mra* (*m*urein cluster *a*) (26). Later, the structural gene of PBP-3 was also located in this area. Different names were given to this gene: *pbpB* (44), *ftsI* (50), and *sep* (5). Spratt (42, 44) first isolated thermosensitive mutants with thermosensitive PBP-3 which at nonpermissive temperatures formed unseptated filament-shaped multinuclear cells. Based on this result and on other auxiliary evidences obtained by antibiotic experiments, he concluded that PBP-3 is responsible for the formation of the septum in *E. coli*.

Great difficulties, however, have been encountered in demonstrating the *in vitro* enzyme activity of PBP-3. The enzyme activities for formation of crosslinked peptidoglycan observed previously by Izaki *et al.* (*12, 13*) in *E. coli* membrane did not seem to involve activities of septum formation, because the crosslinking reaction observed was nearly insensitive to cephalexin, which has an affinity to PBP-3 and induces filamentous cells. After purification of PBP-1Bs by Nakagawa *et al.* (*18b, 19a, 26a, 27, 28*) the enzymatic activities forming crosslinked peptidoglycan of Izaki *et al.* (*12, 13*) were attributed to those of PBP-1Bs. Ishino and Matsuhashi (*8*) using a membrane preparation containing an excessively large amount of PBP-3 first demonstrated enzyme activities forming crosslinked peptidoglycan which are different from that of PBP-1Bs. The formation of peptidoglycan (transglycosylase reaction) was sensitive to enramycin and vancomycin, similar to PBP-1Bs, but the formation of crosslinkage (transpeptidase reaction) was very sensitive to apalcillin and cephalexin. Apalcillin is known to have a specifically high affinity to PBP-3 and induces long filamentous cells in *E. coli* and *Pseudomonas aeruginosa* (*33–35*). At least, however, an aliquot of these *in vitro* enzyme activities could be due to PBP-1A, because the membrane also contained this PBP. Finally in 1981, Ishino and Matsuhashi (manuscript submitted for publication) succeeded in demonstrating peptidoglycan synthetic activities in purified preparations of PBP-3.

The purified preparations carried out synthesis of crosslinked peptidoglycan from the lipid-linked precursor, N-acetylglucosaminyl-N-acetylmuramyl (pentapeptide)-PP-undecaprenol. The transglycosylase activity was completely inhibited by 1 μg per ml of moenomycin and the transpeptidase activity (crosslinking) was inhibited strongly by penicillin G, apalcillin or cephalexin, the β-lactam antibiotics which predominantly bind to PBP-3 and induce unseptated filamentous cells in *E. coli*. The concentrations of these β-lactam antibiotics required for inhibiting the transpeptidase activity of PBP-3 were 1/15 to 1/50 of those of PBP-1B. These results may explain how these β-lactam antibiotics induce filamentous cells of *E. coli* at concentrations lower than required for lysing the cells.

As far as we know, this is the first demonstration of septum-forming reactions *in vitro* by purified enzyme.

ENZYMATIC ACTIVITIES AND POSSIBLE FUNCTIONS OF LOWER MOLECULAR WEIGHT PBPs

1. PBP-4, a Protein Functioning as DD-Alanine Carboxypeptidase, DD-Endopeptidase, and Transpeptidase

Mutants of *E. coli* lacking PBP-4 were isolated (*11, 20*). The mutations *dacB* (*20*), located at 68.6 min on the *E. coli* chromosome map (*2*) caused deletion of very penicillin-sensitive enzymatic activities of DD-alanine carboxypeptidase, DD-endopeptidase, and transpeptidase and thus PBP-4 was identified with the DD-carboxypeptidase-endopeptidase system of Pollock *et al.* (*38*), Nguyen-Disteche *et al.* (*30*), and Nguyen-Distèche *et al.* (*31*), or with the D-alanine carboxypeptidase IB and IC of Tamura, Imae, and Strominger (*55*).

The *dacB* mutants grew normally and no phenotypical changes in cell shape or sensitivities to antibiotics were observed (*20*). Thus, it seems that PBP-4 is not the indispensable protein for proliferation of bacteria but its function is either compensable for by other PBP(s) or of secondary importance.

A unique property of *E. coli* PBP-4 is its DD-endopeptidase activity, which catalyzes splitting the D-alanyl-meso-diaminopimelyl (D-center) linkage of peptidoglycan or its lysozyme digests. A penicillin-insensitive enzyme with a similar DD-endopeptidase activity was also found in *E. coli* (*19, 20*) and was purified as shown in Table III. This enzyme is unique in that it is inhibited strongly by DNA (*59*) and this may

TABLE III. Purification of Penicillin-insensitive DD-Endopeptidase from *E. coli*

Step	Total protein (mg)	Total activity (U)	Specific activity (U/mg)	Purification		Yield (%)
Cell extract	1,650	338	0.21	—	—	(100)
100,000 × *g* supernatant	1,182	414	0.35	(1)	—	122
Ammonium sulfate fraction and dialysis	605	938	1.63	4.7	(1)	291
DEAE-cellulose	22.2	1,093	49.3	141	30	323
DNA-cellulose	0.45	348	767	2,190	466	102
Adsorption to and elution from *Micrococcus luteus* sacculi	0.10	207	2,069	5,910	1,260	61

Enzyme assay procedures by measuring the release of N-acetylglucosaminyl-N-acetylmuramyl-(L-Ala-D-glu-meso-[^{14}C]A$_2$pm-D-Ala) (referred to as [^{14}C]-disaccharide-tetrapeptide) from bis ([^{14}C]-disaccharide-tetrapeptide) (crosslinked) is as previously described (*59*). One enzyme unit was defined as the activity splitting 1 nmol of bis (disaccharide-tetrapeptide) per min at 37°C under the assay conditions (*59*).

Purification procedures. Cells (15 g wet weight) of *E. coli* K12 strain JST752 (*amiA* (*32*)) from the late exponential phase of growth were sonicated and 100,000 × *g* supernatant (60 min) was obtained. The ammonium sulfate fraction (35–60% saturation) of the supernatant was dissolved in 10 ml of 50 mM Tris HCl buffer, pH 7.6, and dialyzed overnight against the same buffer solution at 4°C. Fractionation on a column of DEAE-cellulose was as previously described (*59*). The flow-through fraction from the DEAE-cellulose column was concentrated by the polyethylene glycol method, dialyzed against 20 mM Tris acetic acid buffer, pH 6.0, subjected to affinity chromatography on a DNA-cellulose column (ϕ1.2 × 10 cm), and eluted with the same buffer, pH 6.0, with a concentration gradient of KCl from 0 to 0.5 M (total 150 ml eluting buffer). The active fractions were concentrated, dialyzed against the same buffer, pH 6.0, and the enzyme activity was adsorbed to 6.7 mg of *M. luteus* peptidoglycan (*41*) which was prewashed with the same buffer, pH 6.0, and then eluted with the buffer, pH 6.0, containing 0.08 M KCl and concentrated, and dialyzed against 50 mM Tris acetic acid buffer, pH 6.0. The enzyme may be kept frozen at −20°C. The presumably same enzyme was also purified by others (*15*).

suggest the possibility of an important function of this enzyme in duplication processes of *E. coli*. These results were later confirmed by others (*15*). Unlike PBP-4, the penicillin-insensitive DD-endopeptidase seemed to have no DD-carboxypeptidase and transpeptidase activity. It is highly tempting to suppose that PBP-4 and penicillin-insensitive DD-endopeptidase are functioning together as crosslinkage-splitting enzymes in duplication of the peptidoglycan sacculus and that the latter endopeptidase is responsible for the penicillin-induced cell lysis. It is also possible that PBP-4 functions not only as a hydrolytic enzyme but also as transpeptidase in construction of peptide crossbridges under certain conditions.

2. PBP-5 and PBP-6, Peptidoglycan DD-Alanine Carboxypeptidases?

PBP-5 and 6 were originally found as a doublet band on SDS/acrylamide gel electrophoresis after extensive purification (*55*). However, the genes coding for the two proteins are different (*21*). The structural gene of PBP-5, *dacA* (*19, 21, 46a*), was located between *lip* and *leuS* (see the previous section, p. 211) but that of PBP-6 is unknown. PBP-5 catalyzes the major activity of moderately penicillin-sensitive D-alanine carboxypeptidase 1A (*21*) measured with UDP-N-acetylmuramyl pentapeptide as substrate. Separation of PBP-5 and PBP-6 on a column was achieved by Amanuma and Strominger (*1*). These proteins are surely the most probable candidate for the enzyme functioning in removal of terminal D-alanine from the pentapeptide chains in the newly formed peptidoglycan (peptidoglycan DD-alanine carboxypeptidase activity).

  dacA mutants grew normally under a wide range of growth conditions, but were found to be supersensitive to many β-lactam antibiotics (*53*). Double-mutants, *dacA* and *dacB*, also grew normally and were supersensitive to β-lactam antibiotics. This suggests some importance of PBP-5 in the duplication of the normal peptidoglycan sacculus in *E. coli*.

PBPs IN GRAM-NEGATIVE BACILLI OTHER THAN *E. COLI*

1. Enterobacteria and Related Bacteria

Proteus (*37*) and several other bacteria (*45*) classified in Enterobacteriaceae and *P. aeruginosa* (*33–35*) were found to have PBPs similar to those of *E. coli*. They have PBPs which can be readily correlated respectively with PBP-2 and 3 of *E. coli* by specific binding of mecillinam or the β-lactam antibiotics that induce unseptated multinuclear filamentous cells. PBP-5s could be identified by their weak β-lactamase activity. Probably the functions of PBPs in these bacteria are similar to those of *E. coli*. There are reports suggesting that PBPs in *Vibrio* (*62*) and *Haemophilus influenzae* (*39*) are also similar to those in *E. coli*.

2. PBPs in Gram-negative Bacilli Not Closely Related to Enterobacteria

PBPs in *Caulobacter crescentus* have been reported (*18*). PBPs in species of *Thermus* (*18b*), *Cytophaga*, and *Flavobacterium* are shown in Fig. 4. PBPs in *Thermus* species (*18b*) are unique in that they are stable at 90°C. It seems to be impossible to correlate

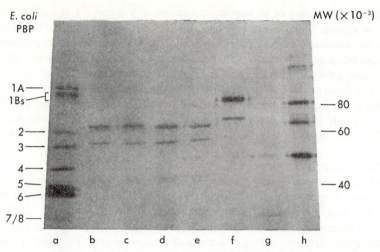

FIG. 4.   PBPs in rod-shaped bacteria not closely related to Enterobacteriaceae.
Fluorogram of SDS/acrylamide gel electrophoresis is shown. Experimental procedures
are practically as described previously (54). a, *E. coli* K12 strain W3110 (reference);
b, *Thermus thermophilus* strain HB8; c–e, three independently isolated strains of
Thermus sp.; f, *Cytophaga johnsonae* strain NCIB9059; g, *Flavobacterium flavescence*
strain AJ2453; h, *Bacillus subtilis* strain 6160 (gram-positive rod).

PBPs in these bacteria with those of *E. coli* by their pattern of SDS/polyacrylamide
gel electrophoresis and specificity of binding of β-lactam antibiotics. By the binding-
competition test, in which β-lactam antibiotics are added together with [^{14}C]peni-
cillin G, the highest molecular weight PBP of *Thermus thermophilus* strain HB8
(70 K) showed high affinities to most β-lactam antibiotics like penicillin G (standard),
apalcillin, cephaloglycin, cephaloridine, cephalexin, or cefmetazole, and the second-
highest molecular weight PBP (60 K) seemed to have a lower affinity to apalcillin
and cephalexin. The lowest molecular weight PBPs (45 K) seemed to have appreciably
high affinities only to penicillin G and cloxacillin among the above-mentioned antibiotics. No D-alanine carboxypeptidase activity as measured by the release of D-
alanine from UDP-N-acetylmuramyl pentapeptide was detected in membranes of
Thermus species (18b).

Genetic and biochemical investigations of individual PBPs are necessary in order
to identify the functions of PBPs of this group of bacteria.

DISCUSSION

The peptidoglycan sacculus is a rigid structure covering the whole cell of bacteria.
In gram-negative bacteria, the sacculus is supposed to consist of a single layer of
peptidoglycan network. Activities of peptidoglycan lytic enzymes which nick the

peptidoglycan network at a specific position on the sacculus have been supposed to be necessary in order to ensure that the peptidoglycan synthetic enzymes function. By assuming a cooperative mechanism of nicking enzymes and synthetic enzymes, the following hypothetical scheme for the duplication of the peptidoglycan sacculus in *E. coli* will be proposed. The total processes are divided tentatively into the following four steps: (1) initiation of elongation of sacculus, (2) elongation of sacculus, (3) septum formation, and (4) postfissional separation of sacculi.

The presumptive first step, initiation of elongation of the sacculus, may be started by the action of a specific nicking enzyme(s) at the center of the sacculus, the growing point. This may allow the insertion of small pieces of newly formed peptidoglycan (initiation piece) into the nick by specific synthetic enzyme activities: transglycosylase and transpeptidase. The most plausible candidate of this synthetic enzyme(s) may be PBP-2. Inactivation of nicking enzyme activities may disturb the synthetic enzyme activities' function of forming initiation pieces, causing inhibition of elongation of the sacculus so that the sacculus divides to form a spherical shape without elongation. Inactivation of the synthetic enzyme activities may cause cell lysis and/or inhibition of elongation of the sacculus. In both cases spherical cells may be formed. Inactivation of nicking enzyme activities will also cause resistance of the cell to mecillinam, because PBP-2, the mecillinam-sensitive protein, cannot function.

In the second step, elongation of the sacculus, cooperative actions of specific nicking enzymes and synthetic enzymes, PBP-1A and 1B(s), will cause elongation of the sacculus until its length reaches twice the original length. Inhibition of both PBP-1A and 1B(s) causes a bulge-formation at the growing point of the cell followed by cell lysis. Inhibition of the nicking enzyme activities could cause interference with elongation of the sacculus. However, another possible phenotype of the cell caused by inhibition of nicking enzyme activities may be tolerance to the lysis by β-lactam antibiotics which preferentially inhibit PBP-1A and PBP-1Bs.

There seems to be no doubt that PBP-3 is involved in the process of septation, because inhibition of PBP-3 causes formation of unseptated filamentous cells (*42*), which is followed by lysis of the cells. It is, however, unknown whether any PBPs other than PBP-3 are involved in septation. Inhibition of presumptive nicking enzyme activities in this step may probably cause either formation of filamentous cells or tolerance of the cells to the β-lactam antibiotics which inhibit septum formation and cause subsequently lysis by binding to PBP-3.

Nothing is known about the mechanism of separation of sacculi in *E. coli*. In gram-positive pneumococci (*58*) and staphylococci (ref. *7* and manuscript in preparation) the enzyme responsible for the postfissional cell-separation and lysis caused by penicillin seemed to be owing to the N-acetylmuramyl-L-alanine amidase activity. The amidase activity exists abundantly in *E. coli* cells. However, its function in *E. coli* is unknown, because the mutation in the gene *amiA* (52 min) (ref. *32* and manuscript in preparation), which is responsible for the action of N-acetylmuramyl-L-alanine amidase, did not cause inhibition of cell separation or tolerance to β-lactam antibiotics.

Our present knowledge about lytic enzymes is still too insufficient. In recent years, a novel muramidase that splits the β-1,4-muramyl glycosidic linkage of peptidoglycan with formation of a 1,6-cyclic muramyl terminus was reported (7, *59a*). Penicillin-insensitive DD-endopeptidase and its inhibition by DNA were found as described in the previous section (see p. 215) (*59*). Several *E. coli* mutants which are tolerant to the lysis caused by several β-lactam antibiotics were isolated (*16, 32*). Cloning of the tolerance genes and identification of the gene products may provide most useful information about the functions of nicking enzyme activities.

There is, however, no evidence so far to conclude that specific nicking enzyme activities exist and are differentiated as proposed for PBPs (*18c*) for steps of the duplication of the sacculus. Study of the function of nicking enzymes will surely provide a most interesting target of investigation on cell wall synthesis, cell duplication, and the mode of action of β-lactam antibiotics.

Acknowledgments

The authors are very much obliged to Drs. S. Mitsuhashi, H. Hashimoto, and M. Inoue, Gumma University Medical School, for their encouragement, help, and advice during the present investigations and to Dr. H. Shimizu in the Basic Research Laboratories, Toray Ind. Inc., for providing us with pure sacculi of *Micrococcus luteus*.

REFERENCES

1. Amanuma, H. and Strominger, J. L. 1980. *J. Biol. Chem.*, **255**, 11173–11180.
1a. Anderson, J. S., Matsuhashi, M., Haskin, M. A., and Strominger, J. L. 1965. *Proc. Natl. Acad. Sci. U.S.A.*, **53**, 881–889.
2. Bachmann, B. J. and Low, K. B. 1980. *Microbiol. Rev.*, **44**, 1–56.
3. Blumberg, P. M. and Strominger, J. L. 1974. *Bacteriol. Rev.*, **38**, 291–335.
4. Clarke, L. and Carbon, J. 1976. *Cell*, **9**, 91–99.
5. Fletcher, G., Irwin, C. A., Henson, J. M., Fillingim, C., Malone, M. M., and Walker, J. R. 1978. *J. Bacteriol.*, **133**, 91–100.
6. Hashizume, T., J., Ishino, F., and Matsuhashi, M. 1981. *Antimicrob. Agents Chemother.*, in preparation.
7. Höltje, J.-V., Mirelman, D., Sharon, N., and Schwarz, U. 1975. *J. Bacteriol.*, **124**, 1067–1076.
8. Ishino, F. and Matsuhashi, M. 1979. *Agric. Biol. Chem.*, **43**, 2641–2642.
9. Ishino, F., Mitsui, K., Tamaki, S., and Matsuhashi, M. 1980. *Biochem. Biophys. Res. Commun.*, **97**, 287–293.
10. Iwaya, M., Jones, C. W., Khorana, J., and Strominger, J. L. 1978. *J. Bacteriol.*, **133**, 196–202.
11. Iwaya, M. and Strominger, J. L. 1977. *Proc. Natl. Acad. Sci. U.S.A.*, **74**, 2980–2984.
12. Izaki, K., Matsuhashi, M., and Strominger, J. L. 1966. *Proc. Natl. Acad. Sci. U.S.A.*, **55**, 656–663.

13. Izaki, K., Matsuhashi, M., and Strominger, J. L. 1968. *J. Biol. Chem.*, **243**, 3180–3192.

14. Kamiryo, T. and Strominger, J. L. 1974. *J. Bacteriol.*, **117**, 568–577.

15. Keck, W. and Schwarz, U. 1979. *J. Bacteriol.*, **139**, 770–774.

16. Kitano, K. and Tomasz, A. 1979. *J. Bacteriol.*, **140**, 955–963.

17. Koyama, T., Yamada, M., and Matsuhashi, M. 1977. *J. Bacteriol.*, **129**, 1518–1523.

18. Koyasu, S., Fukuda, A., and Okada, Y. 1980. *J. Biochem.*, **87**, 363–366.

18a. Kunugita, K., Tamaki, S., and Matsuhashi, M. 1981. *In* "β-Lactam Antibiotic-Mode of Action, New Developments and Future Prospects," ed. by M. R. J. Salton, Academic Press, New York, in press.

18b. Matsuhashi, M., Doi, M., Ishino, F., Nakagawa, J., Matsuhashi, M., Ohta, T., and Ohshima, T. 1979. *Seikagaku (Tokyo)*, **51**, 831.

18c. Matsuhashi, M., Ishino, F., Nakagawa, J., Mitsui, K., Nakajima-Iijima, S., and Tamaki, S. 1981. *In* "β-Lactam Antibiotic-Mode of Action, New Developments and Future Prospects," ed. by M. R. J. Salton, Akademic Press, New York, in press.

19. Matsuhashi, M., Maruyama, I. N., Takagaki, Y., Tamaki, S., Nishimura, Y., and Hirota, Y. 1978. *Proc. Natl. Acad. Sci. U.S.A.*, **75**, 2631–2635.

19a. Matsuhashi, M., Noguchi, H., and Tamaki, S. 1979. *Chemotherapy (Tokyo)*, **27**, 827–840.

20. Matsuhashi, M., Takagaki, Y., Maruyama, I. N., Tamaki, S., Nishimura, Y., Suzuki, H., Ogino, U., and Hirota, Y. 1977. *Proc. Natl. Acad. Sci. U.S.A.*, **74**, 2976–2979.

21. Matsuhashi, M., Tamaki, S., Curtis, S. J., and Strominger, J. L. 1979. *J. Bacteriol.*, **137**, 644–647.

22. Matsuhashi, M., Tamaki, S., Nakajima, S., Nakagawa, J., Tomioka, S., and Takagaki, Y. 1979. *In* "Microbial Drug Resistance," ed. by S. Mitsuhashi, Japan Sci. Soc. Press, Tokyo/Univ. Park Press, Baltimore, Vol. 2, pp. 389–404.

23. Matsuhashi, S., Kamiryo, T., Blumberg, P. M., Linnett, P., Willoughby, E., and Strominger, J. L. 1974. *J. Bacteriol.*, **117**, 578–587.

24. Matsuzawa, H., Hayakawa, K., Sato, T., and Imahori, K. 1973. *J. Bacteriol.*, **115**, 436–442.

25. Matsuzawa, H., Matsuhashi, M., Oka, A., and Sugino, Y. 1969. *Biochem. Biophys. Res. Commun.*, **36**, 682–689.

26. Miyakawa, T., Matsuzawa, H., Matsuhashi, M., and Sugino, Y. 1972. *J. Bacteriol.*, **112**, 950–958.

26a. Nakagawa, J. and Matsuhashi, M. 1980. *Agric. Biol. Chem.*, **44**, 3041–3044.

27. Nakagawa, J., Matsuzawa, H., and Matsuhashi, M. 1979. *J. Bacteriol.*, **138**, 1029–1032.

28. Nakagawa, J., Tamaki, S., and Matsuhashi, M. 1979. *Agric. Biol. Chem.*, **43**, 1379–1380.

29. Nakajima, S., Matsuzawa, H., Tamaki, S., and Matsuhashi, M. 1979. Abstr.

222   MATSUHASHI ET AL.

the Annual Meeting of the American Society for Microbiology, 1979, p. 173.
30. Nguyen-Distèche, M., Ghuysen, J.-M., Pollock, J. J., Reynolds, P., Perkins, H. R., Coyette, J., and Salton, M. R. J. 1974. *Eur. J. Biochem.*, **41**, 447–455.
31. Nguyen-Distèche, M., Pollock, J. J., Ghuysen, J.-M., Puig, J., Reynolds, P., Perkins, H. R., Coyette, J., and Salton, M. R. J. 1974. *Eur. J. Biochem.*, **41**, 457–463.
32. Nikaido, T., Tomioka, S., and Matsuhashi, M. 1979. *Agric. Biol. Chem.*, **43**, 2639–2640.
33. Noguchi, H., Matsuhashi, M., and Mitsuhashi, S. 1979. *Eur. J. Biochem.*, **100**, 41–49.
34. Noguchi, H., Matsuhashi, M., Nikaido, T., Itoh, J., Matsubara, N., Takaoka, M., and Mitsuhashi, S. 1979. *In* "Microbial Drug Resistance," ed. by S. Mitsuhashi, Japan Sci. Soc. Press, Tokyo/Univ. Park Press, Baltimore, Vol. 2, pp. 361–387.
35. Noguchi, H., Matsuhashi, M., Takaoka, M., and Mitsuhashi, S. 1978. *Antimicrob. Agents Chemother.*, **14**, 617–624.
36. Normark, S. 1969. *J. Bacteriol.*, **98**, 1274–1277.
37. Ohya, S., Yamazaki, M., Sugawara, S., and Matsuhashi, M. 1979. *J. Bacteriol.*, **137**, 474–479.
38. Pollock, J. J., Nguyen-Distèche, M., Ghuysen, J.-M., Coyette, J., Linder, R., Salton, M. R. J., Kim, K. S., Perkins, H. R., and Reynolds, P. 1974. *Eur. J. Biochem.*, **41**, 439–446.
39. Saito, K., Ubukata, K., and Konno, M. 1978. Abstr. the 26th Annual Meetings of the Japan. Soc. Chemother., No. 169.
39a.Sekiguchi, R. and Yokota, K. 1979. Abstr. the 52th Annual Meetings of the Japan. Soc. Bacteriol., p. 3-II-9.
40. Shepherd, S. T., Chase, H. A., and Reynolds, P. E. 1977. *Eur. J. Biochem.*, **78**, 521–532.
41. Shimizu, H., Tamura, G., and Arima, K. 1979. *Agric. Biol. Chem.*, **43**, 1483–1492.
42. Spratt, B. G. 1975. *Proc. Natl. Acad. Sci. U.S.A.*, **72**, 2999–3003.
43. Spratt, B. G. 1977. *Eur. J. Biochem.*, **72**, 341–352.
44. Spratt, B. G. 1977. *J. Bacteriol.*, **131**, 293–305.
45. Spratt, B. G. 1977. *J. Antimicrob. Chemother.*, **3** (Suppl. B), 13–19.
46. Spratt, B. G. 1978. *Nature*, **274**, 713–715.
46a.Spratt, B. G., Boyd, A., and Stoker, N. 1980. *J. Bacteriol.*, **143**, 569–581.
47. Spratt, B. G., Jobanputra, V., and Schwarz, U. 1977. *FEBS Lett.*, **79**, 374–378.
48. Spratt, B. G. and Pardee, A. B. 1975. *Nature*, **254**, 516–517.
49. Suzuki, H., van Heijenoort, Y., Tamura, T., Mizoguchi, J., Hirota, Y., and van Heijenoort, J. 1980. *FEBS Lett.*, **110**, 245–249.
50. Suzuki, H., Nishimura, Y., and Hirota, Y. 1978. *Proc. Natl. Acad. Sci. U.S.A.*, **75**, 664–668.
51. Tamaki, S., Matsuzawa, H., and Matsuhashi, M. 1980. *J. Bacteriol.*, **141**, 52–57.

52. Tamaki, S., Matsuzawa, H., Nakajima-Iijima, S., and Matsuhashi, M. 1980. *Agric. Biol. Chem.*, **44**, 2683–2693.
53. Tamaki, S., Nakagawa, J., Maruyama, I. N., and Matsuhashi, M. 1978. *Agric. Biol. Chem.*, **42**, 2147–2150.
54. Tamaki, S., Nakajima, S., and Matsuhashi, M. 1977. *Proc. Natl. Acad. Sci. U.S.A.*, **74**, 5472–5476.
55. Tamura, T., Imae, Y., and Strominger, J. L. 1976. *J. Biol. Chem.*, **251**, 414–423.
56. Tamura, T., Suzuki, H., Nishimura, Y., Mizobuchi, J., and Hirota, Y. 1980. *Proc. Natl. Acad. Sci. U.S.A.*, **77**, 4499–4503.
57. Tipper, D. J. and Strominger, J. L. 1965. *Proc. Natl. Acad. Sci. U.S.A.*, **54**, 1133–1141.
58. Tomasz, A. and Waks, S. 1975. *Proc. Natl. Acad. Sci. U.S.A.*, **72**, 4162–4166.
59. Tomioka, S. and Matsuhashi, M. 1978. *Biochem. Biophys. Res. Commun.*, **84**, 978–984.
59a. Taylor, A., Das, B. C., and van Heijenoort, J. 1975. *Eur. J. Biochem.*, **53**, 47–54.
60. Westling-Häggström, B. and Normark, S. 1975. *J. Bacteriol.*, **123**, 75–82.
61. Wise, E. M. and Park, J. T. 1965. *Proc. Natl. Acad. Sci. U.S.A.*, **54**, 75–81.

RECOGNITION OF PENICILLINS BY β-LACTAMASE: THE ROLE OF THE SIDE CHAIN

Nathan CITRI

Institute of Microbiology, Hebrew University-Hadassah Medical School*

I have been asked to contribute a brief review of our work on the role of the N-acyl substituent in the recognition of substrate by β-lactamase.

For clarity, I shall limit my review to the interaction of penicillins with a single species of β-lactamase I (EC 3.5.2.6) isolated from the culture supernatant of *Bacillus cereus* strain 569/H. This is not to say that the phenomena described below are uniquely related to some unusual properties of that β-lactamase. On the contrary, there are indications, both from our and other laboratories, that some other β-lactamases which have been adequately examined appear to follow a similar pattern of response to their substrates. The differences which did emerge are in detail rather than in principle, and in the choice of methodological tools most appropriate for the enzyme under study.

If penicillin is defined as an N-acyl derivative of 6-aminopenicillanic acid (APA) (*8*), all differences among penicillins stem from differences in the structure of the N-acyl substituent ("side chain"). And when penicillins are examined as substrates for β-lactamase, we do indeed observe that they differ in their affinity for the enzyme and in the rate at which they are hydrolyzed at saturation. Hence the side chain of the substrate does influence the binding and catalytic constants of the enzymic reaction. This is not unexpected, and in fact has been at first perceived as an obvious case of steric hindrance. The idea was that a bulky side chain will hinder the access of the substrate to the catalytic site and thus confer on the penicillin a degree of resistance to β-lactamase. It still persists as part of the disturbing myth that semi-synthetic penicillins are "tailor-made" to meet the increasing demands of antibacterial therapy. (Imagine the tailor who, unconcerned with the shape of his client, proffers many thousands of useless sartorial creations before producing anything acceptable.)

The effect of the side chain on the properties of a penicillin can be deduced by reference to the unsubstituted APA molecule. When that is done for all penicillins

* Jerusalem, Israel.

which have been studied as substrates of β-lactamase the result is surprising. As a rule the side chain improves the binding of the spbstrate, although it may either retard or accelerate the rate of hydrolysis of the β-lactam ring. In other words, there are two types of known N-acyl substituents: one, termed the A-type, which interferes with the β-lactamase reaction, and another, termed the S-type, which promotes it. In looking for a mechanism consistent with the contrasting effects of the two types of side chains it is clear that steric hindrance in the accepted sense plays no role in protecting the β-lactam ring (9). (The K_m is similarly lowered by both types of side chain). It is almost inevitable that we postulate *a priori* a conformational change induced in the enzyme by the presence of a side chain. The change induced by an S-type side chain would improve the catalytic efficiency of the enzyme, whereas that induced by an A-type side chain would have the opposite effect.

What then is the evidence for two types of conformational transitions corresponding to the two types of N-acyl substituents in the substrate? The simplest kind of evidence is illustrated schematically in Fig. 1. We select conditions which allow us to follow the rate of inactivation of the enzyme by heat, urea, proteolysis, or iodination (5, 7, 10). The rate of inactivation is then examined in the presence of saturating substrate concentrations. With an A-type substrate (*i.e.*, a penicillin carrying an A-type side chain) the rate of inactivation is dramatically accelerated. Conversely, all S-type substrates protect the enzyme against inactivation. The unsubstituted APA has no effect. Furthermore, in the presence of both types (A and S)

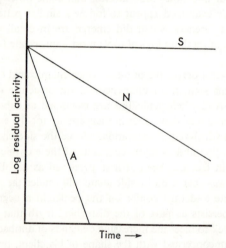

FIG. 1.   The rate of inactivation of β-lactamase is determined by the side chain of the substrate.

Inactivation by either heat, urea, iodination, or proteolytic enzymes is accelerated (A) by penicillins with A-type side chains and retarded or prevented (S) by penicillins with S-type side chains. The rate of inactivation observed in the absence of substrates (N) is not affected by APA, which has no side chain.

the rate of inactivation is intermediate and consistent with the relative affinities of the substrates for the enzyme and their molar ratios. This is as expected, since both ligands compete for the same binding site (5, 7).

It is fortunate that reversible conformational transitions, induced by closely related substrates (compare the structure of benzylpenicillin, an S-type, and methicillin, an A-type penicillin) can be so readily detected and differentiated by simple and in part independent, criteria. This in itself does not indicate that the changes in conformation extend beyond the binding site: the rates of inactivation, serve to detect and greatly amplify changes which are important in the function, rather than the morphology, of the enzyme. The topology and extent of the conformational changes can be deduced from a more recent report on the effect of A substrates (methicillin and cloxacillin) on the hydrogen exchange in β-lactamase (12). About half of the hydrogen atoms probed in the enzyme were affected and their half-life changed from 20 hr to 45 min. By contrast, benzylpenicillin had no detectable effect on hydrogen exchange. This is consistent with the view that the powerful effect of S-type side chains on the stability and catalytic efficiency of the enzyme is topologically restricted to the binding site.

Returning to the scheme in Fig. 1, we note that the rate of inactivation in the presence of a saturating class-A substrate follows first-order kinetics. At subsaturating substrate concentrations a family of slopes is obtained for which first-order rate constants can be derived. A double-reciprocal plot of such rate constants against the respective substrate concentrations yields an equilibrium constant, termed K_{CR} and representing that substrate concentration which induces a half-maximal change in the conformation of the enzyme (6, 22). And, since the change is induced by the formation of an enzyme-substrate complex, it was expected to be half-maximal at half-saturation ($K_{CR} = K_{diss}$). Yet the K_{CR} values turned out to be consistently lower than the corresponding dissociation constants derived from appropriately corrected K_m or K_i values (22). That was taken to mean that part of the free enzyme was reacting as if in an enzyme-substrate complex, presumably because there was a significant lag between the dissociation of that complex and the recovery of the native conformation of the enzyme. Here was the first indication of a hysteretic behavior (11) of β-lactamase in responding to A penicillins. Indeed, close examination of the kinetics of the catalytic reaction revealed that, unlike S substrates which are hydrolyzed at a constant rate, substrates of type A show biphasic kinetics (19): an initial, decelerating phase followed by a linear phase (Fig. 2). In a subsequent study (9) we have shown that the affinity for such substrates undergoes a parallel change; the decrease in k_{cat} is accompanied by a corresponding decrease in K_m. The significance of these time-dependent changes became obvious when we found that both initial parameters are unrelated to the structure of the side chain and, in fact, approximate those of the unsubstituted APA (9). (The much lower K_{cat} and K_m values, characteristic of each substrate, are reached in the second phase, which is the source of the conventionally derived parameters found in the literature). It became evident that in the initial encounter the enzyme fails to respond to an A-type side chain by

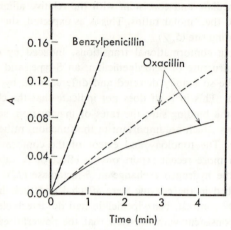

FIG. 2. The side chain determines the course of hydrolysis of a penicillin by β-lactamase.

The kinetics are linear with benzylpenicillin, a typical S-type penicillin, but biphasic with oxacillin, and all other A-type penicillins. Antibodies to β-lactamase, which have no effect on the hydrolysis of benzylpenicillin (broken line) prevent the kinetic shift and thus appear to stimulate the hydrolysis of oxacillin (9).

a perceptible change in conformation. The progressive conformational adjustment and the eventual acquisition of the final reaction parameters require the turnover of many substrate molecules in the course of the decelerating phase of the catalytic reaction. The cumulative impact of the side chain is, of course, consistent with the hysteretic properties of the enzyme. The gradual acquisition of binding and catalytic parameters specific for class A substrates implied that the enzyme is flexible enough to progressively adapt to the structural complications introduced by A-type substituents (see below). Indeed, when the conformational freedom of β-lactamase is restrained, the adaptation is prevented. A very effective constraint can be attained by the use of homologous antibodies. The enzyme molecule can accommodate two antibody molecules, of which one binds away from the active site and thus has no effect on the hydrolysis of S penicillins. When combined with that antibody alone (23), the enzyme, now partly stabilized in the native conformation (24), fails to display the biphasic kinetics of hydrolysis of A substrates and retains the initial parameters of binding and catalysis (Fig. 2). When first discovered by Pollock (18) the antibody was perceived as, and termed, "stimulating" and its effect was attributed to an ability to mold and thus improve the conformation of the enzyme (18). Such ability, even if known to exist, is of course not necessary, and restriction of the conformational freedom by other, nonspecific means, such as immobilization (13) or crosslinking (14) has since been shown to have a similar effect. With a suitable bifunctional reagent it is even possible to crosslink the enzyme in the presence of a substrate and obtain a catalytically active derivative which retains indefinitely some of the conformational changes induced by that substrate (15). Although at this stage too crude to provide us with much insight, such derivatives demonstrate that it is possible to alter the properties of an enzyme in a predictable or even desirable way by learning to control its specific conformational responses.

The isolation of substrate-guided derivatives provides direct evidence that the conformational states corresponding to the A and S substrates are indeed different. Yet there is nothing obvious in the chemical structure of a side chain that will make it recognizable as belonging to the A or S class. What is more, the rotation of a side chain of either class about the C-N bond is similarly hindered, with a preferred orientation that is virtually independent of its structure (1, 21). The structural basis for the contrasting effects of A- and S-type penicillins has been found, perhaps surprisingly, in the energetics of rotation *within* the side chain. Independent studies by Blanpain and Durant (1–4) and by Samuni and Meyer (21) have provided evidence for energy barriers within A-type side chains which are not seen in S-type side chains. This evidence is based on computed conformational energy maps (21) and on crystallographic (1–4) and NMR (1) data obtained for representative substrate molecules. A careful analysis of the data has led Blanpain et al. to the illuminating conclusion that the feature distinguishing an A-type penicillin is the *rigidity*, rather than the *shape*, of its side chain. It provides a tangible reason for the strenuous, protracted conformational adjustment reflected in the biphasic hydrolysis of such substrates. And when optimal binding of each inflexible and, implicitly, unique structure is finally attained, it is at the expense of the catalytic efficiency and general stability of the enzyme.

The conformational response of β-lactamase to its varied substrates is but one example of the widely documented, and possibly general, phenomenon of conformational adaptability in enzymes (6, 16, 17). The biological meaning of that phenomenon is not understood, but in view of the observations reported above we were led to assume that enzyme specificity may ultimately depend on the conformational adaptability of the enzyme molecule (6). In other words, the native conformation of the active site is capable of recognizing the basic structural features common to all its substrates and competitive inhibitors, but may need to adapt the structural details in which they differ among themselves. The adaptation may be virtually instant, as in β-lactamase and class S substrates (and probably most other enzyme-substrate systems) or it may be a cumulative process as described above for class A substrates. In biological terms a distinction between native and acquired specificity makes good sense. It provides a plausible solution to the perplexing problem of the origin of enzyme specificity.

The evolution of an enzyme with a β-lactam binding site presents no conceptual difficulty. That basic level of specificity is inherent in the native structure, and determined by the sequence, and consequent folding, of the protein. It is hardly conceivable, and there is no need to assume, that the parameters specifying the interaction of the enzyme with each present or future semi-synthetic penicillin are similarly predetermined (6, 20). The precise discrimination among nearly identical β-lactam derivatives appears to depend on the conformational freedom which evolution has carefully preserved and which allows the enzyme to respond to the structural details of the substrate. If we maintain that this is the source of the fine specificity of the enzyme, we must look for evidence that the response in conformation is equally specific.

To illustrate, let us consider the family of isoxazolyl penicillins (Fig. 3) where minor modifications within the side chain are known to alter the K_m and k_{cat} values acquired in the catalytic reaction (9). We attribute the altered parameters to an altered conformation and thus imply that each member of that family induces a distinct conformational change in the enzyme. Direct evidence for such subtle conformational

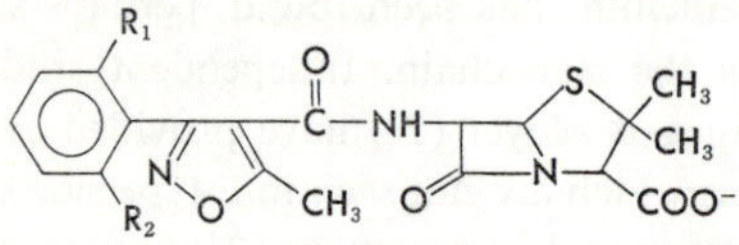

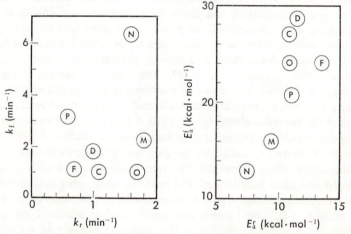

FIG. 3. The general structure of an isoxazolyl penicillin.

The four members of the isoxazolyl family included in our studies are; oxacillin ($R_1=R_2=H$); cloxacillin ($R_1=H$; $R_2=Cl$); dicloxacillin ($R_1=R_2=Cl$); and fluocloxacillin ($R_1=F$; $R_2=Cl$).

FIG. 4. Individual A-type penicillins can be identified by their effect on the conformation of β-lactamase.

The position of each penicillin is specified (on the left) by 8–10 determinations of the conformational transition rate constants, k_f and k_r, described in the text. It is also specified (on the right) by 4–6 replicate determinations of the activation energies of the corresponding conformational transitions. For further details see ref. 20. O, oxacillin; C, cloxacillin; F, fluocloxacillin; D, dicloxacillin; M, methicillin; N, nafcillin; P, pyrazocillin.

differences is unavailable, and probably unattainable by existing methods, but their existence can be inferred, and even quantitatively expressed, by making use of the following observations.

As shown above, the conformational adjustment to an A-type substrate is time dependent. In addition, no further lag is seen when that substrate is replaced with another substrate of the same type, indicating that conformational states induced by A-type substrates are very similar if not identical. However, replacement with an S-type substrate requires a major conformational adjustment which is time dependent (9).

We have thus two kinds of conformational transitions which can be quantitated: a transition from native to A-type conformation and a transition from A-type to S-type (benzylpenicillin-induced) conformation. The rate constants of these transitions (k_f and k_r, respectively) depend entirely on the precise structure of the A-type side chain, as do the corresponding activation energies of the conformational transitions (Fig. 4). Of particular interest are the parameters discriminating among the closest members of the isoxazolyl family of penicillins (Fig. 3). The exquisite precision of the conformational response is certainly adequate to explain the fine specificity of β-lactamase. It remains to be seen whether the specificity of other biologically active proteins is ultimately determined by conformational adaptability. But, in our present state of knowledge, it is difficult to conceive of an alternative to such "openended specificity" as the course favored by evolution.

REFERENCES

1. Blanpain, P. C., Nagy, J. B., Laurent, G. H., and Durant, F. V. 1980. *J. Med. Chem.*, **23**, 1283–1292.
2. Blanpain, P. C., Melebeck, M., and Durant, F. V. 1977. *Acta Cryst. B*, **33**, 580–582.
3. Blanpain, P. C., Laurent, G.H., and Durant, F. V. 1977. *Bull. Soc. Chim. Belg.*, **86**, 767–775.
4. Blanpain, P. C. and Durant, F. V. 1977. *Cryst. Struct. Commun.*, **6**, 711–716.
5. Citri, N. 1971. *In* "The Enzymes," ed. by P. D. Boyer, 3rd, Ed. Academic Press, New York, Vol. 4, pp. 23–46.
6. Citri, N. 1973. *Adv. Enzymol.*, **37**, 397–648.
7. Citri, N. and Garber, N. 1962. *J. Pharm. Pharmacol.*, **14**, 784–797.
8. Citri, N. and Pollock, M. R. 1966. *In* "Advances in Enzymology," ed. by F. F. Nord, John Wiley and Sons, Inc., New York, Vol. 28, pp. 237–323.
9. Citri, N., Samuni, A., and Zyk, N. 1976. *Proc. Natl. Acad. Sci. U.S.A.*, **73**, 1048–1052.
10. Citri, N. and Zyk, N. 1965. *Biochim. Biophys. Acta.*, **99**, 427–441.
11. Frieden, C. 1970. *J. Biol. Chem.* **245**, 5788–5799.
12. Kiener, P. A. and Waley, S. G. 1977. *Biochem. J.*, **165**, 279–285.
13. Klemes, Y. and Citri, N. 1979. *Biotechnol. Bioeng.*, **21**, 897–905.
14. Klemes, Y. and Citri, N. 1979. *Biochim. Biophys. Acta*, **567**, 401–409.

15. Klemes, Y. and Citri, N. 1980. *Biochem. J.*, **187**, 529–532.
16. Koshland, D. E., Jr. 1958. *Proc. Natl. Acad. Sci. U.S.A.*, **44**, 98–104.
17. Koshland, D. E., Jr. and Neet, K. E. 1968. *Annu. Rev. Biochem.*, **37**, 359–410.
18. Pollock, M. R. 1964. *Immunology*, **7**, 707–723.
19. Samuni, A. and Citri, N. *Biochem. Biophys. Res. Commun.*, **62**, 7–11.
20. Samuni, A. and Citri, N. 1979. *Mol. Pharmacol.*, **16**, 250–255.
21. Samuni, A. and Meyer, A. Y. 1978. *Mol. Pharmacol.*, **14**, 704–709.
22. Zyk, N. and Citri, N. 1967. *Biochim. Biophys. Acta*, **146**, 219–226.
23. Zyk, N. and Citri, N. 1968. *Biochim. Biophys. Acta*, **159**, 317–326.
24. Zyk, N. and Citri, N. 1968. *Biochim. Biophys. Acta*, **159**, 327–339.

6 PHARMACOKINETICS

GASTROINTESTINAL ABSORPTION OF β-LACTAM ANTIBIOTICS

Akira Tsuji*[1] and Tsukinaka Yamana*[2]

Department of Pharmaceutics, Faculty of Pharmaceutical Sciences[1] *and Hospital Pharmacy,*[2] *Kanazawa University*

A great deal of information is now available concerning the comparative serum levels after oral admintstration of a variety of penicillins (1, 15) and cephalosporins (2, 11) to humans. But it is not always easy to discuss and compare the gastrointestinal (GI) absorption rate and its mechanism from only the serum level data because complex kinetic processes such as dissolution of solid antibiotics, degradation in the GI, absorption through the GI membrane, distribution into tissues, and elimination from the body may determine the serum levels (see Fig. 1).

For example, let us compare the blood levels of three similar types of penicillins, oxacillin, cloxacillin, and dicloxacillin. Early comparisons of blood levels of these three compounds, following oral administration of 500 mg doses, showed that dicloxacillin produced a dramatically higher blood-time profile than cloxacillin, which, in turn, was higher than that of oxacillin (6). Understandably, this was initially interpreted as being a difference in oral absorption. But when these same three antibiotics were given by continuous i.v. infusion, the same relative order was observed with dicloxacillin dramatically higher than cloxacillin which was somewhat higher than oxacillin (17). Therefore, absorption cannot be the sole cause for the observed differences in the plasma-time profiles after oral administration. A similar relationship between plasma-time profiles after oral and i.v. administration was observed for phenoxypenicillin derivatives, penicillin V, phenethicillin, and propicillin (15).

β-Lactam antibiotics are susceptible to acid degradation and attack by β-lactamase in the GI tract (see Fig. 1). Since such degradation and GI absorption processes compete at the absorption site, the GI absorption of β-lactam antibiotics is difficult to study even in experiments utilizing suitable animal GI tracts. In this chapter, we would like to describe the GI absorption characteristics established in our laboratory using rats as experimental animals for β-lactam antibiotics. The initial discussion will present their physicochemical properties, the GI absorption kinetics,

[1],[2] Takara-machi 13-1, Kanazawa 920, Japan.

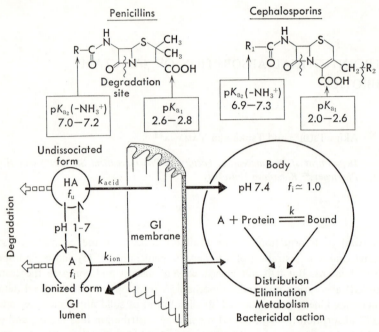

FIG. 1. Chemical structure and the dissociation constants of β-lactam antibiotics and schematics of the compartments relating to GI absorption, degradation, and blood levels of the orally-administered antibiotics.

the mechanism interpreted by the pertinent mathematical model, and the structure-absorption rate relationship for quantitative drug design of β-lactam antibiotics, excluding amphoteric ones. At the end of the chapter, the kinetic results of the absorption of amino-acid-like β-lactam antibiotics suggesting some types of carrier-mediated absorption and a short review of these absorption mechanisms that have been published in the last 5 years will be given.

BACKGROUND REGARDING GI ABSORPTION OF β-LACTAM ANTIBIOTICS

The mucosal surface of the GI tract acts as a lipoidal barrier to drug absorption. To characterize absorption of foreign compounds through such a barrier, Schanker and his colleagues (18) proposed the pH-partition hypothesis which states that the degree of absorption of weakly acidic and basic drugs depends on their lipid solubility and the degree of ionization. This hypothesis predicts very poor absorption by the small intestine of acidic drugs having pK_a values lower than 3.

Penicillins and cephalosporins are acidic antibiotics of which the pK_a values of the carboxylic acid moiety are about 2 to 3, as listed in Table I (23, 25, 31, 33, 40).

TABLE I. Physicochemical Properties of β-Lactam Antibiotics

β-Lactam antibiotics	Degradation half-life at pH 1 and 35°C (min)[a]	Dissociation constant at 37°C[b]		Partition coefficient at 37°C[c]	
		pK_{a1}	pK_{a2}	$\log P_u$ (octanol-water)	P_{app} (2-methyl-propanol-water)[d]
Penicillins					
Carindacillin	25	2.94		3.77	9.12
Carfecillin	25	2.91		2.96	4.17
Dicloxacillin		2.76		2.91	4.07
Floxacillin		2.76		2.61	2.57
Cloxacillin	13	2.78		2.43	2.40
Oxacillin	10	2.73		2.31	1.78
Propicillin	13	2.76		2.70	3.02
Phenethicillin	26	2.80		2.20	1.55
Penicillin V	25	2.79		1.95	1.10
Penicillin G	0.7	2.75		1.70	0.501
Methicillin	0.5	2.77		1.30	0.363
Carbenicillin	6.3	3.06(35°C)			
Sulbenicillin	12	2.45(35°C)		0.59[e]	
Ampicillin	250	2.67	6.95		0.373
Amoxicillin	220	2.67	7.11		0.130
Cyclacillin	85	2.64	7.18		0.866
Epicillin	250	2.77(35°C)	7.17(35°C)		0.438
Cephalosporins					
Cephalothin	1,500	2.22(35°C)		0.95	0.417
Cefazolin	140	2.54(35°C)		0.39[e]	
Cephaloridine	2,300	1.67(35°C)			
Cephaloglycin	2,100	2.03	6.89		
Cefatrizine	19,000	2.62	6.99		0.145
Cephalexin	36,000	2.67	6.96		0.193
Cephradine	38,000	2.63	7.35		0.268
Cefadroxil	44,000	2.69	7.22		0.081

[a] Data from refs. *25, 31, 33, 34, 39,* and *40.* [b] Data from refs. *23, 25, 31, 33, 34, 39,* and *40.*
[c] Data from refs. *23* and *34.* [d] Determined at pH 7.4. [e] Data from ref. *41.*

These antibiotic drugs exhibit a wide range of lipid solubility, depending on the nature of the side chains. The partition coefficients between oil and water are summarized in Table I (*23, 34, 41*). But we must mention that their lipid solubilities

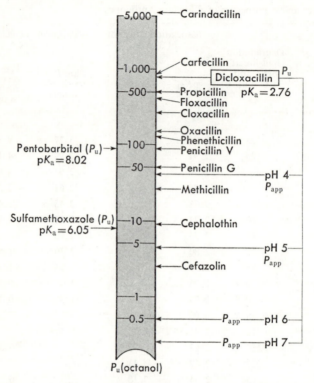

FIG. 2. Partition coefficients between octanol and water for the undissociated forms of β-lactam antibiotics and other drugs and the apparent partition coefficient of dicloxacillin as a function of pH.

largely depend on the pH of the GI lumen solution. This phenomenon is typically illustrated in Fig. 2 for dichloxacillin. At intestinal pH 6–7, all of the β-lactam antibiotics have very low lipid solubility compared with other drugs ingested orally (see Fig. 2).

Some basic information on the absorption mechanism for β-lactam antibiotics has been accumulated (5, 7, 9, 12, 13, 16, 24, 26, 27, 29, 30, 32, 37). However, at the time when we first started to study this matter in 1976, it was not clearly understood as yet whether the absorption follows the pH-partition hypothesis or another specialized mechanism.

There are some questions regarding GI absorption of β-lactam antibiotics which can be summarized as follows (see also Fig. 1):

    1) What factors of the physicochemical properties of these antibiotics determine the GI absorption rates?

2) Do the absorption rates obey the pH-partition hypothesis?

3) At intestinal pH, these antibiotics must be completely ionized. If the small intestine plays a major role in antibiotic absorption, is there any significant absorption of the ionized species?

4) Aminopenicillins such as ampicillin and aminocephalosporins like cephalexin have zwitterionic structures. In spite of being completely ionized at all pH values and very poorly lipid-soluble (Table I), these amino-β-lactam antibiotics are well absorbed by the GI. What mechanism underlies the absorption of poorly lipid-soluble amino-acid type antibiotics? Does this absorption mechanism exclusively differ from that of antibiotics without an amino group?

METHODOLOGY

To answer the above questions, we employed the *in situ* GI loop absorption technique by utilizing rats as our experimental animals. The precise meaning of absorption is associated with the technique employed. It has been suggested that the term "absorption" should be reserved for the whole process of movement of a drug substance from the lumen of the GI into the mesenteric venous blood or the lymphatic channels.

The *in situ* absorption method used (*24, 26, 27, 29, 30, 32*) was essentially based on that developed by Schanker *et al.* (*18*) except for utilization of a pH-control system. The perfusion solution pH was kept constant at the desired value by means of a pH-stat. This absorption experimental technique has the potential advantages of accurate pH control and suitable changes in the perfusion volume. The antibiotics remaining in the lumen solution and those accumulated in GI wall were determined by the sensitive UV spectrophotometric assay developed by Bundgaard and Ilver (*3*), spectrofluorometrical methods (*10, 28*), high-performance liquid chromatographic (HPLC) analysis, and/or microbiological assay.

β-LACTAM ANTIBIOTICS WITHOUT AMINO GROUP

1. Kinetics of Competing Degradation and Absorption

Figure 3 shows the disappearance of various penicillins from solution perfused at 37°C and a flow rate of 10 ml/min through the rat stomach and small intestine (*26, 27*), indicating that the total disappearance followed the first-order kinetics. However, it should be emphasized that the first-order rate constant, k_{app}, thus computed from these slopes may be the sum of the rate constants for absorption and degradation.

Penicillins can be easily degraded in an acidic environment by intramolecular attack by the side chain amide on the β-lactam to produce the corresponding penicillenic, penillic, and penicilloic acids. The reaction rates are known to depend on the polar nature of the side chain, as listed in Table I (*25, 33, 39, 40*). Although the β-lactam moiety of cephalosporins is relatively acid stable (*40*) (see Table I), the initial degradation product corresponding to penicilloic acid is not stable and is readily fragmented in aqueous solution. Additionally, the ester bond of acetylcephalosporin such as cephalothin and cephaloglycin is easily hydrolyzed in acidic solution to produce deacetylcephalosporin and its lactone (40).

Because of these circumstances, the quantitative determination of the degradation products resulting from β-lactam antibiotics seems to be experimentally difficult or impossible. How do we distinguish the total disappearance rate constant, k_{app}, into the absorption rate constant, k_a, and the degradation rate constant, k_d?

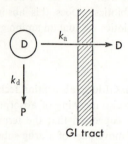

SCHEME I.   Simultaneous absorption and nonenzymatic degradation.

D, intact drug; P, product; k_a, absorption rate constant; k_d, degradation rate constant.

Scheme I represents the simultaneous absorption from the GI tract and the nonenzymatic degradation of the drug in the perfusion solution. Under suitable conditions (26), the total disappearance of the drug amount in the perfusion solution can be expressed as Eq. 1:

$$-\frac{dA}{dt}=k_a(C-C_b)+k_d A \tag{1}$$

where A represents the amount of drug; C and C_b represent the drug concentrations in the perfusion solution and in blood, respectively; k_a means the absorption clearance having a unit of volume $\times$ time^{-1}; and k_d is the first-order rate constant of degradation. Under the experimental conditions of the constant volume, V, of the drug solution and $C \gg C_b$, Eq. 1 becomes:

$$-\frac{dC}{dt}=\left(\frac{k_a}{V}+k_d\right)C \tag{2}$$

By integration:

$$\log\left(\frac{C_0}{C}\right)=-\frac{k_{app}}{2.303}t \tag{3}$$

where C_0 is the concentration at time zero and k_{app} is:

$$k_{app}=k_a\frac{1}{V}+k_d \tag{4}$$

The experimental results shown in Fig. 3 (*26, 27*) agree with the prediction from Eq. 3 that the semilogarithmic plots of C/C_0 against time show a straight line to give the apparent first-order rate constant, k_{app}.

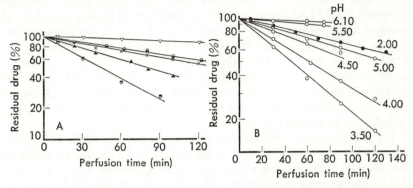

FIG. 3.   First-order plots of percent of β-lactam antibiotics remaining in the *in situ* GI recirculating perfusion experiments at pH 4.0 (A) and at various pH values (B). The drug solution was perfused at a flow rate of 10 ml/min. The small intestine used was a 100-cm distance from the pylorus. Key for A (volume of the intestinal perfusion solution): ◓ carindacillin, 80 ml; ▲ propicillin, 70 ml; × penicillin G, 50 ml; ◒ penicillin V, 60 ml; ▽ cephalothin, 50 ml. Key for B (volume of the perfusion solution): ● propicillin, 50 ml (from the stomach); ○ propicillin, 50 ml (from the intestine). Data from refs. *26* and *27*.

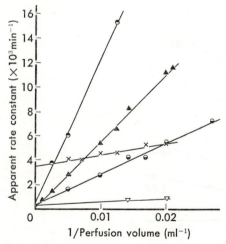

FIG. 4.   Effect of the volume of the perfusion solution on the absorption of β-lactam antibiotics by the *in situ* rat small intestine at pH 4.0 and 37°C. See the legend for Fig. 3. ◓ carindacillin; ▲ propicillin; × penicillin G; ◒ penicillin V; ▽ cephalothin. Data from ref. *26*.

Equation 4 predicts that the plots of k_{app} against the reciprocal of the volume of the drug solution, $1/V$, give a straight line. The absorption clearance, k_a, can be determined from the slope and the degradation rate constant, k_d, from the intercept value. Figure 4 illustrates the plots of the results from the rat intestinal absorption experiments at pH 4 (26). For all β-lactam antibiotics, good straight lines with various slopes and intercepts were obtained in agreement with Eq. 4. The different intercept values equal to the degradation rate constants reflect their acid stabilities depending on their polar nature of the side-chain (see Table I). Penicillin G is the most unstable and has the smallest intestinal absorption rate in the series of penicillins. Cephalothin is rather acid stable, but has the lowest absorbability of β-lactam antibiotics. The quantitative relationship between the structure and the absorption rate of β-lactam antibiotics will be discussed later.

For the rat stomach recirculation experiments with propicillin at various pH values, similar results were obtained as shown in Fig. 5 (27). The k_d values determined from the intercepts were almost equal to those determined *in vitro* at the same pH. The results suggest that nonenzymatic degradation of penicillin in the perfusion solution through the rat stomach depends only on the bulk pH values.

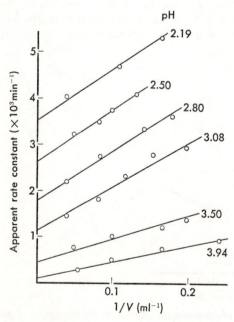

FIG. 5. Effect of the volume of the perfusion solution on the absorption of propicillin by the *in situ* rat stomach at various pH values and 37°C. See the legend for Fig. 3. Data from ref. 27.

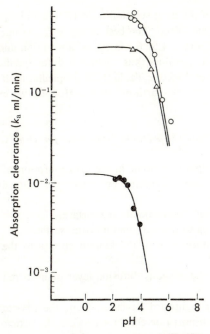

FIG. 6.   Plots of the *in situ* rat GI absorption clearance, k_a, of propicillin *versus* the pH of the perfusion solution at 37°C.
● experimental points from the stomach at a flow rate of 10 ml/min; ○ experimental points from the intestine at a flow rate of 10 ml/min; △ experimental points from the intestine at a flow rate of 10 ml/min for 2.5 min and with perfusion stopped for 10 min. The small intestine used was a 100-cm distance from the pylorus. The solid lines were generated from Eq. 8 and the parameters computed by the nonlinear least squares method. Data from ref. *27*.

2. Deviation from the pH-partition Hypothesis

Figure 6 illustrates the absorption clearances, k_a, of propicillin from the rat stomach and small intestine against the pH of the perfusion solution (*27*).

The intestinal absorption rates of propicillin were about 100 times faster than the gastric absorption rates at every pH. This large difference is undoubtedly due to the relative surface areas of the two absorption sites.

From these pH-rate profiles, it is apparent that the major absorbable species of propicillin is its undissociated form. If the pH-partition hypothesis underlies propicillin absorption, the theory expressed as Eq. 5 gives the $K_{a_{app}}$ value.

$$k_a = k_u \frac{a_H}{a_H + K_{a_{app}}}$$ (5)

where a_H is the hydrogen-ion activity of the drug solution ($a_H = 10^{-pH}$) and k_u is the absorption clearance for the undissociated drug. The best fitting $pK_{a_{app}}$ value with these data at a perfusion rate of 10 ml/min is 4.61 for intestinal absorption and 3.49 for gastric absorption. However, the $pK_{a_{app}}$ values thus computed differ significantly by 1 to 2 pK_a units from the true pK_a of 2.76 (see Table I) for propicillin itself. This discrepancy is not well interpreted by the pH-partition theory. How do we explain this pK_a difference?

3. Possible Explanation of Deviation from pH-partition Hypothesis for Drug GI Absorption

Discrepancies from the pH-partition hypothesis occur in the GI absorption of some drugs. Each of these phenomena has been interpreted by one of the following explanations:

1) The existence of the virtual pH at the GI membrane surface.
2) The existence of the drug binding to the intestinal mucosal surface.
3) The contribution of the absorption rate of the ionized species to the total absorption rate of the drug.
4) The existence of the barrier of the aqueous diffusion layer or unstirred layer on the lumen side of the GI.

Interestingly, we found a very similar rightward deviation from the pH-partition hypothesis in the *in vitro* two-phase transport rate constant between the octanol and water-pH profiles of various penicillins (27). The first two possibilities cannot explain the shifts of such pH-rate curves of penicillins observed *in vitro*, since the presence of such complicated physiological factors can be completely excluded in this case. Therefore, there is no reason to apply both the virtual pH resulting from the secretion of H⁺ ions by the mucosal cells and the binding hypothesis for the harmonious interpretation of both *in situ* and *in vitro* phenomena observed for penicillins.

In situ kinetic evidence of the absorption of the ionized species of some drugs was successful in explaining of the deviation from the pH-partition hypothesis in intestinal absorption. The ionized penicillin species can be absorbed by the rat intestine to a considerable extent in the neutral and alkaline pH regions (30), but this contribution to the total intestinal absorption curve below pH 5 had no significant effect on the pH-intestinal absorption curve. Similar to the *in situ* result, below pH 5 the two-phase transport of the ionized species of penicillins can be regarded as almost negligible (27).

Therefore, attribution of both *in situ* and *in vitro* deviation from the pH-partition hypothesis for penicillins to the hydrodynamic diffusion theory involving the aqueous diffusion layer seems to be the most reasonable explanation.

4. Mathematical Diffusion Model for β-Lactam Antibiotic Absorption

Scheme II shows a two-compartment diffusion model related to drug transport and GI absorption proposed by Suzuki, Higuchi, and Ho (22). The first compartment showing the mucosal side or aqueous phase consists of a bulk aqueous drug solution

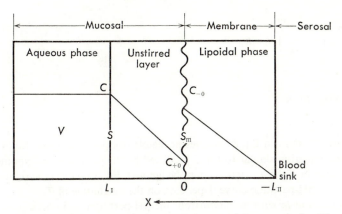

SCHEME II.   Schematic model of the transport of drug across the GI tract.
The bulk aqueous solution with an aqueous diffusion layer on the mucosal side is followed by a heterogeneous membrane consisting of lipoidal pathway and thereafter by a sink on the serosal side.

phase and an unstirred layer of thickness L_I, and it is in series with the second compartment consisting of a lipid phase or membrane of thickness L_{II}. If there is a perfect sink on the second side after the lipoidal barrier and only the undissociated species can permeate through the lipid membrane, this diffusion model yields the apparent transfer and absorption clearances, k_a, expressed as Eq. 6 under quasi-steady-state conditions (27):

$$k_a = \frac{SD_{aq}}{L_I}\left[\frac{1}{\left[1+\dfrac{K_a}{(a_H)_s}\right]T+1}\right] \tag{6}$$

where

$$T = \frac{L_{II}D_{aq}}{L_I D_{IIp} Pl_u R} \tag{7}$$

where D_{aq} is the diffusion coefficient of the drug in water and D_{IIp} is that in oil or membrane; Pl_u represents the partition coefficient of the undissociated antibiotic between oil or membrane and aqueous solution; S is the surface area at the aqueous diffusion layer and R means the ratio of the true interfacial area (S_m) of the oil or membrane surface to S; and $(a_H)_s$ is the hydrogen ion activity at the surface of the lipoidal phase or membrane.

In a well-buffered solution, as in the present *in situ* and *in vitro* experiments, the pH at the lipoidal surface would not differ substantially from that in the bulk of the solution (20). Hence $(a_H)_s = a_H$. Rearrangement of Eq. 6 yields:

$$k_a = k_u' \frac{a_H}{\left(1 + \dfrac{1}{T}\right) a_H + K_a} \tag{8}$$

where

$$k_u' = \frac{S D_{IIp} P l_u R}{L_{II}} \tag{9}$$

If T is large, the T^{-1} term in Eq. 8 becomes negligible compared to 1 and Eq. 8 can be reduced to an equation similar to Eq. 5 predicted by the pH-partition hypothesis. But if T is not large or if the T^{-1} term cannot be ignored, Eq. 8 predicts the rightward deviation from the pH-partition curve depending on the magnitude of T.

If both *in situ* and *in vitro* deviation from the pH-partition hypothesis presently observed for penicillins were to be substantially attributed to the aqueous diffusion layer theory described by Eq. 8, a change in the T value should produce a change in the shift of the pH-absorption profile. The increasing thickness of the aqueous diffusion layer, L_I, should lower the T value and thereby not only decrease the absorption rate but also yield a rightward shift of the pH-rate curve from the dissociation curve. Figure 6 shows the *in situ* intestinal absorption rate-pH profiles of propicillin under two different hydrodynamic conditions (27); one was carried out at a flow rate of 10 ml/min for 2.5 min with a static situation for 10 min, and the other at a constant flow rate of 10 ml/min. When the drug solution was less agitated, the intestinal absorption rates were significantly decreased and the profile shifted rightward. Similar agitation effects were also observed in the *in vitro* transfer rate-pH curves (27). Both results are in good agreement with the prediction from Eq. 8.

It is concluded from all the experimental evidence obtained in our studies that the deviation from the pH-partition hypothesis of penicillins was interpreted successfully by the absorption mechanism of penicillins through the aqueous diffusion layer of the membrane side of the GI, the membrane transport being restricted by the lipophilicity of the undissociated species.

5. Kinetic Evidence for Absorption of Ionized Species

Figure 7 illustrates the plots of the *in situ* absorption clearance of a series of penicillins from the solution perfused at a flow rate of 2 ml/min through the 30-cm long small intestine against the pH of the drug solution (30).

Between pH 6.5 and 9, the penicillin absorption was independent of the lumen solution pH, with an average clearance of 0.012 ml/min for the ionized species of penicillins, which was almost identical among penicillin molecules and cefazolin (30). Below pH 6, the absorption clearances increased significantly with a decrease in the lumen solution pH, depending on the lipophilicity of the undissociated species. Therefore, k_a can be expressed as:

$$k_a = k_{acid} + k_{ion} \tag{10}$$

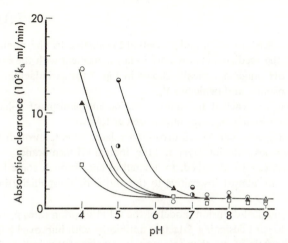

FIG. 7. Plots of the *in situ* rat intestinal absorption clearance, k_a, of penicillins *versus* the pH of the perfusion solution at 37°C.
The perfusion solution (9 ml) was recirculated at a flow rate of 2 ml/min. The small intestine used was a 30-cm distance from the pylorus. The points are experimental values and the solid lines were generated from Eq. 11. Data from refs. *30* and *34*.
□ penicillin V; ▲ propicillin; ○ dicloxacillin; ◑ carfecillin; ◒ carindacillin.

where k_{acid} and k_{ion} are the apparent absorption clearances for the undissociated and ionized species of β-lactam antibiotics, respectively.

6. Structure-absorption Rate Relationship and Application to Quantitative Drug Design
We establihsed the structure-absorption rate relationship for k_{acid} of penicillins and cephalosporins to yield Eq. 11, converted by use of the proper physicochemical treatment (*30*) of Eq. 8.

$$k_a(\text{ml/min}) = \frac{a}{\sqrt{MW}} \left[\frac{P_u f_u}{b + P_u f_u} \right] + k_{ion} \qquad (11)$$

where MW is the molecular weight of the undissociated form of antibiotics; P_u is the partition coefficient of the undissociated drug between oil (for example, octanol) and water as an index of the lipophilicity of the drug; a and b are the constants; and f_u is the fraction of the undissociated species as a function of pH as expressed in Eq. 12.

$$f_u = \frac{a_H}{a_H + K_a} \qquad (12)$$

Thus, $P_u f_u$ represents the apparent partition coefficient, P_{app}, as a function of the drug solution pH.

$$P_{app} = P_u f_u \qquad\qquad (13)$$

With the parameters of $a=4.62$, $b=35.9$, and $k_{ion}=0.012$ evaluated by the nonlinear least squares calculation, the predicted curves were in fair agreement with the experimental points in a wide pH range as typically shown in Fig. 7 for carindacillin, carfecillin, dicloxacillin, propicillin, and penicillin V.

The conclusions that we reached for the absorption mechanism of β-lactam antibiotics, excluding zwitterionic ones, are summarized as follows:

1) The undissociated species can be absorbed, to a large extent, through both barriers of the aqueous diffusion layer and the lipoidal GI membrane.

2) The ionized species can be absorbed, to a small extent, through some forms of barriers which are almost insensitive to the antibiotic lipophilicity in the first-order fashion.

The preceding mathematical diffusion model of the GI absorption rates provides some significant insights toward designing β-lactam antibiotics with improved passive GI absorption. Taking the ratio of the absorption rate constants of the undissociated

TABLE II.   Absorption Clearance Determined at pH 4.0 in the *In Situ* Absorption Experiments through the Rat Small Intestine and the Related Parameters for β-Lactam Antibiotics

β-Lactam antibiotics	Molecular weight[a]	pK_a[b]	$\log P_u$[b] (octanol-water)	P_{app}[c]	$10^2 k_{acid}$[d] (ml/min)	k_{acid}/k_{acid}^*[e]
Hydrodynamic condition: flow rate of 2 ml/min[f]						
Penicillin V	350. 4	2. 79	1. 95	5. 18	3. 20	1. 00
Phenethicillin	364. 4	2. 80	2. 20	9. 41	4. 87	1. 52
Propicillin	378. 4	2. 76	2. 70	27. 3	9. 93	3. 04
Oxacillin	401. 4	2. 73	2. 31	10. 4	5. 75	1. 80
Cloxacillin	435. 9	2. 78	2. 43	15. 3	4. 85	1. 52
Floxacillin	453. 9	2. 76	2. 61	22. 2	7. 64	2. 39
Dicloxacillin	470. 3	2. 76	2. 91	44. 2	13. 1	4. 09
Hydrodynamic condition: flow rate of 10 ml/min[g]						
Carindacillin	494. 6	2. 94	3. 77	471. 8	117	4. 68
Propicillin	378. 4	2. 76	2. 70	27. 3	54	2. 16
Penicillin V	350. 4	2. 79	1. 95	5. 18	25	1. 00
Penicillin G	334. 4	2. 75	1. 70	2. 66	8	0. 32
Cephalothin	396. 4	2. 22(35°C)	0. 95	0. 15	2	0. 08

[a] As free acid.   [b] Determined at 37°C and at ionic strength of 0.15.   See Table I.   [c] $P_u f_u$ where $f_u = a_H/(a_H + K_a)$.   [d] Determined at pH 4. Data from refs. *26* and *30*.   [e] A ratio relative to penicillin V.   [f] The small intestine used was a 30-cm distance from the pylorus.   [g] The small intestine used was a 100-cm distance from the pylorus.

species of a derivative or analogue modification of β-lactam antibiotics, k_{acid}, to that of the reference standard antibiotic, k^*_{acid}, we get:

$$\frac{k_{acid}}{k^*_{acid}} \sqrt{\frac{MW}{MW^*}} = \left[\frac{P_{app}}{P^*_{app}}\right]\left[\frac{b'+1}{b'+\dfrac{P_{app}}{P^*_{app}}}\right] \tag{14}$$

where b' equals b/P^*_{app}. Table II summarizes the results obtained for β-lactam antibiotics under different conditions, where we took penicillin V as a reference standard because it has the proper lipophilicity and acid stability (see Table I) for oral use.

Plots of $k_{acid}\sqrt{MW}/k^*_{acid}\sqrt{MW^*}$ against P_{app}/P^*_{app} are illustrated in Fig. 8. The theoretical curve was generated with the best fitting parameter of $b'=4.6$, being in good agreement with the experimental points of all β-lactam antibiotics used. The partition coefficients, P_u, for cephalothin and cefazolin are about one-tenth to one-thirteenth lower than that of penicillin V (Table I). Poor absorbability of the two orally ingested cephalosporins may be attributed to the considerable reduction of the absorption clearance, k_{acid}, both in the stomach and upper intestine.

Using Eq. 14, one can predict upon knowing the absorption clearance of the reference antibiotic, how much additional lipophilicity is required to improve the rate of the object antibiotic drug. Generally speaking, the absorption rate of an anti-

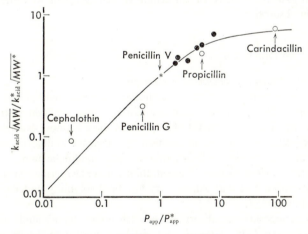

FIG. 8.   Plots of $k_{acid}\sqrt{MW}/k^*_{acid}\sqrt{MW^*}$ against P_{app}/P^*_{app} for the data listed in Table II.

The solid line was generated from Eq. 14 with the nonlinear least squares best fitting parameter of $b'=4.6$ for the data determined at a flow rate of 10 ml/min. ○ experimental points determined at a flow rate of 10 ml/min (see Table II); ● experimental points determined at a flow rate of 2 ml/min.

biotic having poor lipid solubility in its acid form may possibly be increased rate by means of a suitable chemical modification to increase the lipophilicity. But it must be emphasized that a drug may be "overdesigned" by excessively extending the lipophilicity. All factors such as pH, pK_a, molecular size, and hydrodynamic condition being constant, Eq. 14 predicts that the absorption of β-lactam antibiotics almost reaches a plateau in a compound having about 50 times greater lipophilicity than penicillin V. This phenomenon is due to the fact that the aqueous diffusion layer in front of the mucosal membrane is the rate-limiting barrier and not the biomembrane pathways.

We have found a good example to understand the drug modification approach to improve the GI absorption of β-lactam antibiotics. Since carbenicillin is very acid unstable and has low lipid solubility (see Table I), this compound is poorly absorbed by the GI tract after administration by the oral route and its use is limited to parenteral administration. A series of α-carboxyl esters of carbenicillin has been synthesized in attempt to improve these disadvantages and to increase carbenicillin oral bioavailability (4). These esters are designed to undergo hydrolysis in the body to liberate carbenicillin. Carindacillin, one of these carbenicillin prodrugs, has a similar acid stability (33) and about 100 times greater lipophilicity compared to penicillin V (Table I) to produce a dramatic increase in the intestinal absorption rates, but only to the extent of 4.7 times, as seen in Table II. A similar prodrug, carfecillin, also has a similar acid stability (33) and 10 times greater lipophilicity compared to penicillin V (Table I). The theory (Eq. 14) predicts a 3.7-time the increase in the absorption rate, indicating that the lipophilicity of carfecillin is well designed to sufficiently improve carbenicillin absorption.

AMINO-β-LACTAM ANTIBIOTICS

1. Absorption Sites and Evidence for Saturable Absorption

Aminopenicillins, such as amoxicillin and cyclacillin, and aminocephalosporins, such as cephalexin and cephradine are known to be absorbed well after oral administration to humans (1, 2, 11, 15). However, the GI absorption of these amino-β-lactam antibiotics could not be predicted from the mechanism by which the antibiotics are absorbed by passive lipoidal barrier diffusion of the highly lipophilic undissociated species described in the previous section. These antibiotics have zwitterionic structures that are completely ionized and that exhibit very low lipid solubility under GI circumstances, as listed in Table I.

What mechanism underlies the absorption of such poorly lipid soluble amino-acid like antibiotics? From 1976 to the present, we have studied to determine the difference in absorption characteristics and the mechanism between β-lactam antibiotics with and without amino groups. Utilizing rats as experimental animals, we have found clear evidence indicating a common absorption mechanism specialized for amino-β-lactam antibiotics (24, 29, 32, 34).

The left curves in Fig. 9 depict the reported serum levels after oral administration

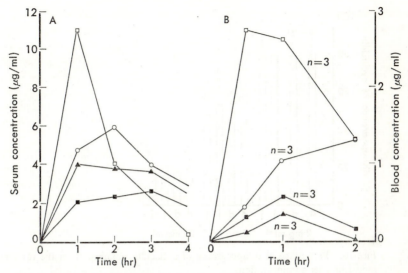

FIG. 9.   Comparative blood levels of aminopenicillins.
A: man (oral). Dose: 500 mg. B: rat (introduodenal). Dose: 100 mg/kg. ▲ ampicillin;
○ amoxicillin; ■ epicillin; □ cyclacillin. Data from refs. *36* and *34* for humans and
rats, respectively.

of 500 mg of cyclacillin (*36*), amoxicillin (*14*), ampicillin (*14*), and epicillin (*14*) in
humans. The right curves show the mean whole-blood levels after intraduodenal
administration of the same antibiotics in rats at a dose of 10 mg/kg. The blood level
ranking order was cyclacillin, amoxicillin, epicillin, closely followed by ampicillin. This order is almost identical to the order in humans. When these aminopenicillins were administered into the rat stomach, they were not detectable in serum
analyzed by microbiological assay. This result indicates that the aminopenicillins,
although sufficiently acid stable (see Table I), were less absorbable by the stomach.
It is easy to speculate that the absorption of amino-β-lactam antibiotics occurs in
the small intestine but not in the stomach, as claimed previously by Lode (*8*) for the
absorption of ampicillin and cephalexin in humans.

Judging from these observations, it can be said that the rat is suitable as an
experimental animal in elucidating the absorption mechanism of amino-β-lactam
antibiotics in humans.

In order to explore the mechanism responsible for absorption of amino-β-lactam
antibiotics, the effect of dose concentration on the percent of disappearance from
the rat small intestinal loops was examined. If the percent of disappearance is not
affected by the initial dose concentration, the apparent first-order absorption may
proceed as observed for other β-lactam antibiotics described previously. But, if it is
really affected, a contribution of some specialized mechanism is suggested. As seen
in Fig. 10, it is very interesting to note that the percent of disappearance of cyclacillin

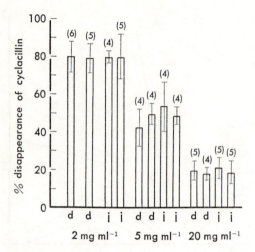

FIG. 10. Percentage of disappearance of cyclacillin obtained from the rat intestinal loop 1 hr after administration.

Each dose was dissolved in pH 7.4 isotonic phosphate buffer and injected in a volume of 1 ml into a 5-cm intestinal loop. In each experiment, two loops were prepared. The first loop was made at 2 cm from the pylorus, with 1 cm of intestine separating the consecutive loop in the duodenum. For the study in the jejunum, the loops were prepared at 15 cm from the pylorus. The points represent the mean disappearance with standard deviation shown as a bar. Experimental number is shown in parentheses. d, duodenum; j, jejunum. Data from ref. 29.

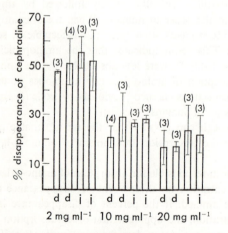

FIG. 11. Percentage of disappearance of cephradine obtained from the rat intestinal loop 1 hr after administration.

See the legend for Fig. 10. Data from ref. 32.

as a typical result for aminopenicillins depends remarkably on the initial dose concentration in the small intestinal portions (*29*). The results show that the percent of disappearance at a low dose of 2 mg/ml was extremely large, to the extent of about 80%, while that at a high dose of 20 mg/ml was reduced markedly, to the extent of about 20%. The drug accumulation in the intestinal wall was found to be negligible and to be 3% during the absorption experimental period (*34*).

Figure 11 illustrates a clear dose-dependent disappearance feature for cephradine as a typical example for aminocephalosporins (*32*). Similar interesting phenomena were also observed for other amino-β-lactam antibiotics (*19, 24, 32, 34*).

These remarkable dose-dependent absorptions strongly suggest that the absorption of amino-β-lactam antibiotics is likely to follow some forms of specialized and saturable transport mechanisms.

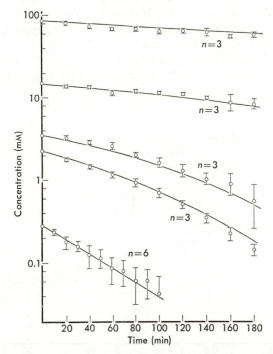

FIG. 12.   Time-courses of the disappearance of cyclacillin as a function of dose from the isotonic phosphate buffer perfused through the rat small intestine.
The perfusion solution (9 ml) was recirculated at pH 7.0, 37°C and at a flow rate of 2 ml/min. The small intestine used was a 30-cm distance from the pylorus. The remaining antibiotic was assayed by HPLC and/or microbiological assay. The points represent the mean concentration and vertical bars represent the standard deviations. The curves were generated from Eq. 15 with the non-linear least squares best fitting parameters listed in Table III. Data from refs. *29* and *34*.

2. Evidence for Competing Michaelis-Menten and First-order Kinetics

To confirm kinetically the speculated saturable absorption, experiments using the *in situ* recirculating perfusion technique were conducted at 37°C in the various dose-concentration ranges. The pH of the perfusion solution was maintained at 7.0 by means of a pH-stat.

Figure 12 illustrates the time-courses for the disappearance of cyclacillin from the rat intestinal perfusates (*29, 34*). The data showing time-dependency and initial dose-concentration dependency can be described by Eq. 15 involving a Michaelis-Menten and simple first-order kinetic terms:

$$-\frac{dC}{dt} = \frac{V_{max}C}{K_m + C} + (k_1 + k_2)C \tag{15}$$

where C is the cyclacillin concentration remaining in the perfusate at time t; V_{max} is the maximum rate of disappearance and K_m is the Michaelis-Menten constant; and k_1 and k_2 are the first-order rate constants of absorption and degradation of cyclacillin, respectively. The nonlinear least squares analysis of the data in Fig. 12, to be fitted to Eq. 15, provided the parameters (*34*): $V_{max} = 1.47 \pm 0.09$ mM/hr, $K_m = 1.23 \pm 0.08$ mM, and $k_1 + k_2 = 0.111 \pm 0.014$ hr^{-1}. The solid lines in Fig. 12

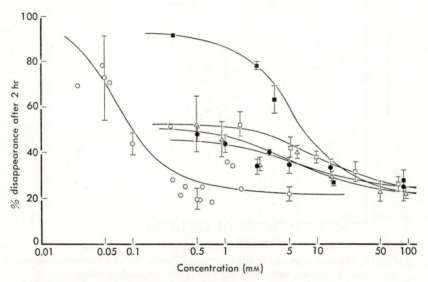

FIG. 13. Percentage of disappearance after 2 hr against the initial concentrations of amino-β-lactam antibiotics at pH 7.0 from the rat small intestine using the *in situ* recirculating perfusion technique.

See the legend for Fig. 12. The curves were generated from Eq. 15 with the nonlinear least squares best fitting parameters listed in Table III. ○ amoxicillin; ■ cyclacillin; ● cephalexin; △ cephradine; □ cefadroxil. Data from refs. *24, 29, 32,* and *34*.

TABLE III.   Kinetic Parameters for the *In Situ* Rat Intestinal Absorption of Aminopenicillins and Aminocephalosporins at pH 7.0[a]

$$-\frac{dC}{dt} = \frac{V_{mxa}C}{K_m+C} + (k_1+k_2)C$$

Amino-β-lactam antibiotics	Michaelis-Menten kinetic parameters[b]		First-order rate constant[b]	
	K_m (mM)	V_{max} (mM hr^{-1})	V_{max}/K_m (hr^{-1})	k_1+k_2 (hr^{-1})
Ampicillin	c	c	c	0.12
Amoxicillin	0.00751$\pm$0.00048	0.0170$\pm$0.0012	2.26	0.12
Cyclacillin	1.23$\pm$0.08	1.47$\pm$0.09	1.20	0.111$\pm$0.014
Cephalexin	3.88$\pm$0.16	0.674$\pm$0.170	0.17	0.138$\pm$0.016
Cephradine	3.34$\pm$0.14	0.808$\pm$0.097	0.24	0.119$\pm$0.015
Cefadroxil	6.89$\pm$0.15	1.93$\pm$0.18	0.28	0.115$\pm$0.008

[a] The perfusion solution (9 ml) was recirculated at a flow rate of 2 ml/min.   The small intestine used was a 30-cm distance from the pylorus.   [b] The values were evaluated by the nonlinear least-squares analysis of experimental points in Figs. 12 and 13.   Data from refs. *24, 29, 32,* and *34.*   [c] Undetectable.

were generated using Eq. 15 with the best-fitting parameters, indicating that Eq. 15 reasonably describes all the experimental data.

Percentage disappearances of amoxicillin, cephalexin, cephradine, cefadroxil, and also cyclacillin after 2 hr are illustrated in Fig. 13 as a function of their initial dose-concentration *(24, 29, 32, 34)*. These curves show very similar shapes, indicating that great losses from the lumen solution occur at a low dose, while there are small losses at a high dose. The generated curves from Eq. 15 with the best-fitting parameters listed in Table III are in fairly good agreement with all the experimental data for each antibiotic.

3. Absorption Mechanism

Our present observations of common phenomena showing Michaelis-Menten kinetics in the disappearance from the lumen solution can lead to the most reasonable conclusion. That is, some types of carrier-mediated transport mechanisms by way of active transport and/or facilitated diffusion underlie the absorption of poorly lipid soluble and completely ionized amino-β-lactam antibiotics in the rat. Such carrier systems may be localized only in the small intestinal porition but not in the stomach.

Some evidence has been reported to show that cyclacillin *(5)* and cephradine *(37)* were actively transported across the everted rat intestine. But, at high dose of cyclacillin of 2 mg/ml, Dixon and Mizen *(5)* could not find such active transport, being consistent with the previous observation from Penzotti and Poole *(13)* in a similar experiment. Such active transport was also not the case for a number of other penicillins including amoxicillin ahd ampicillin (*5, 7, 13, 37*) and cephalosporins including cephaloglycin (*13*) and cephalexin (*9, 13, 37, 42*), which are apparently passively diffused across the intestinal wall. Kimura *et al.* (*7*) demonstrated by using the *in situ* perfusion technique that the absorption of amoxicillin and cyclacillin from the rat small intestine was saturable, being consistent with our results (*24, 29*), and inhibited by short-term pretreatment of the intestine with a low concentration of $HgCl_2$. The simultaneous perfusion of two types of dipeptides inhibited the absorption of cyclacillin but not of amoxicillin (*7*). Kimura and others (*7*) claimed the presence of two carrier systems for the active transport of cyclacillin in the intestinal mucosa, one of which can be blocked by amoxicillin and the other by dipeptides, and proposed that amoxicillin may be transported by the facilitated diffusion mechanism, the carrier of which seems to be common to one of the carrier systems for cyclacillin transport. Although Kimura *et al.* (*7*) and also we could not find any evidence for carrier-mediated transport of ampicillin, recently Shindo and his colleagues (*19*) obtained evidence of a saturable absorption of ampicillin from the rat intestinal loop by a successful and skilful technique.

It may be safe to say from the accumulated observations in the last 5 years (*5, 7, 9, 13, 19, 24, 29, 32, 34, 37*) that amino-β-lactam antibiotics are transported by the mixed ways of active and simultaneously proceeding facilitated and simple diffusions. The significance of the contribution of each transport rate-term of various amino-β-lactam antibiotics (Table III) may be pooled parameters for parallel Michaelis-Menten paths, probably including active and facilitated transport across the intestinal membrane, and also if present, metabolic degradations of the antibiotics both in the GI lumen and tract. Our most recent observation for cyclacillin (*34*) showed that, when the area under the time-blood concentration curve (AUC) after three different administration routes in rats at the dose of 10 mg/kg was compared, the AUC after intraduodenal administration was almost equal to those after intra-portal and intravenous doses. The results strongly indicate that metabolisms both in the gut wall and liver are negligible and that the disappearance of this compound from the lumen solution may be exclusively due to the absorption by way of major Michaelis-Menten and minor simple first-order kinetic pathways.

Whether such a carrier-mediated transport system is present or not in the human intestine has not been clarified as yet. It is conceivable, however, that the complete absorption of amoxicillin (*21*), cephalexin, and cephradine (*2*), and 80% absorption of cyclacillin (*38*) after oral administration in humans may be due to the contribution of a saturable carrier system rather than the other possibility of membrane transport of very poorly lipid-soluble and zwitterionic amino derivatives of β-lactam antibiotics.

Acknowledgment

The authors gratefully acknowledge the collaboration of their associates, Dr. Etsuko Miyamoto and Mrs. Emi Nakashima.

REFERENCES

1. Bergan, T. 1978. *Antibiot. Chemother.*, **25**, 1–122.
2. Brogard, J. M., Comte, F., and Pinget, M. 1978. *Antibiot. Chemother.*, **25**, 123–162.
3. Bundgaard, H. and Ilver, K. 1972. *J. Pharm. Pharmacol.*, **24**, 790–794.
4. Clayton, J. P., Cole, M., Elson, S. W., Hardy, K. D., Mizen, L. W., and Sutherland, R. 1975. *J. Med. Chem.*, **18**, 172–177.
5. Dixon, C. and Mizen, L. W. 1977. *J. Physiol.*, **269**, 549–559.
6. Granvenkemper, C. F., Bennett, J. V., Brodie, J. L., and Kirby, W. M. M. 1965. *Arch. Intern. Med.*, **116**, 340–345.
7. Kimura, T., Endo, H., Yoshikawa, M., Muranishi, S., and Sezaki, H. 1978. *J Pharm. Dyn.*, **1**, 262–267.
8. Lode, H. 1975. *In* "Chemotherapy, Proceedings of International Congress on Chemotherapy," ed. by J. D. Williams and A. M. Geddes, Plenum Press, New York, Vol. 4, pp. 199–203: through *Chem. Abstr.*, **86**, 165045g (1972).
9. Miyazaki, K., Ogino, O., Nakano, M., and Arita, T. 1977. *Chem. Pharm. Bull. (Tokyo)*, **25**, 246–252.
10. Miyazaki, K., Ogino, O., Sato, H., Nakano, M., and Arita, T. 1977. *Chem. Pharm. Bull. (Tokyo)*, **25**, 253–258.
11. Nightingale, C. H., Greene, D. S., and Quintiliani, R. 1975. *J. Pharm. Sci.*, **64**, 1899–1927.
12. Perrier, D. and Gibaldi, M. 1973. *J. Pharm. Sci.*, **62**, 1486–1490.
13. Penzotti, S. C., Jr. and Poole, J. W. 1974. *J. Pharm. Sci.*, **63**, 1803–1806.
14. Philipson, A., Sabath, L. D., and Posner, B. 1975. *Antimicrob. Agents Chemother.*, **8**, 311–320.
15. Rolinson, G. N. and Sutherland, R. 1973. *In* "Advances in Pharmacology and Chemotherapy," ed. by G. Garrattini, A. Goldin, F. Hawking, and I. J. Kopin, Academic Press, New York, Vol. 11. pp. 151–220.
16. Rollo, J. M. 1972. *Can. J. Physiol. Pharmacol.*, **50**, 986–998.
17. Rosenblatt, J. E., Kind, A. C., Brodie, J. L., and Kirby, W. M. M. 1968. *Arch. Intern. Med.*, **121**, 345–348.
18. Schanker, L. S., Tocco, D. J., Brodie, B. B., and Hogben, C. A. M. 1958. *J. Pharmacol. Exp. Ther.*, **123**, 81–88.
19. Shindo, H., Fukuda, K., Kawai, K., and Tanaka, K. 1978. *J. Pharm. Dyn.*, **1**, 310–323.
20. Smolen, V. F. 1973. *J. Pharm. Sci.*, **62**, 77–79.
21. Spyker, D. A., Rugloski, R. J., Vann, R. L., and O'Brien, W. M. 1977. *Antimicrob. Agents Chemother.*, **11**, 132–141.
22. Suzuki, A., Higuchi, W. I., and Ho, N. F. H. 1970. *J. Pharm. Sci.*, **59**, 644–651.
23. Tsuji, A., Kubo, O., Miyamoto, E., and Yamana, T. 1977. *J. Pharm. Sci.*, **66**, 1675–1678.

24. Tsuji, A., Nakashima, E., Kagami, I., Honjo, N., and Yamana, T. 1977. *J. Pharm. Pharmacol.*, **29**, 707–708.
25. Tsuji, A., Nakashima, E., Hamano, S., and Yamana, T. 1978. *J. Pharm. Sci.*, **67**, 1059–1066.
26. Tsuji, A., Miyamoto, E., Kagami, I., Sakaguchi, H., and Yamana, T. 1978. *J. Pharm. Sci.*, **67**, 1701–1704.
27. Tsuji, A., Miyamoto, E., Hashimoto, N., and Yamana, T. 1978. *J. Pharm. Sci.*, **67**, 1705–1711.
28. Tsuji, A., Miyamoto, E., and Yamana, T. 1978. *J. Pharm. Pharmacol.*, **30**, 811–813.
29. Tsuji, A., Nakashima, E., Kagami, I., Asano, T., Nakashima, R., and Yamana, T. 1978. *J. Pharm. Pharmacol.*, **30**, 508–509.
30. Tsuji, A., Miyamoto, E., Kubo, O., and Yamana, T. 1979. *J. Pharm. Sci.*, **68**, 812–816.
31. Tsuji, A., Nakashima, E., and Yamana, T. 1979. *J. Pharm. Sci.*, **68**, 308–311.
32. Tsuji, A., Nakashima, E., Asano, T., Nakashima, R., and Yamana, T. 1979. *J. Pharm. Pharmacol.*, **31**, 718–720.
33. Tsuji, A., Miyamoto, E., Terasaki, T., and Yamana, T. 1979. *J. Pharm. Sci.*, **68**, 1259–1263.
34. Tsuji, A., Nakashima, E., and Yamana, T. Unpublished results.
35. Tsuji, A., Miyamoto, E., and Yamana, T. Unpublished results.
36. Ueda, Y., Matsumoto, E., Nakamura, N., Saito, A., Noda, K., Furuya, C., Omori, M., Shimojo, S., Hanaoka, H., Utsunomiya, M., and Fujinoki, T. 1970. *Japan. J. Antibiot.*, **23**, 48–52.
37. Umeniwa, K., Ogino, O., Miyazaki, K., and Arita, T. 1979. *Chem. Pharm. Bull. (Tokyo)*, **27**, 2177–2182.
38. Warren, G. H. 1976. *Chemotherapy*, **22**, 154–182.
39. Yamana, T., Tsuji, A., and Mizukami, Y. 1974. *Chem. Pharm. Bull. (Tokyo)*, **22**, 1186–1197.
40. Yamana, T. and Tsuji, A. 1976. *J. Pharm. Sci.*, **65**, 1563–1573.
41. Yamana, T., Tsuji, A., Miyamoto, E., and Kubo, O. 1977. *J. Pharm. Sci.*, **66**, 747–749.
42. Yasuhara, M., Miyoshi, Y., Yuasa, A., Kimura, T., Muranishi, S., and Sezaki, H. 1977. *Chem. Pharm. Bull. (Tokyo)*, **25**, 675–679.

CEPHALOSPORIN PHARMACOKINETICS

Charles H. Nightingale,[1],[2] Margaret A. French,[1],[2] and Richard Quintiliani[3],[4]

Department of Pharmacy Services, Hartford Hospital,[1] University of Connecticut School of Pharmacy,[2] and Division Infectious Diseases, Hartford Hospital[3] and University of Connecticut School of Medicine[4]

Over the past few years a relatively large number of cephalosporins became available for general physician use: cephalothin, cephaloridine, cephaglycin, cephalexin, cefazolin, cephapirin and cephradine, cefamandole, cefoxitin, cefadroxil, cefaclor, cefuroxime, and cefotaxime. Many new agents are in various stages of development and are expected to be released for general use within the next 3–5 years. Clinicians have found it difficult to distinguish any particular merit of one of these drugs over another, given their similarities in names and properties. This monograph is intended to present a comparison of the pharmacokinetics of these agents and is intended as an update of our past work (*99, 119*). Excellent reviews on this subject have also been published by Brogard *et al.* (*20*), Anderson (*1*), and Barza and Miao (*9*).

ORAL AGENTS (CEPHALEXIN, CEPHRADINE, CEFADROXIL, CEFACLOR)

The pharmacokinetics of the oral cephalosporins are shown in Table I where it is obvious that more similarities exist between these drugs than differences.

1. Cefalexin and Cephradine
1) Absorption and elimination
The oral cephalosporins, cephalexin and cephradine (Fig. 1), differing in structure by only 2 hydrogen atoms in a six-membered ring, not unexpectedly have almost identical pharmacokinetic properties, microbiological activities, and clinical effectiveness.

We recently studied the pharmacokinetics of these agents in normal volunteers after the administration of one g (2×500-mg capsules) of cephalexin, one g (2×500-mg capsules) of cephradine, and a one-g (1×1.0) tablet of cephalexin in a three-way

[1],[3] Hartford, Connecticut 06115, U.S.A.
[2] Storrs, Connecticut 06268, U.S.A.
[4] Farmington, Connecticut 06032, U.S.A.

TABLE I. Pharmacokinetic Parameters of the Oral Cephalopsorins

Parameter	Cephalexin									
	(61)	(99)	(20)	(45)	(32)	(112)	(87)	(149)	(138)	Mean±S.D.
α (hr⁻¹)	4.57	4.12	—	—	—	—	—	—	—	4.35±0.32
β (hr⁻¹)	0.91	0.86	—	0.90	0.83	1.21	0.67	0.71	0.69	0.85±0.17
k_a (hr⁻¹)	1.90	1.92	0.85	3.35	1.44	4.78	2.79	2.10	2.30	2.38±1.15
k_{12} (hr⁻¹)	1.16	1.13	—	—	—	—	—	—	—	1.15±0.02
k_{21} (hr⁻¹)	2.66	2.24	—	—	—	—	—	—	—	2.45±0.30
k_e (hr⁻¹)	1.63	1.60	—	—	—	—	—	—	—	1.62±0.02
Lag time (hr)	0.43	0.31	—	0.37	0.43	0.30	—	0.20	—	0.34±0.09
$t1/2\alpha$ (hr)	0.15	0.17	—	—	—	—	—	—	—	0.16±0.01
$t1/2\beta$ (hr)	0.78	0.84	0.76	0.77	0.84	0.57	1.04	0.99	1.00	0.84±0.15
V_c (liters)	9.50	12.39	—	—	—	—	—	—	—	10.95±2.04
V_{dss} (liters)	13.70	19.50	—	—	—	—	—	—	—	25.60±8.63
$V_{d\beta}$ (liters)	16.70	24.31	—	—	—	—	—	—	—	20.51±5.38
V_{dext} (liters)	21.40	32.46	—	22.2	21.1	—	—	—	—	24.29±5.47

Parameter	Cephradine					
	(149)	(20)	(45)	(32)	(112)	Mean±S.D.
α (hr⁻¹)	—	—	—	—	—	—
β (hr⁻¹)	0.78	0.83	0.77	0.76	1.14	0.86±0.16
k_a (hr⁻¹)	1.80	1.25	2.50	1.31	3.73	2.12±1.03
k_{12} (hr⁻¹)	—	—	—	—	—	—
k_{21} (hr⁻¹)	—	—	—	—	—	—
k_e (hr⁻¹)	—	—	—	—	—	—
Lag time (hr)	0.20	—	0.33	0.43	0.30	0.32±0.09
$t1/2\alpha$ (hr)	—	—	—	—	—	—
$t1/2\beta$ (hr)	0.91	0.83	0.90	0.91	0.61	0.83±0.13
V_c (liters)	—	—	—	—	—	—
V_{dss} (liters)	—	—	—	—	—	—
$V_{d\beta}$ (liters)	—	—	—	—	—	—
V_{dext} (liters)	—	20.10	18.40	22.30	—	20.27±1.96

( ) Literature references.

crossover study (45). The results of this analysis (Fig. 2) show that no significant pharmacokinetic differences exist between cephalexin or cephradine. The extent of absorption, effect of food, peak serum concentrations, time to reach the peak, rates of absorption and elimination, clearances, urinary recovery, urinary concentrations, and protein binding ($\leq 20\%$ (140)) are either indistinguishable or the differences, e.g., protein binding, are not important with these two cephalosporins.

Parameter	Cefadroxil				
	(76)	(112)	(78)	(87)	Mean±S.D.
α (hr^{-1})	—	—	—	—	—
β (hr^{-1})	0.50	0.55	0.44	0.43	0.48±0.06
k_a (hr^{-1})	—	2.44	3.08	1.37	2.30±0.86
k_{12} (hr^{-1})	—	—	—	—	—
k_{21} (hr^{-1})	—	—	—	—	—
k_e (hr^{-1})	—	—	—	—	—
Lag time (hr)	—	0.37	0.35	—	0.36±0.01
$t1/2\alpha$ (hr)	—	—	—	—	—
$t1/2\beta$ (hr)	1.39	1.27	1.66	1.61	1.48±0.18
V_c (liters)	—	—	—	—	—
V_{dss} (liters)	—	—	—	—	—
$V_{d\beta}$ (liters)	—	—	—	—	—
V_{dext} (liters)	20.65	—	—	—	20.65

Parameter	Cefaclor					
	(149)	(132)	(82)	(138)	(74)	Mean±S.D.
α (hr^{-1})	—	—	—	—	—	—
β (hr^{-1})	1.10	0.87	1.22	0.80	0.92	0.98±0.17
k_a (hr^{-1})	2.30	—	—	2.40	—	2.35±0.07
k_{12} (hr^{-1})	—	—	—	—	—	—
k_{21} (hr^{-1})	—	—	—	—	—	—
k_e (hr^{-1})	—	—	—	—	—	—
Lag time (hr)	0.20	—	—	—	—	2.0
$t1/2\alpha$ (hr)	—	—	—	—	—	—
$t1/2\beta$ (hr)	0.63	0.80	0.58	0.90	0.75	0.73±0.13
V_c (liters)	—	—	—	—	—	—
V_{dss} (liters)	—	—	—	—	—	—
$V_{d\beta}$ (liters)	—	—	—	—	—	—
V_{dext} (liters)	—	—	—	—	—	—

Although the study described above (45) clearly establishes the lack of pharmacokinetic differences between cephalexin and cephradine, it also illustrates the excellent serum concentrations that can be achieved with these drugs. The peak serum concentrations of approximately 32 mcg/ml far exceeds that obtained with cephradine, cephalothin, and cephapirin after an equal dose administered by the intramuscular route (99).

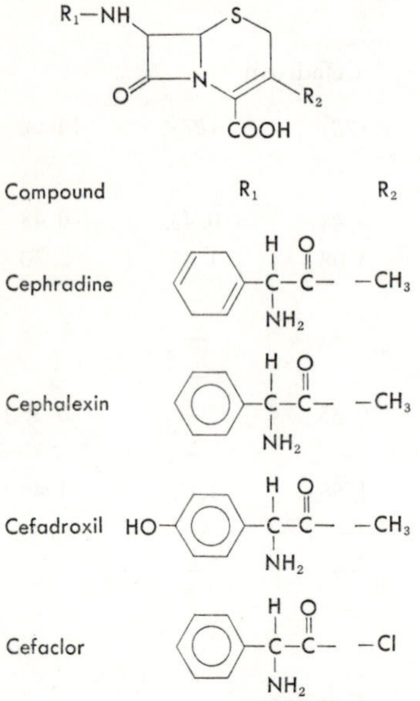

FIG. 1. Chemical structures of oral cephalosporins.

This observation prompted another study in which we compared the pharmacokinetics of cephalexin and cephradine after the administration of a 2.0-g dose in a multiple dose regimen (*32*). Again it was found that the pharmacokinetics of these drugs are identical. Of possible clinical relevance was the attainment of a peak serum concentration of approximately 50 mcg/ml, a concentration that is essentially similar to that observed after a 1.0-g intravenous dose of cephradine, cephalothin, or cephapirin (*32*).

The peak serum levels obtained even after a 1-g dose of these oral cephalosporins ($\sim$32 mcg/ml) are almost 10 times their usual minimum inhibitory concentrations (MICs) for penicillin-resistant staphylococci ($\sim$3.4 mcg/ml). Therapeutic results theoretically should be similar to those obtained with the parenteral cephalosporins in the treatment of staphyloccal infections. Supporting this impression was a recent study (*144*) in which excellent clinical results were obtained in the therapy of staphylococcal osteomyelitis and suppurative arthritis in children with an initial one-week course of a parenteral cephalosporin.

The only apparent difference between these agents is the affect of food on the absorption process in children and infants. When these drugs are administered to adults, it is well established that the rate of absorption (as reflected in the peak serum concentration and the time to reach the peak) is altered but the extent of absorption, as measured by the area under the serum concentration time curve (AUC), is not. This was recently also shown to be true in the case of cephradine absorption in infants and children (*53*), but not for cephalexin (*89*). For the latter drug, the AUC was also

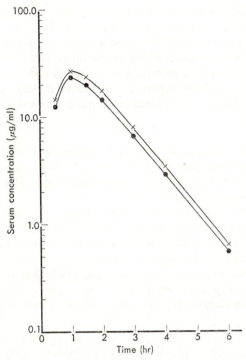

FIG. 2.   Cephalexin (●) and cephradine (×) serum concentrations after a 1.0-g oral dose.

reduced. This is a surprising finding given the almost identical molecular structure and the tendency for cephradine to convert into cephalexin in solution. Further study is necessary to explain this finding.

2) Distribution

The usefulness of cephalexin or cephradine in the treatment of tissue infections depends upon their ability to penetrate into the tissue. Two recent studies (*77, 137*) indicate that cephalexin levels in synovial fluid, joint tissues, and mandibular alveolar bone were high enough to be clinically useful. A review of the literature (*20, 99*) however, reveals that although both agents are widely distributed into a variety of tissues, their concentrations are not particularly high. For example, levels of 2 to 40 mcg/ml are observed in the bile after a 500-mg dose (*20, 99*). This is a relatively low concentration compared to equal doses of cefazolin or cefamandole. Like all cephalosporins, spinal fluid levels are low (*20, 99*) and this class of agents is generally not recommended in the treatment of central nervous system (CNS) infections. Levels in amniotic fluid (*94, 99, 119*), breast milk (*20, 94, 99*), aqueous humor (*20, 99*), and saliva (*99*) were also not outstanding, although a recent report demonstrated exudate levels of approximately 50% of serum concentrations for cephalexin (*71*), and that cephradine lung tissue concentrations were 42% of serum levels (*81*). Rapid transport of cephradine into the fetus (10 min) from maternal blood has been observed (*34*).

Although not well established, it appears that tissue levels are proportional to serum concentrations. This is not unexpected considering the drugs' lack of protein binding. Other similar oral agents with a prolonged serum half-life should yield sustained tissue concentrations greater than cephalexin-cephradine. Recently a sustained release cephalexin dosage form was developed but is not commercially available (*133*).

3) Clinical considerations

Both cephalexin and cephradine have similar activity against the same microorganisms (*Staphylococcus aureus*, Group A streptococcus, *Escherichia coli*, *Proteus mirabilis*, *Klebsiella pneumoniae*, and *Haemophilus influenzae*); they are used orally to treat the same types of infections from these pathogens.

No evidence can be found to indicate that treatment failures with one drug would result in treatment successes with the other. If one drug is effective, it is likely that the other will also be effective and, similarly, if one drug fails, it is likely that the other will fail; in essence there are no therapeutic differences.

Thus, based upon all measurable parameters (*e.g.*, microbiological activity, pharmacokinetic characteristics, therapeutic effectiveness, and toxicity), it is concluded that these drugs are not significantly different agents and should be considered equivalent antibiotics.

2. Cefaclor

1) Absorption and elimination

From a pharmacokinetic view, only minor differences between cefaclor and cephalexin-cephradine exist. Cefaclor, like the other oral cephalosporins, exhibits negligible protein binding (<20%). Examination of Table I reveals that cefaclor has a somewhat shorter half-life than cephalexin-cephradine but this difference is only about 6 min. Dosage adjustments because of this difference are not required. It is also evident that the percent of the dose excreted in the urine is lower with cefaclor (54 %) than with cephalexin-cephradine (~90%) in adults (*82, 87, 138, 149*), as well as children (*45, 119*). This is not due to metabolic loss of the drug in the body; rather it is caused by an instability which appears to be pH dependent (*47*), *i.e.*, stability decreases with increasing pH. These differences between cefaclor and cephradine-cephalexin in blood and urine concentrations are not large and are probably of little clinical significance in light of cefaclor's enhanced microbiological activity. Other pharmacokinetic studies (*55, 92*), although noncomparative, support these findings. Cefaclor's absorption rate, extent of absorption, effect of food on absorption, and protein-binding characteristics are similar to cephalexin-cephradine. McCracken *et al.* (*88*) reported somewhat less of a food effect on cefaclor absorption compared to cephalexin in children.

The molecular instability of cefaclor results in a lack of accumulation when this drug is used to treat patients with impaired renal function or chronic renal failure. In chronic renal failure, the half-life ratio ($t1/2$ renal failure: $t1/2$ normal) of cephalexin increases to 16 (*142*). With cefaclor the ratio increases to only 3.6 (*17, 85, 132, 142*). The relationship between cefaclor elimination and creatinine clearance has been characterized by several authors (*17, 142*). Hemodialysis was found to decrease the elimination half-life by only 25–30% (*15, 85, 132*).

2) Distribution

The tissue penetration of cefaclor cannot be fully evaluated at this time. Only two reports are available, and neither one is a comparative study. In one report (*88*), cefaclor saliva and tear levels were determined in infants and children after a 15-mg/kg dose. Tear levels were reported to be >1.0 mcg/ml while saliva levels were stated to be equal to serum concentrations, although the authors did not demonstrate that the saliva concentrations were not due to residual drug in the mouth after oral administration of suspended solid particles (suspension) of cefaclor.

The other report concerns cefaclor penetration into sputum after 0.5- and 1-g doses (*138*). At the peak, the ratio of cefaclor serum: sputum concentrations was 26 : 1 and 33 : 1 for the 0.5-g and 1.0-g doses, respectively. The mean peak sputum concentrations were 0.4 and 0.6 mcg/ml for the low and high doses. Non-peak saliva concentrations were as much as four times lower (0.14 mcg/ml) than the peak concentrations. Conclusions concerning the penetration ability of cefaclor cannot be made at this time due to a paucity of data and lack of comparative studies. Its pharmacokinetic profile in serum and urine compared to cephalexin-cephradine suggests that tissue penetration will be equal to, or less than, that of older agents.

3) Clinical considerations

While cefaclor, cephradine, and cephalexin have similar wide spectra of antimicrobial activity, cefaclor has greater *in vitro* activity against various species including *E. coli, K. pneumoniae, P. mirabilis*, and *H. influenzae* (*16, 134*). For this reason cefaclor cannot be considered as a therapeutic alternative to cephalexin-cephradine.

3. Cefadroxil

1) Absorption and elimination

Cefadroxil differs from cephalexin by the addition of a *para*-hydroxyl group on the aromatic ring (Fig. 1). The only property (Table I) affected by *p*-hydroxylation of the cephalexin molecule is a decrease in the rate of elimination (*72, 76, 78, 87, 112*). This results in prolonged and higher serum and urine concentration (Fig. 3, Table I) of cefadroxil (*69, 72, 78, 87, 112*). The mechanisms for this change in elimination are not clear. Significant protein-binding differences do not exist between these agents and must be ruled out as a possible mechanism. The prolonged excretion of cefadroxil compared to cephalexin does not mean that more cefadroxil is eliminated *via* the urine. The urinary recovery of both drugs is essentially the same. After 12 hr, urinary recoveries of 89%, 85%, and 100% have been reported for cefadroxil, cephalexin, and cephradine, respectively. The kinetics of excretion of these drugs however, is not similar. After administration of equivalent doses, cefadroxil urinary concentrations are initially (0–3 hr) lower (1,200 mcg/ml compared to 2,000 mcg/ml) than

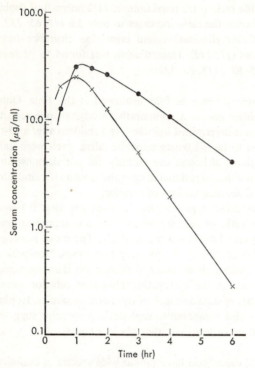

FIG. 3.   Cefadroxil (●) and cefaclor (×) serum concentrations after a 1.0-g oral dose.

that of cephalexin and cephradine after a 0.5-g dose, but at all other time intervals, cefadroxil concentrations are higher (1,100 mcg/ml compared to 600 mcg/ml at 3–6 hr post dosing and 170 mcg/ml compared to 70 mcg/ml, 6–12 hr fast dosing, respectively) (*69, 72, 112*).

Since cephalexin has a short half-life, it is essentially all eliminated within a 6-hr period. After 6 hr, urinary concentrations are negligible, and if microbiologic activity is still desired after this time, then another dose of the drug is necessary. In fact, the usual dose of cephalexin in uncomplicated urinary tract infections (UTI) is 500-mg every 6 hr. Since cefadroxil is not completely eliminated from the body in 6 hr due to its longer half-life (it is only eliminated *via* the kidneys), appreciable urine concentration persists for 6–12 hr. Using equal doses (2 g per day), it should be possible to achieve adequate urine concentrations for the treatment of uncomplicated UTI with the administration of 1 g cefadroxil every 12 hr. This has been found to be true (*71, 148*). No clinical difference exists in the treatment of uncomplicated UTI with equal daily doses (2 g) of cephalexin (0.5-g q6 hr) or cefadroxil (1-g q12 hr). The advantage of this new oral cephalosporin is therefore one of patient compliance. It is assumed that compliance is greater when less self-administrations per day are required by the patient. An additional advantage of this drug is that its absorption is less affected by the presence of food (*54, 112*) in the stomach compared to cephalexin and cephradine. Since the entire dose of the drug is recovered in the urine regardless of meals, it is doubtful that this difference is of real clinical significance in UTI.

Cefadroxil, like cephalexin-cephradine, will accumulate in patients with impaired renal function. The half-life ratio of anuric patients' $t1/2$ to normals is 10–18 (*38, 76*) which is similar to that of cephalexin (*76, 142*). The relationship between drug half-life and renal function has been well characterized (*38*). Dosage adjustment is not necessary until creatinine clearance falls to less than 25 ml/min. Hemodialysis (6–8 hr) has decreased serum concentrations by 75% (*76*).

2) Distribution

Like cefaclor, cefadroxil penetration into tissue cannot be evaluated since sufficient data have not been published. Saliva levels in infants and children were reported in one study (*54*).

3) Clinical considerations

Para-hydroxylation has not altered cefadroxil's microbiological spectrum compared to cephalexin. Both agents share equal activity against *E. coli*, *Klebsiella* species, and *P. mirabilis* and are not active against most strains of *Enterobacter*, *P. morganii*, *P. vulgaris*, and *Pseudomonas* (*27, 69*). The mild side effects seen with cephalexin are equally observed with cefadroxil (*71, 148*) and both share the same stability to β-lactamase inactivation (*27*).

PARENTERAL AGENTS (CEPHALOTHIN, CEPHAPIRIN, CEFOXITIN, CEFAMANDOLE, CEFAZOLIN, CEFOTAXIME, CEFUROXIME, CEPHRADINE)

The parenteral cephalosporins can be historically classified into the older "first-generation" agents (cephalothin, cephapirin, and cefazolin) and the newer "second-generation" agents (cefoxitin, cefamandole, and cefuroxime). Cefotaxime is considered a "third generation" cephalosporin because of its enhanced activity against *Psuedomonas*. The pharmacokinetic parameters of these drugs after intravenous administration are shown in Table II and after intramuscular administration in Table III. It can be seen that considerable similarities exist between the metabolized cephalosporins (cephalothin, cephapirin) and marked differences exist between cefazolin and the other agents.

1. Cephalothin-Cephapirin

1) Metabolism and elimination

The metabolized cephalosporins (Fig. 5) have similar pharmacokinetic properties (Tables II and III). Both drugs are bound to serum proteins to a moderate extent: 69.4% (*20, 109, 140*) and 55.7% (*6, 20, 109*) for cephalothin and cephapirin, respectively. Limited pharmacokinetics have been reported in children (*20, 127*). The biological half-life after intravenous administration is 32 and 41 min and after intra-

TABLE II.   Pharmacokinetic Parameters of the Parenteral Cephalosporins

Parameter	Cephalothin				Cephapirin				
	(99)	(84)	(12)[a]	Mean±S.D.[b]	(99)	(84)	(12)[a]	(28)	Mean±S.D.[b]
α (hr⁻¹)	7.28	6.0	7.15	6.95±1.93	5.32	5.7	4.69	5.52	5.31±0.44
β (rh⁻¹)	1.56	1.3	1.42	1.50±0.48	1.00	1.2	0.91	1.91	1.05±0.12
k_{12} (hr⁻¹)	2.01	1.5	1.77	1.82±0.83	0.99	1.4	1.07	1.14	1.15±0.18
k_{21} (hr⁻¹)	2.73	2.1	2.21	2.52±0.88	1.37	1.9	1.34	1.52	1.53±0.26
k_{10} (hr⁻¹)	4.09	3.7	4.59	4.12±0.87	3.96	3.6	3.19	3.94	3.67±0.36
$t1/2\alpha$ (hr)	0.10	0.12	0.10	0.11±0.03	0.13	0.12	0.15	0.13	0.13±0.01
$t1/2\beta$ (hr)	0.56	0.53	0.49	0.53±0.28	0.71	0.58	0.76	0.64	0.67±0.08
V_c (liters)	7.76	10.15	7.28	8.08±2.68	9.27	9.88	8.84	10.31	9.58±0.65
V_{dss} (liters)	14.29	17.40	13.11	14.61±5.59	15.87	17.60	15.90	18.04	16.85±1.13
V_d (liters)	22.20	28.88	23.53	23.54±8.48	34.94	29.64	30.99	37.28	33.21±3.52

Parameter	Cefoxitin				Cefamandole				
	(99)	(135)	(44)[a]	Mean±S.D.	(23)	(8)[a]	(113)	(66)	Mean±S.D.
α (hr⁻¹)	6.32	5.36	5.80	5.82±0.48	2.66	3.13	3.13	3.74	3.21±0.45
β (hr⁻¹)	1.04	0.88	0.89	0.94±0.09	0.74	0.72	0.80	0.97	0.81±0.11
k_{12} (hr⁻¹)	2.19	1.80	2.04	2.01±0.20	—	0.73	0.82	0.72	0.76±0.06
k_{21} (hr⁻¹)	2.27	1.65	1.84	1.92±0.32	—	1.14	1.39	1.40	1.31±0.15
k_{10} (hr⁻¹)	2.89	2.79	2.81	2.83±0.05	—	1.98	1.90	2.58	2.15±0.37
$t1/2\alpha$ (hr)	0.11	0.12	0.12	0.12±0	0.26	0.22	0.20	0.19	0.22±0.03
$t1/2\beta$ (hr)	0.67	0.79	0.78	0.76±0.07	0.94	0.96	0.87	0.71	0.87±0.11
V_c (liters)	6.88	0.82	7.07	7.38±0.71	—	5.01	(0.12 liters/kg) 9.41	4.17	6.20±2.81
V_{dss} (liters)	13.52	16.1	14.91	14.80±1.29	—	8.22	(0.19 liters/kg) 14.90	6.30	9.81±4.51
V_d (liters)	19.12	25.3	22.32	22.25±3.09	—	13.78	(0.28 liters/kg) 22.00	11.09	15.62±5.68

[a] Data re-analyzed using a two compartment model.   [b] Means obtained by individually

muscular administration is 47 and 51 min for cephalothin and cephapirin, respectively. These relatively short $t1/2$'s are due to metabolism to desacetyl compounds as well as elimination *via* the kidneys. The metabolites possess 20% and 54% of the microbiological activity of the parent drugs for cephalothin and cephapirin, respectively (20).

It should be stressed that the pharmacokinetic parameters shown in Tables II and III are somewhat artifactual since they were obtained from studies where drug

Parameter	Cefazolin			Cephradine	
	(99)	(12)[a]	Mean±S.D.[b]	(99)	Mean±S.D.
α (hr^{-1})	3.97	3.07	4.30±2.56	6.39	±1.39
β (hr^{-1})	0.40	0.46	0.42±0.08	0.99	±0.38
k_{12} (hr^{-1})	1.73	0.93	1.72±1.31	2.26	±0.13
k_{21} (hr^{-1})	1.67	1.83	2.00±1.28	2.81	±1.54
k_{10} (hr^{-1})	0.97	0.77	1.00±0.32	2.32	±0.10
$t1/2\alpha$ (hr)	0.24	0.23	0.23±0.14	0.11	±0.03
$t1/2\beta$ (hr)	1.80	1.51	1.74±0.36	0.76	±0.30
V_c (liters)	4.44	4.74	4.10±1.68	9.23	±1.88
V_{dss} (liters)	8.48	7.15	8.32±1.92	16.04	±2.22
V_d (liters)	10.27	7.93	12.38±4.43	21.20	±3.03

Parameter	Cefotaxime				Cefuroxime			
	(153)	(73)	(18)	Mean±S.D.	(58)	(49)	(41)	Mean±S.D.
α (hr^{-1})	2.7	2.67	—	2.69±0.02	2.36	2.83	4.31	3.17±1.02
β (hr^{-1})	0.4	0.68	—	0.54±0.20	0.49	0.62	0.56	0.56±0.06
k_{12} (hr^{-1})	1.0	0.79	—	0.90±0.15	0.70	0.77	1.76	1.08±0.59
k_{21} (hr^{-1})	0.8	1.22	—	1.01±0.30	0.99	1.55	1.60	1.38±0.34
k_{10} (hr^{-1})	1.3	1.66	—	1.48±0.25	1.18	1.12	1.50	1.27±0.20
$t1/2\alpha$ (hr)	—	0.26	0.29	0.28±0.02	0.29	0.25	0.16	0.23±0.07
$t1/2\beta$ (hr)	1.72	1.04	1.14	1.30±0.37	1.41	1.12	0.62	1.05±0.40
V_c (liters)	—	9.1	10.7	9.90±1.13	8.09	9.80	5.47	7.79±2.18
V_{dss} (liters)	—	14.3	—	14.30	13.78	14.64	11.46	13.29±1.64
V_d (liters)	—	21.8	—	21.8	19.39	17.83	14.86	17.30±2.40

averaging all data found in review articles (1).

concentrations were determined by microbiological analysis. These studies did not separate the biologically active metabolites from the parent compound. Since concentrations of parent drug-metabolite mixtures were calculated using standard solutions of the parent compound, the concentration-time relationship is over estimated (127) and therefore, the pharmacokinetic parameters are also in error (127). The serum concentration-time curve for cephalothin-cephapirin (Fig. 5) should be considered as a "microbiologically active" concentration-time curve. For comparative

TABLE III. Absorption-I.M.

	Cephalothin				
	(20)	(84)	(109)	(1)	Mean±S.D.
Serum peak (μg/ml) (500 mg dose)	7.3	10.7	8.6	—	9.6±2.00
Serum peak (μg/ml) (1,000 mg dose)	18	—	—	—	18
t max (hr)	1.0	0.46	0.75	—	0.62±0.33
k_a (hr^{-1})	—	—	—	—	—
t1/2 abs. (min)	—	—	—	—	—
t1/2 (i.m.) (hr)	0.6	0.73–0.82	0.97	—	0.78±0.16
24 hr urine (% recovery)	—	—	51.2	50–70	57.1±11.2
Bioavailability (%)	—	98	—	—	98

	Cephapirin				
	(20)	(84)	(109)	(1)	Mean±S.D.
Serum peak (μg/ml) (500 mg dose)	10	9.5	14.0	—	11.3±2.00
Serum peak (μg/ml) (1,000 mg dose)	25	16.9	—	—	20.0±4.40
t max (hr)	0.5–1.0	0.37–0.6	0.75	—	0.55±0.25
k_a (hr^{-1})	—	—	—	—	—
t1/2 abs. (min)	—	—	—	—	—
t1/2 (i.m.)(hr)	0.8±1.0	0.67–0.82	0.98	—	0.85±0.14
24 hr urine (% recovery)	—	—	69.5	69–72	70.2±1.60
Bioavailability (%)	—	98	—	—	98

	Cefoxitin				
	(20)	(135)	(1)	(141)	Mean±S.D.
Serum peak (μg/ml) (500 mg dose)	11	13	—	—	12.0±1.40
Serum peak (μg/ml) (1,000 mg dose)	22	22–30.3	—	28.8±2.27	24.8±4.80
t max (hr)	0.3	0.17–0.46	—	0.43±0.03	0.31±0.15
k_a (hr^{-1})	—	—	—	1.39	1.39
t1/2 abs. (min)	—	—	—	30	30
t1/2 (i.m.)(hr)	0.7–1.0	0.8–1.5	—	0.75±0.09	1.0±0.40
24 hr urine (% recovery)	—	—	90–99	—	90–99
Bioavailability (%)	—	95% with and without lidocaine	—	—	95

	Cefamandole					
	(20)	(109)	(1)	(64)	(96)	Mean±S.D.
Serum peak (μg/ml) (500 mg dose)	12–15	12	—	12.2	—	13.0±1.70
Serum peak (μg/ml) (1,000 mg dose)	20–35	20	—	20.6	20	23.8±7.50
t max (hr)	1	1.0–1.5	—	—	0.5	1.0±0.40
k_a (hr^{-1})	6.47	—	—	—	—	6.47
$t1/2$ abs. (min)	6	—	—	—	—	6
$t1/2$ (i.m.)(hr)	1.0–1.2	1.7	—	—	1.0–1.5	1.28±0.31
24 hr urine (% recovery)	—	—	80–100	71.3% $\bar{p}$-8 hr	—	—
Bioavailability (%)	—	—	—	—	—	—

	Cefazolin					Cephradine		
	(20)	(109)	(1)	(13)	Mean±S.D.	(20)	(109)	Mean±S.D.
Serum peak (μg/ml) (500 mg dose)	37	31.5	—	—	34.3±3.90	—	9.51	9.51
Serum peak (μg/ml) (1,000 mg dose)	68	—	—	68.3	68.2±0.20	12	—	12
t max (hr)	1	0.75	—	1.19	0.98±0.22	1.0	0.75	0.88±0.18
k_a (hr^{-1})	1.91	—	—	2.22	2.07±0.22	1.1	—	1.1
$t1/2$ abs. (min)	24	—	—	—	24	36	—	36
$t1/2$ (i.m.)(hr)	1.5	2.07	—	2.71	2.09±0.61	1.5	1.24	1.37±0.18
24 hr urine (% recovery)	—	73.3	80–88	—	80.4±7.40	—	91.9	91.9
Bioavailability (%)	—	—	—	—	—	100	—	100

	Cefotaxime					Cefuroxime			
	(19)	(73)	(60)	(18)	Mean±S.D.	(49)	(41)	(68)	Mean±S.D.
Serum peak (μg/ml) (500 mg dose)	11.80	—	—	—	11.80	25.7	21.2	—	23.45±3.18
Serum peak (μg/ml) (1,000 mg dose)	20.50	—	33.9	35.9	30.1±8.37	40.0	32.2	—	36.1±5.52
t max (hr)	—	—	0.5–1	—	0.5–1	0.57	0.83	0.78	0.73±0.14
k_a (hr^{-1})	—	—	—	—	—	—	—	—	—
$t1/2$ abs. (min)	—	—	—	—	—	—	—	—	—
$t1/2$ (i.m.)(hr)	1.27	0.93	—	—	1.10±0.24	1.18	1.48	1.18	1.28±0.17
24 hr urine (% recovery)	36	—	—	—	36	95	—	84.5	89.8±7.4
Bioavailability (%)	—	—	—	—	—	100	—	—	100

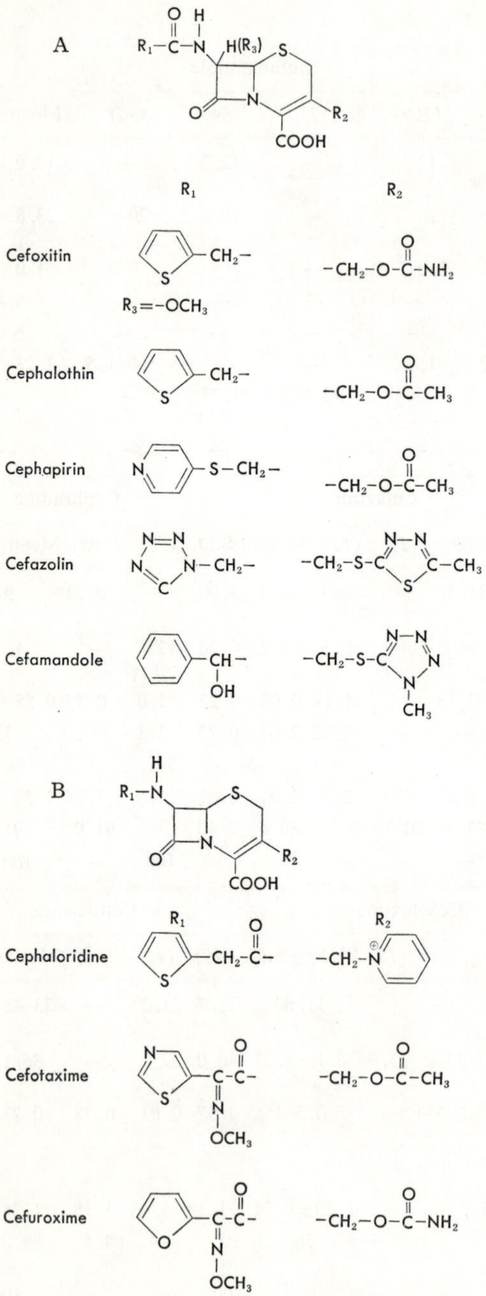

FIG. 4. Chemical structures of parenteral cephalosporins.

purposes Flg. 5 can be utilized to described the decline of microbiological activity as a function of time.

The metabolism of these drugs by esterases occurs in virtually all tissues with minor metabolism in serum. Both the metabolites and parent compounds are eliminated from the body *via* the kidneys. Active secretion accounts for the majority of metabolite excretion (*28, 93*). The desacetyl metabolites of cephalothin and cephapirin are also excreted renally with 43% of a dose of cephalothin and 45.3% of a dose of cephapirin appearing in the urine after 6 hr as the metabolite. This is 44% and 48%, respectively, of the total drug recovered (*28, 102*). In uremic patients, 4.7% of a cephalothin dose was recovered after 14 hr and 78.2–94.4% of the total drug recovered was the metabolite (*102*).

Cephalothin, using a microbiological assay method, has been found to have a mean $t1/2$ of 3.7 hr in patients with creatinine clearance values of <10 ml/min (*53*). Interestingly though, in the same study, when investigated with high pressure liquid chromatography (HPLC) assay, the desacetyl metabolite was found to be accumulating in these patients given 1-g q12 hr. Further, there was no apparent decline in the metabolite concentration at 14 hr after a dose. In contrast, with normal renal function, the $t1/2$ of unmetabolized cephalothin was 0.47 hr and no desacetyl metabolite was detected at 6 hr after dosing. Hemodialysis has little affect on the clearance of cephalothin with reported $t1/2$sec during dialysis at 3.3 hr (*99*) and 2.6 hr (*2*)—not very different than that in severe renal insufficiency. Serum concentrations have been reported to be reduced by 50% with peritoneal dialysis (*2*).

At a mean creatinine clearance of 12.6 ml/min, the $t1/2$ of cephapirin was reported as 1.59 hr, while during hemodialysis the $t1/2$ was found to be 1.8 hr (*99*).

2) Distribution

There have been few studies which compare the tissue penetration of cephalothin and cephapirin. In two recent studies comparing the tissue penetration characteristics of these drugs in adults (*118*) and children (*64*) undergoing open heart surgery, it was found in adults that cephapirin achieved slightly higher levels than those with cephalothin in pericardial fluid and the right atrial appendage, whereas in children these levels were identical.

Several new cephalosporin tissue penetration studies have been reported, such as in the prostate and seminal vesicles (*129*), ascitic fluid (*20*), bronchial secretions (*20*), pleural fluid (*20*), spinal fluid (*20*), and placental cord blood (*20*), in addition to previously reviewed work (*99*). Although tissue concentration comparisons between the metabolized and nonmetabolized cephalosporins are difficult to assess because of experimental differences in study design and methodology, it appears that the metabolized drugs in general exhibit lower tissue concentrations than the nonmetabolized agents (aqueous humor (*138*), ascitic fluid (*20*), heart (*5, 43, 118*), bone (*36, 46, 110, 136, 150*), synovial fluid (*20, 99, 136*), and amniotic fluid (*138*)). This is partially due to the fact that at equal doses the serum concentrations are lower compared to the nonmetabolized drugs. A little appreciated aspect of tissue metabolism is that this phenomenon occurs both *in vivo* as well as *in vitro*. Recently we determined that the usual procedures of homogenization, centrification, and assay in uterine tissue causes almost total conversion of cephalothin to its metabolite (*101*). This confirms earlier findings in bone tissue (*46*) where cephalothin recoveries were unacceptably low, forcing us to change our method of extraction. In virtually every study reporting tissue concentrations of cephalothin and cephapirin, recovery values were not provided nor was any mention made of special techniques to prevent drug metabolism during sample handling. We must assume that no special measures were taken. In addition almost all workups used the microbiological method of analysis. In our estimation, cephalothin, in the absence of measures to prevent *in vitro* metabolism, will be converted by tissue esterases to the desacetyl form during the extraction procedure. Measurement of the parent compound and metabolite concentration by microbiological techniques using parent compound standard solutions will grossly underestimate cephalothin concentrations if *in vitro* conversion to the metabolite is not prevented. It is highly likely that most cephalothin tissue penetration studies reported artifactual data that underestimated the true tissue penetration of cephalothin. Insufficient data are available concerning cephapirin to conclude whether this is also a problem with this drug, however, the similarities in pharmacokinetics (as measured by microbiological assay) suggest that cephapirin tissue concentrations are also underestimated.

Cephalothin and cephapirin do not penetrate well through noninflamed meninges (*20, 99*). Penetration through inflamed meninges is somewhat better but does not yield reliably high cerebrospinal fluid(CSF) levels to comfortably treat serious infection. These drugs are generally not recommended for the treatment of CNS infections.

3) Clinical considerations
From a therapeutic view both drugs are equally effective in the treatment of infections from gram-positive bacteria such as staphylococci (*S. aureus* and *S. epidermidis*), Group A streptococcus, anaerobic streptococci, and *Streptococcus pneumoniae* and from gram-negative organisms such as *E. coli, P. mirabilis, H. influenzae,* and *K. pneumoniae.*

It may be best not to use the metabolized cephalosporins in patients with renal failure. The desacetyl metabolite is cleared renally but the pharmacokinetics have not yet been fully characterized. This metabolite appears to accumulate (*102*) and the potential for toxicity or development of resistant organisms is unknown.

Based upon all measurable parameters (*e.g.*, microbiological activity, pharmacokinetic characteristics, therapeutic effectiveness, and toxicity), it can be concluded that these drugs are not significantly different agents.

2. Cefotaxime
Cefotaxime is a "third generation" cephalosporin with an enhanced microbiological spectrum, and a degree of stability to β-lactamase (*95*). It is a semi-synthetic cephalosporin (Fig. 5) available for parenteral use, as oral absorption is poor. A single 500-mg or 1-g i.m. dose in normal volunteers gave peak serum concentrations of 11.7 μg/ml

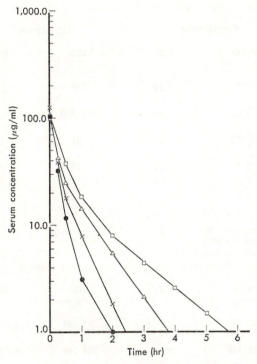

FIG. 5. Cephradine (△), cephalothin (×), cephapirin (●), and cefotaxime (□) serum concentrations after a 1.0-g i.v. bolus dose.

and 20.5 µg/ml, respectively. The half-life by this route was about 1.1 hr. When given by i.v. bolus a 500-mg, 1-g, or 2-g dose gave serum concentrations of 38.9 µg/ml, 101.7 µg/ml, and 214.4 µg/ml. One g infused over 30 min gave a serum concentration at the end of infusion of 41.1 µg/ml (75).

The half-life calculated from i.v. dosing was about 1.05 hr (18, 31, 73, 75, 154) (see Table II). The half-life in children was found to be the same as in adults but was 3 hr in neonates (70, 79). In one premature infant, on the first day of life, the cefotaxime half life was found to be 8 hr (70).

1) Excretion

Since this drug is partially eliminated *via* the renal route as well as by metabolism to the desacetyl compound, it is expected that renal dysfunction will prolong cefotaxime's half-life. This was shown to occur in several studies (31, 146, 154). The prolongation of the half-life was related to the decrease in creatinine clearance: GFR <30 ml/min, $t1/2$ is 1.87 hr; GFR <5, $t1/2$ is 4.2 hr (154). The volume of distribution decreased with decreasing renal function from 27.3 to 19.2 liters (154). Peritoneal dialysis resulted in a 0–42% decrease in $t1/2$ (154) while hemodialysis of 8 anephric patients resulted in

TABLE IV. Renal Excretion

	Cephalothin		Cephapirin	
	Value	Ref.	Value	Ref.
TBC-normal ml/min/1.73 m²	472	99	580	1
RCL-normal ml/min/1.73 m²	274	99	342–360	1,6
% normally excreted unchanged in 24 hr	50–70	99	41	99
% excreted in 24 hr in renal failure	<5 ml/min 2.5	20	19	20
t1/2-MRF	1.4	2	1.6	99
t1/2-SRF	3.7	102	—	—
Hemodialysis t1/2	2.6–3.3	2,99	1.8	99
Peritoneal dialysis t1/2	↓ Serum concentration by 50%	2	20% removed in 6 hr	2

	Cefoxitin		Cefotaxime	
	Value	Ref.	Value	Ref.
TBC-normal ml/min/1.73 m²	247–331	20	207–383	18,73,154
RCL-normal ml/min/1.73 m²	225–329	20,44	101–164	18,73,75
% normally excreted unchanged in 24 hr	84–100	44,99	61–68	18,79,154
% excreted in 24 hr in renal failure	<10 ml/min 26.6	44	5–27	146,154
t1/2-MRF	—	—	1.4–1.9	146,154
t1/2-SRF	15.0±5.3	2,44,50	2.4–6.2	146,154
Hemodialysis t1/2	3.9±0.2	44,50	1.5–2.2	146,154
Peritoneal dialysis t1/2	—	—	No change	154

TBC, total body clearance; RCL, renal clearance; MRF, moderate renal function (Cl$_{CR}$ 10–35

an elimination half-life of 3 hr (146). Accumulation could be avoided by increasing the dosing interval. If the GFR was 20–50, 10–20, or 5–10 ml/min the suggested dosing interval is 8, 12, and 24 hr, respectively. Evidence for active secretion was observed when the cefotaxime clearance was reduced from 223 to 174 ml/min by the administration of probenecid (18).

2) Metabolism

It has been found that cefotaxime is converted to desacetyl metabolite in the liver and possibly other organs (152, 154). The extent of metabolism ranges from 35–56% (73, 90, 152). Renal dysfunction will cause the metabolite to accumulate in the blood

	Cefamandole		Cefazolin	
	Value	Ref.	Value	Ref.
TBC-normal ml/min/1.73 m²	193-303	*20, 96, 115*	52-63	*20, 99*
RCL-normal ml/min/1.73 m²	160-250	*8, 20, 96, 135*	42-64	*20, 99*
% normally excreted unchanged in 24 hr	65-96	*8, 20, 67*	80-100	*20, 99*
% excreted in 24 hr in renal failure	8.6-30	*20, 39*	22.1±14	*99*
t1/2-MRF	3.0±0.3	*2*	14.9±2.9	*2*
t1/2-SRF	10.4±2.4	*3, 4, 29, 39, 91*	35.3±9.6	*2, 24*
Hemodialysis t1/2	5.6±1.1	*3, 4, 28, 29, 91*	5.5±1.9	*2, 24*
Peritoneal dialysis t1/2	8.7±2.4	*1, 29*	32.5	*2*

	Cephradine		Cefuroxime	
	Value	Ref.	Value	Ref.
TBC-normal ml/min/1.73 m²	435	*99*	146-152	*56, 58*
RCL-normal ml/min/1.73 m²	367	*99*	143-148	*49, 58*
% normally excreted unchanged in 24 hr	79-96	*99*	94-97	*49, 56, 58*
% excreted in 24 hr in renal failure	—		35	*59*
t1/2-MRF	—		16.1	*59*
t1/2-SRF	—		15-22	*59, 83*
Hemodialysis t1/2	—		3.3-3.75	*83*
Peritoneal dialysis t1/2	—		13.5	*83*

ml/min); SRF, severe renal function (Cl$_{CR}$<5 ml/min).

and hepatic necrosis was found to decrease metabolite production. Bile, which is a normal route of excretion for desacetyl cefotaxime, has high metabolite/parent compound ratios: 243/36 and 193/16 in common and gallbladder bile, respectively (*90*).

3) Distribution

The distribution of cefotaxime has not been extensively studied. Bile levels were found to be equal to or greater than serum concentrations (*90, 153*) with a biliary t1/2 of 118 min (*153*).

The concentration of the drug in CSF in animals and humans has been reported to be low (*75, 90*). However, the drug has been used to treat 14 children (2 days–7

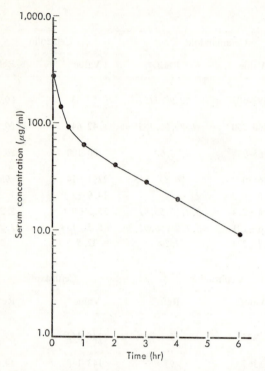

FIG. 6.   Cefazolin serum concentrations after a 1.0-g i.v. bolus dose.

years) with meningitis caused by sensitive organisms (*11*). The majority of children (9/14) were given other antibiotics as well to which the organisms were usually sensitive. Early in therapy, the CSF: serum concentration ratios at 2 hr after a 20–100-mg/kg dose were found to be 0.25–4.77. Actual cefotaxime concentrations by microbiological assay were 1.4 to 27.2 mg/ml. These concentrations seemed to decrease as therapy continued and the cells in CSF declined.

Concentrations were found to be adequate in bone (5.4–20 mcg/g) (*128, 153*) and as high as 50% of serum concentrations after multiple dosing (*108*). Peak concentrations in other fluids were also found to be good: secretions of postsurgical wounds after hip replacement, 20.8 mcg/ml (*153*); peritoneal fluid, 28.6 mcg/ml (*153*), pus, 50% of serum (*i.e.*, 7.4 mcg/ml) (*90*); and pleural fluid, 7.2 mcg/ml with an estimated pleural fluid $t1/2$ 5–6 hr (*80*). Variable sputum levels were reported. One study (*90*) reported values of 0.6–23.4 mcg/ml concentrations, while another study reported sputum/serum ratios of 0.01 increasing to 0.17 from 0.5 to 8 hr postdosing (2.0 g i.v.) (*60*). It was also reported that bronchial secretion ratios increased from 0.0009 to 0.25 from 0.25 hr to 8 hr after dosing.

4) Clinical considerations

Obviously the advantage of this agent is its enhanced microbiological activity against gram-negative bacteria and anaerobes. This is important for the empiric treatment of hospital-acquired infections, especially if *Pseudomonas* is suspected as the causative organism. Cefotaxime has excellent activity against *Neisseria meningitidis* and *H. influenzae*. Its penetration into the CNS is such that concentrations in the CSF can be achieved that are far in excess of the MIC for these organisms. This characteristic may prove to be an advantage for this drug in the treatment of CNS infections caused by these organisms, compared to treatment with the older cephalosporins. Further extensive study, however, is required.

3. Cefamandole-Cefoxitin

Recently two new "second-generation" cephalosporins, cefamandole and cefoxitin became available for general use. Cefoxitin is often referred to as a cephamycin rather than a cephalosporin antibiotic; yet the differences in its basic nuclei are so small that it seems reasonable to consider this drug as another cephalosporin derivative.

Examination of Table II and Fig. 7 reveals that although the pharmacokinetic parameters of cefoxitin and cefamandole are not identical, they are sufficiently similar to each other and different from cephalothin-cephapirin or cefazolin that it is also reasonable to discuss these drugs together.

1) Elimination

Both drugs have half-lives that are shorter than that of cefazolin but closer to that of cephalothin-cephapirin. The half-life for cefamandole and cefoxitin after intravenous administration is 55 and 45 min, respectively, and after intramuscular injection the apparent half-lives are 78 and 60 min, respectively. Since the protein binding for cefamandole is relatively high, *i.e.*, approximately 77% (*20, 101*), it is surprising that the half-life is not longer as is the case with cefazolin (83% binding; $t1/2$, 1.8 hr). This is because with cefamandole the majority of renal elimination occurs by secretion which is not dependent on the degree of protein binding (*65*). Cefoxitin is only 50–60% protein bound (*20*) and probably undergoes a smaller amount of active secretion. As a result, the half-life is shorter and serum concentrations as a function of time are somewhat, but probably not significantly, reduced (Fig. 5).

As a consequence of their high renal clearance, urinary concentrations of the cephalosporins are great and even in renal failure, sufficient to give values many times above the MICs of the common urinary tract pathogens. For example, in patients with creatinine clearance values of 5–20 ml/min, 30% of a dose of cefamandole was excreted in the urine in 24 hr and the concentrations in the urine ranged from 230 ± 33 μg/ml initially to 66 ± 15 μg/ml at 24 hr (*39*). In patients with similar creatinine clearance values, the lowest concentration of cefamandole has been reported as 53 μg/ml (*119*). Rather than comparing concentrations which are dependent on urine volume, the percent of dose excreted can be compared. For all the unmetabolized

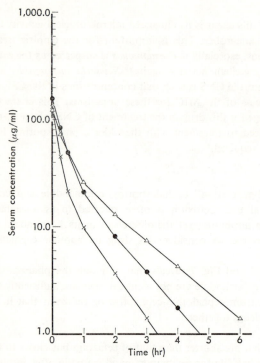

FIG. 7.   Cefoxitin ($\times$), cefamandole ($\bullet$), and cefuroxime ($\triangle$) serum concentrations after a 1.0-g i.v. bolus dose.

cephalosporins, the percent of dose excreted in 24 hr even with severe renal failure is around 20% (Table IV).

The $t1/2$ of these antibiotics in various degrees of renal failure is reported with much variability. This is probably because at creatinine clearance values <20 ml/min, very small changes in clearance will markedly prolong $t1/2$ (*35, 39, 44*). In spite of this, most studies group patients into relatively broad categories, and a mean $t1/2$ for the group is calculated, *e.g.*, 5–20 ml/min or <10 ml/min may be one category. Further, creatinine clearance is not always measured and the number of patients is often small. With these limitations it is difficult to assess the literature in this area.

With cefamandole given i.m. the mean $t1/2$ in 9 patients in moderate renal function (MRF) (creatinine clearance 10–35 ml/min) was calculated as 3.0 ± 0.3 hr (*2*) (Table IV). In patients with severe renal function (SRF) (creatinine clearance <5 ml/ min), the mean $t1/2$ can be calculated from various references (27 patients) to be 10.4 ± 2.4 hr (*3, 4, 29, 39, 91*). The affect of hemodialysis on cefamandole relative to cefazolin is interesting. The mean $t1/2$ during dialysis for cefamandole (including twin coil and single pass dialyzers, as no appreciable difference was seen) was calculated to be 5.64 ± 1.11 hr (*3, 4, 29, 39, 91*) (29 patients). This is very similar to cefazolin's hemodialysis $t1/2$, and both drugs are highly protein bound. However, *relative to $t1/2$ in SRF*, hemodialysis appears less pronounced with cefamandole, *i.e.*, decreasing $t1/2$ by about 50% *vs.* 84% for cefazolin. Peritoneal dialysis seems to affect $t1/2$ very little with cefamandole, since the $t1/2$ during dialysis is reported as 11.75 ± 2.05 in 2 patients (*91*).

In 5 patients with creatinine clearance between 10–30 ml/min, the mean $t1/2$ of cefoxitin was found to be 6.3 hr. This changed to 13.2 hr in 5 other patients with creatinine clearance <10 ml/min but not requiring hemodialysis (*44*). In patients with SRF, the mean $t1/2$ between dialysis was calculated as 15.0 ± 5.3 hr (*2, 44, 50*). During hemodialysis, the mean $t1/2$ was 3.89 ± 0.15 hr (*44, 50*).

2) Distribution
The difference in protein binding between cefamandole and cefoxitin does not appear to result in significantly different tissue levels of these drugs. This was observed in atrial appendage tissue in patients undergoing open heart surgery (*107*). It was observed that cefamandole and cefoxitin had approximately the same tissue concentrations and tissue half-life. Other authors have also observed good heart tissue (*5, 43, 107*) but poor aqueous humor (*7*) concentration with cefamandole; cefoxitin exhibited penetration into breast milk (*51*). Like the other cephalosporins, cefamandole and cefoxitin do not penetrate well into noninflamed meninges in adults (*86, 143*) or children (*147*). Cefoxitin, presumably because it is less protein bound, achieves higher concentrations in noninflamed meninges than cefamandole (*86*). Treatment of patients with CNS infections with cefoxitin resulted in measurable CSF concentrations, but the levels were not within the therapeutic range. In children, cefamandole was found to penetrate into CSF in low (1.2 mcg/ml) concentrations (*147*). Neither cefamandole nor cefoxitin is recommended for the treatment of CNS infections in children or adults.

Walker and Gahal (*147*) reported the typical age-$t1/2$ relationship for cefamandole. In infants <3 months of age the $t1/2$ was approximately 2 hr. This declined to approximately 1.5 hr in children >1 year.

3) Clinical considerations
Both cefoxitin and cefamandole generally exhibit microbiological activity against gram-positive organisms that is somewhat inferior to cephalothin-cephapirin and cefazolin (*34*). This, along with their shorter half-life (at least as compared to cefazolin), makes these drugs a poor choice in treating infections caused by organisms which are susceptible to the older cephalosporins. The rationale is that compared to cefazolin, higher or more frequent dosing is required to compensate for the shorter half-life and lesser microbiological activity resulting in greater expense to the patient (*10*). Although treatment failures may not necessarily result from using these drugs in place of cefazolin, no advantage is offered the patient, and the use of these agents should be discouraged if older cephalosporins exhibit equal microbiological activity. Cefoxitin has enhanced activity against *B. fragilis* and its use in below-the-diaphragm infections and surgery as presumptive therapy or as a prophylactic agent is not unreasonable, especially if this drug is used as a sole agent replacing several other

antibiotics. Likewise, the use of cefamandole is not unreasonable in certain situations where advantage can be taken of its enhanced microbiology, *e.g.*, in the treatment of chronic lung disease where there is a high likelihood of *H. influenzae* infections occurring.

On comparing cefamandole with first-generation cephalosporins, no one would doubt its superior microbiologic activity against a number of gram-negative bacteria. For instance, cefamandole demonstrates activity against certain unusual Enterobacteraceae, like indole-positive *Proteus* (*P. morganii, P. rettgeri*), *Enterobacter* spp., *Citrobacter*, and *Providencia*. These organisms are almost always resistant to first-generation cephalosporins. Cefamandole also displays somewhat greater activity than these drugs toward *H. influenzae* and *E. coli.*

Thus, it would initially seem reasonable that cefamandole would have its greatest usage in the treatment of serious hospital-acquired infection, since gram-negative bacteria emerge as the usual pathogens in this situation. This would be true if it were not for its lack of any appreciable activity against *P. aeruginosa*. Patients who typically acquire pseudomonas infections also acquire infections from the usual Enterobacteriaceae mentioned above and *vice versa*. These patients usually have impaired host defenses, have had a recent extensive intraabdominal surgical procedure, have received prior antibiotic therapy, and often have indwelling foreign bodies (bladder catheter, polyethylene intravenous catheters, and tracheostomies) or a combination of these factors. Consequently, in most patients of this type who develop a hospital-acquired infection, an aminoglycoside must be used to provide coverage against *P. aeruginosa.*

Once an aminoglycoside is introduced, there no longer remains any reason to administer a cephalosporin with enhanced gram-negative bacterial activity since these aminoglycosides exhibit even greater activity against the same organisms covered by cefamandole. The combination of cefamandole and an aminoglycoside merely duplicates bacterial coverage and increases costs, since cefamandole is more expensive than the first-generation cephalosporins (*97*). In fact, in combination therapy with an aminoglycoside, it usually is considered more appropriate to use a penicillin derivative, like ticarcillin, carbenicillin, or ampicillin, than a cephalosporin, because the penicillin derivatives achieve better coverage for the organisms (anaerobes, streptococci) that are "missed" by the aminoglycoside.

4. Cefazolin

It has been demonstrated that cefazolin pharmacokinetics can be described by a two compartment open model (*99*). Recently it was demonstrated that a physiological perfusion model could also describe cefazolin disposition and this model was successfully used to predict cefazolin bone concentrations (*62*). Recently the bactericidal activity of cephalosporins was described in an *in vitro* model. This approach by Nishida *et al.* (*103*) is novel since it provides a model which can be used to mimic cephalosporin serum concentrations and to predict the rate of bacterial killing as a function of drug concentration. Further expansion of this concept is provided by the excellent work of Tsuji (*145*) who was able to successfully predict the drug dose necessary to maintain a minimum biologically active concentration in infected interstitial fluid.

1) Elimination

In contrast with cephapirin and cephalothin, which are metabolized to a varying degree to the less microbiologically active desacetyl form, cefazolin remains unchanged in the body. Comparative pharmacologic studies in adults show that at equivalent dosage, cefazolin achieves serum concentrations that are significantly greater than those achieved by the other cephalosporins (20, 99, 119). The peak serum concentrations after a 500-mg intramuscular dose of cefazolin is about 34 μg/ml compared with 9.6, 11.3, 9.5, 12.0, and 13.0 μg/ml after a similar injection of cephalothin, cephapirin, cephradine, cefoxitin, and cefamandole, respectively (Table III).

The lower rate of elimination through the kidneys, the higher protein binding in serum, i.e., 83% (63, 99, 109, 140), and the smaller volume of distribution, compared with that of the other cephalosporins (Table II) are mainly responsible for cefazolin's higher and more prolonged blood concentrations (Fig. 6). The serum half-life for cefazolin, after an intravenous dose, is 1.74 hr. Although the high protein binding theoretically has a potential disadvantage in reducing the amount of free or microbiologically active drug, this problem is offset by its longer half-life and higher total serum levels. Owing to these pharmacokinetic properties, cefazolin can frequently be administered half as often and/or in half the amount as the other parenteral cephalosporins.

The area under the serum concentration-time curve (AUC) for *free* drug can be used as an "availability index," for it takes into account all processes such as absorption, distribution, and elimination from the body. Such an analysis was done by Bergan (12) who found that the AUC for cefazolin was slightly higher (54.2) than that for cephalothin (47.6) and cephapirin (49.0). One must conclude, therefore, that the high binding of cefazolin to serum proteins is not a disadvantage compared with the other cephalosporins.

A mean $t1/2$ of 14.9$\pm$2.9 hr for cefazolin in 13 patients with creatinine clearance values of 10–35 ml/min has been calculated by compilation of published data (2). and by adding subsequent data, a mean $t1/2$ of 25.3$\pm$ 9.6 hr (31 patients) can be calculated (Table IV). Hemodialysis, with a twin coil dialyzer, will decrease this $t1/2$ This was also done for patients with creatinine clearance values <5 ml/min (2) to 5.54$\pm$1.86 hr (2, 24) (37 patients). Peritoneal dialysis, on the other hand, affects the $t1/2$ of cefazolin very little (32.5 hr), even though 19% of the dose is recovered in the dialysate (2).

2) Distribution

In a study comparing heart tissue and pericardial fluid levels of the highly protein-bound cefazolin with the negligibly-bound cephradine in patients undergoing open heart surgery (100), it was found that the free (unbound) levels of cephradine in pericardial fluid were higher than those of cefazolin. The free cefazolin concentrations, however, were within the therapeutic range. Since pericardial fluid contains albumin (app. 50% serum concentration) to which cefazolin can bind, it is expected that the total (unbound plus bound) cefazolin concentrations would be greater than the free concentration. This was observed and the fact that atrial appendage homogenate concentrations of cefazolin were higher than that of cephradine suggests that cefazolin also binds to tissue protein. Higher total cefazolin concentrations were also observed in synovial fluid and knee bone (37) as well as hip bone (36), and occurred even though the free serum concentrations of cefazolin were lower than those of cephradine. Other studies demonstrating high cefazolin tissue concentrations have recently been reported in aqueous humor (20), tonsils (99), peritoneal fluid (20), skeletal muscle (139), heart (43), pleural fluid (20, 33), bone (136, 150), and synovial fluid (136). Poor penetration into milk (155) and spinal fluid was observed (10, 20). The apparent volume of distribution of cefazolin was shown to be affected by stress (98). Additional studies were previously reviewed (99, 119).

3) Clinical considerations

In studies comparing the therapeutic effectiveness of cephalosporins and penicillins in the therapy of infection from S. aureus, S. epidermidis, Group A and B streptococci, nonenterococcal Group D streptococci, S. pneumoniae, S. viridans, E. coli, and P. mirabilis the results have been similar and, hence, cephalosporins can be safely relied on to eradicate these bacteria from the following sites: respiratory tract, genitourinary tract, skin, soft tissue, blood, heart, bone, and joints.

There has been considerable controversy regarding the use of cefazolin in serious staphylococcal infections, such as bacterial endocarditis, owing to the in vitro observations (48, 124, 130) that cefazolin is more easily inactivated than cephalothin by staphylococcal β-lactamase. Scientific knowledge about the significance of this difference, however, is incomplete and conflicting. All of these studies involve in vitro testing for antibiotic hydrolysis in the presence and absence of β-lactamase-producing S. aureus. In every case it was shown that cefazolin was inactivated more rapidly than cephalothin, but even with cefazolin the viable bacterial cell count either decreased for 6 to 8 hr or remained relatively constant for 12 hr after incubation of the drug with the β-lactamase-producing organisms. This occurs even though the concentration of cefazolin is rapidly declining due to inactivation. If the viable bacterial cell count decreases for 6 to 8 hr after dosing when the normal dosing interval is 6 to 8 hr, the clinical significance of the more rapid rate of cefazolin hydrolysis must be questioned.

Another factor that confuses the issue is the effect of the growth medium on the rate of inactivation (114). The MICs for cefazolin are higher when the organisms are grown in trypticase soy broth than in Mueller-Hinton broth. Likewise, the rate of antibiotic degradation is lower when the drug is incubated with β-lactamase-producing S. aureus in Mueller-Hinton broth compared with trypticase soy broth, presumably because of the high dextrose content of trypticase soy broth, which may stimulate greater production of β-lactamase. Another recent study (111) showed a large disparity between MICs and the minimum bactericidal concentrations (M-BCs) of antistaphylococcal antibiotics, including cephalothin and cefazolin, in different media. Eighty seven percent of staphylococcal strains tested showed an 8-fold or greater difference in MBC when tested in Mueller-Hinton or in brain heart infusion broth. Moreover, because microorganisms in the body are exposed to serum or interstitial fluid and not to artificial media, the interpretation and extrapolation of these *in vitro* data to the clinical situation may not be possible.

Another factor that obscures this issue is the variability in degree of protein binding among the cephalosporins. Because cefazolin is highly bound *in vivo*, it is possible that while in this form its susceptibility to β-lactamase inactivations is different from that of the free drug. This subject was not addressed in the *in vitro* broth studies but was investigated by Oles *et al.* (*106*) who found that cefazolin inactivation at 37°C in serum without bacteria present was so rapid that the addition of β-lactamase-producing organisms to the incubating serum did not appreciably increase the rate of degradation.

Skeptics of the use of cefazolin in bacterial endocarditis point out that there are three case reports (*26, 116*) of supposed failure of cefazolin in the treatment of staphylococcal endocarditis. However, because these cases occurred in heroin addicts, two of whom had splenic abscesses and one of whom had received 2 weeks of cephalothin before the introduction of cefazolin, they certainly cannot be considered true therapeutic failures. Moreover, even if all three cases are real failures, the number is not surprising, because it is well known that therapeutic failures in staphylococcal endocarditis are not unusual with any antibiotic. In a study of the treatment of experimental staphylococcal endocarditis in rabbits with methicillin, cefazolin, and cephalothin, no difference was observed in the cure rates (*30*).

Clearly the relevance of finding different rates of β-lactamase inactivation with the cephalosporins is still uncertain, but the bulk of scientific information favors the optimistic view that there is as yet no direct evidence for the hypothesis that these differences will result in any greater likelihood of a therapeutic failure if the clinician opts for one cephalosporin over another in the therapy of serious staphylococcal infection.

4) Renal excretion considerations

The mechanism of renal clearance for these cephalosporin antibiotics is glomerular filtration of free drug and active secretion of total drug. A decrease in creatinine clearance will prolong the $t1/2$ of all of these drugs. Evidence for tubular secretion exists in the fact that renal clearance for all, except cefazolin, is far in excess of the normal glomerular filtration rate (see Table IV). Further, probenecid (which blocks the tubular secretion of organic acids) will decrease excretion of all of these compounds, including cefazolin. One g of probenecid has been found to double the peak serum concentrations of cephalothin (*99*); increase the peak serum concentrations of cephradine by 40–70% (*20*); increase the peak serum concentration of cefoxitin by 31/2 times, prolong the $t1/2$ to 83 min (*135*), and decrease renal clearance to 80 ml/min/ 1.73 m² (*20*); increase serum concentrations of cefamandole by about 80% and also decrease renal clearance of this drug (*65, 67, 96*). Two g of cefazolin plus 1 g of probenecid will give an AUC value about equal to a 3-g dose of cefazolin alone (*99*). The renal clearance of cefazolin (protein binding ~85%) is less than the other cephalosporins. Cefamandole also has high protein binding (~80%) and is rapidly renally excreted, probably due to its high degree of active secretion (65).

Arvidsson et al. (6) have recently presented data suggesting that cephapirin is also renally reabsorbed and that this process is saturable.

All of these cephalosporins, except cephalothin and cephapirin, are eliminated unchanged almost exclusively by renal processes. For the unmetabolized cephalosporins urinary recovery in 24 hr is reported from 80–100% of a given dose (Table IV).

A change in dosing does not become critical with cephalosporins until creatinine clearance is <20–30 ml/min. Then 1/2 the normal dose should be given approximately every $t1/2$, (or at the normal interval if this is longer than $t1/2$). This approach avoids possible prolonged periods of relatively low serum concentrations. This also holds true for patients on intermittent hemodialysis. The dose of cephalosporin can be given after dialysis and then approximately every $t1/2$ off dialysis. Peritoneal dialysis does not significantly remove cephalosporins and dosing does not need to be changed from the selected severe renal failure regimen. Dosing can always be individualized by checking serum concentrations.

5) Biliary excretion considerations

In addition to the biliary studies which were previously reviewed (99), several new studies have appeared describing the biliary excretion of cephalosporins in the presence of biliary disease (20, 21, 25, 120–123). Due to differences in experimental design and patient population these studies are extremely difficult to evaluate and compare. Fortunately two comparative studies appeared that are helpful in elucidating the differences in biliary excretion between these agents. Brogard et al. (21) compared cephalexin, cefazolin, and cephalothin biliary concentrations. Peak concentrations after a 1-g i.v. dose were ~28 and 11 mcg/ml for cefazolin and cephalothin, representing 0.13 and 0.03% of the administered dose, respectively. One g of cephalexin administered orally yielded levels of 26 mcg/ml and 0.28% of the dose. Ratzan et al. (122) compared cefamandole, cefazolin, and cephalothin. After a 1-g dose of cefamandole, cefazolin, and cephalothin, bile concentrations were approximately 352, 40, and 10 mcg/ml, representing 0.4%, 0.12%, and 0.025% of the administered dose, respectively. It is clear that cefamandole yields the highest bile levels followed by cefazolin, cephalexin, and cephalothin. In two patients with T-tubes, cefoxitin also produced high (227.6 mcg/ml at 2 hr after a 2-g i.v. dose) biliary concentrations (51).

The higher levels of cefamandole compared with first generation cephalosporins in bile are often mentioned as a therapeutic advantage; yet there is no evidence of any difference in the eradication of biliary tract infection with any cephalosporin. Perhaps the concentration of the cephalosporin in tissue like the gallbladder wall is more important than the actual levels in the bile. For instance, although cefamandole achieves much higher bile levels than those of cefazolin, the concentrations in the gallbladder wall are similar (115).

5. Cephaloridine

This agent shares the similar broad spectrum of activity of cephalothin and cephapirin.

The drug appears, however, to be more stable both *in vitro* and *in vivo* (99). Like most parenteral cephalosporins it is not absorbed from the gastrointestinal tract but is well absorbed after intramuscular injection (20, 99).

1) Elimination

Cephaloridine is not metabolized (99) but eliminated unchaged *via* the kidneys through glomerular filtration and active secretion (20, 99). A serum half-life of approximately 1.4 hr was observed by several authors (20, 99) and is extended in impaired renal function (99). The relationship of the overall elimination rate constant to creatinine clearance was described by Brogard *et al.* (19). Arvidsson *et al.* (6) suggest that cephaloridine undergoes active tubular reabsorption; however, the number of subjects studied is too small to be conclusive.

Biliary excretion was found to be a minor pathway of elimination (0.12%) but good drug concentrations (20 mcg/ml) were observed after a 1-g i.v. dose (11).

2) Distribution

Like all cephalosporins, passage into spinal fluid in patients with noninflammed meninges is poor (20, 99). Penetration into peritoneal and pleural fluid and bronchial secretions was also reported (20, 99).

3) Clinical considerations

Cephaloridine seems to offer no distinct advantages over many of the other cephalosporins. Its outstanding characteristic is its tendency to cause renal toxicity (99). Since this is not true of the other cephalosporins the use of cephaloridine should be discouraged in favor of other agents.

6. Cefuroxime

Cefuroxime is a newer cephalosporin with good β-lactamase stability and an enhanced spectrum of activity. It is available only for parenteral use as oral absorption is poor (49). Intramuscular (i.m.) administration is well tolerated and gives area-under-the-curve values equal to intravenous administration (i.v.) (22, 49, 105). Five hundred-mg and 1,000-mg doses give peaks of around 23 μg/ml and 36 μg/ml, respectively (Table III). It was found in males that excercise after i.m. injection of 750 mg increased the peak serum concentration from 17 to 26 μg/ml; in females, an i.m. injection in the thigh produced a shorter apparent half-life (61 *vs.* 89 min) than an i.m. injection in the buttock (68). These differences are not enough to warrant changes in dosing. Pharmacokinetic parameters determined after i.v. dosing are shown in Table II and Fig. 7.

Cefuroxime's binding to protein has been reported as 33$\pm$5.7% (49) and 41% (57). Distribution in tissues and extravascular fluids would be expected to be good provided the drug is not rapidly cleared. Indeed, cefuroxime gives adequate concentrations in a number of tissues and fluids.

Bronchial secretions obtained from patients with tracheostomies showed concentrations of 2.35 μg/ml 1 hr after a 750-mg dose and 0.58 μg/ml 5.5 hr after the dose (14). Drug concentration in bone 2–2.5 hr after a 750-mg i.m. or i.v. dose ranged from 1.2–5.2 μg/g (40, 42). A 1,000-mg i.m. dose gave bone concentrations at 2 hr of 12.4–13.5 μg/g (40). A skin abrasion technique was used to study the exudate concentration of cefuroxime (52). At 1 hr, the cefuroxime exudate to serum ratio was 0.77; at 3 hr the ratio was 0.90. In comparison, oral cephalexin gave a ratio at 1 hr of 0.77 and 0.72 at 3 hr. Cefoxitin's ratio at 1 hr was 0.92 and undetectable in the exudate at 3 hr. In aqueous humor of patients undergoing cataract removal surgery, at 0.5–6 hr, 1,000-mg i.m., 1,000-mg i.v. or 1,500-mg i.v. gave mean concentrations of 0.9 μg/ml, 1.7 μg/ml, and 1.6 μg/ml, respectively (126).

The status of gallbladder function can influence the concentration of cefuroxime in bile. With a functioning gallbladder at 2.5 hr after 750-mg q8hr, gallbladder bile concentrations of cefuroxime were 1.2–58.0 μg/ml. In nonfunctioning gallbladders, this range was 0.39–21 μg/ml (131). Brogard et al. have calculated the % of dose of cefuroxime excreted in the bile to be 0.13–0.22 (22). With inflammation, cefuroxime enters the CSF better than when there is no inflammation. In 3 infants with meningitis, CSF concentrations were from 2.5–5.3 μg/ml. In another 3 infants without meningitis the range was from 0.4–1.5 μg/ml (125). Others have found CSF concentrations of from 16–40 μg/ml (104) and 20–47.3 μg/ml (151) when inflammation was present.

Cefuroxime is not significantly metabolized. Using an HPLC assay, Foord (49) found 95% of a dose excreted unchanged in the urine in 24 hr. About 90% of this dose is excreted in the first 6 hr (41, 49, 56, 58). There is a component of renal tubular secretion in addition to glomerular filtration of drug with cefuroxime renal clearance greater than creatinine clearance (41, 49, 56). In addition, 0.5 g of probenecid 2 hr before and 1 hr after a dose of cefuroxime will decrease the renal clearance of cefuroxime by 40% (49). This results in a 30% increase in peak height after a 500-mg i.m. dose, a 32% increase in half-life, a 66% increase in AUC, and a 20% decrease in V_D (49).

In analyzing the serum concentration of normal adults with a two-compartment model, the $t1/2\ \beta$ was found to be 1.12 hr (49). In infants 1 day old, the half-life was found to be 5.6 hr and this decreased to 4 hr at 14 days (125).

Renal failure prolongs the half-life of cefuroxime. When EDTA clearance is from 20–59 ml/min the half-life was increased to 1.8 hr (59). Below a GFR of 20 ml/min however, the half life is markedly prolonged to 16.1 (hr) (59). In anuric patients, the half-life is reported as from 15–22 hr (59, 83). Hemodialysis decreases this half-life to 3.3–3.75 hr (59, 83). Peritoneal dialysis is less effective in removing the drug and decreases the half-life to only 13.5 hr (83). Urine concentrations in renal failure are adequate to treat infections (59).

REFERENCES

1. Anderson, K. E. 1978. J. Infect. Dis. (Suppl. 13), 37–46.

2. Andriole, V. T. 1978. J. Infect. Dis., 137, S88–S99.

3. Ahern, M. J., Finkelstein, F. O., and Andriole, V. T. 1976. Antimicrob. Agents Chemother., 10, 457–461.

4. Appel, G. B., Neu, H. C., Parry, M. F., Goldgerger, M. J., and Jacob, G. B. 1976. *Antimicrob. Agents Chemother.*, **10**, 623–625.

5. Archer, G. L., Polk, R. E., Duma, R. J., and Lower, R. 1978. *Antimicrob. Agents Chemother.*, **13**, 924–929.

6. Arvidsson, A., Borga, O., and Alvam, G. 1979. *Clin. Pharmacol. Ther.*, **25**, 870–876.

7. Axelrod, J. L. and Kochman, R. 1978. *Am. J. Ophthalmol.*, **85**, 342–348.

8. Aziz, N. S., Gambertoglio, J. G., Lin, E. T., Grausz, H., and Benet, L. Z. 1978. *J. Pharmacol. Biopharmacol.*, **6**, 153–164.

9. Barza, M. and Miao, P. V. M. 1977. *Am. J. Hosp. Pharm.*, **34**, 621–629.

10. Bassaris, H. R., Quintiliani, R., Maderazo, E., and Nightingale, C. H. 1976. *Curr. Ther. Res.*, **19**, 110.

11. Belohradsky, B. H., Geiss, D., Marget, W., Bruch, K., Kafetzis, D., and Peters, G. 1980. *Lancet,* **i**, 61–63.

12. Bergan, T. 1977. *Chemotherapy*, **23**, 389–404.

13. Bergan, T., Digranes, A., and Schreiner, A. 1978. *Chemotherapy*, **24**, 277–282.

14. Bergogne-Berezin, E., Even, P., Berthelot, G., and Pierre, J. 1977. *Proc. Roy. Soc. Med.*, **70** (Suppl. 9), 34.

15. Berman, S. J., Boughton, W. H., Sugihara, J. G., Wong, E. G. C., Sato, M. M., and Siemsen, A. W. 1978. *Antimicrob. Agents Chemother.*, **14**, 281–283.

16. Bill, N. J. and Washington, J. A. 1977. *Antimicrob. Agents Chemother.*, **11**, 470–474.

17. Bloch, R., Szwed, J. J., Sloan, R. S., and Luft, F. C. 1977. *Antimicrob. Agents Chemother.*, **12**, 730–732.

18. Box, R., White, L., Reeves, D., Ings, R., Bywater, M., and Holt, H. 1980. *Curr. Chemother. Infect. Dis.*, **1**, 155–157.

19. Brogard, J. M., Brandt, C., Dorner, M., and Dammorn, A. 1976. *Chemotherapy*, **22**, 1–11.

20. Brogard, J. M., Comte, F., and Pinget, M. 1978. *Antibiot. Chemother.*, **25**, 123–162.

21. Brogard, J. M., Dorner, M., Pinget, M., Adloff, M., and Lavillaureix, J. 1975. *J. Infect. Dis.*, **131**, 625–633.

22. Brogard, J. M., Kopfershmitt, J., Pinget, M., Arnaud, J. P., and Lavillaureix, J. 1977. *Proc. Roy. Soc. Med.*, **70** (Suppl. 9), 42.

23. Brogard, J. M., Kopferschmitt, J., Spach, M. O., Grudet, O., and Lavillaureix, J. 1979. *J. Clin. Pharmacol.*, **19**, 366–377.

24. Brogard, J. M., Pinget, M., Brandt, C., and Lavillauriex, J. 1977. *J. Clin. Pharmacol.*, **17**, 225–230.

25. Brogard, J. M., Pinget, M., Dauchel, J., Dorner, M., and Lavillauriex, J. 1976. *Med. Chir. Dig.*, **5**, 327–335.

26. Bryant, R. E. and Alford, R. H. 1977. *J. Am. Med. Assoc.*, **237**, 569–570.

27. Buck, R. E. and Price, K. E. 1977. *Antimicrob. Agents Chemother.*, **11**, 324–330.

28. Cabana, B. E., Van Harken, D. R., and Hottendorf, G. H. 1976. *Antimicrob.*

Agents Chemother., **10**, 307–317.

29. Campillo, J. A., Lanao, J. M., Dominguez-Gil, Tabernero, J. M., and Rubina, F. 1979. *Int. J. Clin. Pharmacol. Biopharmacol.*, **17**, 416–420.

30. Carrizosa, J., Santoro, J., and Kaye, D. 1978. *Antimicrob. Agents Chemother.*, **13**, 74–77.

31. Clumeck, N., Vanhoff, R., Vanlaethem, Y., and Butzler, J. P. 1980. *Curr. Chemother. Infect. Dis.*, **1**, 122.

32. Chow, M., Quintiliani, R., Cunha, B. A., Thompson, M., Finkelstein, E., and Nightingale, C. H. 1979. *J. Clin. Pharmacol.*, **19**, 185–194.

33. Cole, D. R. and Pung, J. 1977. *Antimicrob. Agents Chemother.*, **11**, 1033–1035.

34. Craft, I. and Forster, T. C. 1978. *Antimicrob. Agents Chemother.*, **14**, 924–926.

35. Craig, W. A., Welling, P. G., Jackson, T. C., and Kunin, C. M. 1973. *J. Infect. Dis.*, **128** (Suppl.), S347–S353.

36. Cunha, B. A., Gossling, H. R., Pasternak, H. S., Nightingale, C. H., and Quintiliani, R. 1977. *J. Bone Joint Surg.*, **59A**, 856–859.

37. Cunha, B. A., Quintiliani, R., and Nightingale, C. H. Unpublished data.

38. Cutler, R. E., Blair, A. D., and Kelly, M. R. 1979. *Clin. Pharmacol. Ther.*, **25**, 514–521.

39. Czerwinski, A. W. and Pederson, J. A. 1979. *Antimicrob. Agents Chemother.*, **15**, 161–164.

40. Daikos, G. K., Kosmidis, J., Stathakis, C., Anyfantis, A., Plakoutsis, T., and Papathanassiou, B. 1977. *Proc. Roy. Soc. Med.*, **70** (Suppl. 9), 42.

41. Daikos, G. K., Kosmidis, J. C., Stathakis, C. H., and Giamarellou, H. 1977. *J. Antimicrob. Chemocher.*, **3**, 555.

42. Dornbush, K., Hugo, H., and Lindstrom, A. 1980. *Scand. J. Infect. Dis.*, **12**, 49–53.

43. Eigel, P., Tschirkov, A., Satter, P., and Knothe, J. 1978. *Infection*, **6**, 23–28.

44. Fillastre, J. P., Leroy, A., Godin, M., Oksenhendler, G., and Humbert, G. 1978. *J. Antimicrob. Chemother.*, **4** (Suppl. B), 79–83.

45. Finkelstein, E., Quintiliani, R., Lee, R., Bracci, A., and Nightingale, C. H. 1978. *J. Pharm. Sci.*, **67**, 1447–1450.

46. Fitzgerald, R. H., Kelly, P. J., Snyder, R. J., and Washington II, J. A. 1978. *Antimicrob. Agents Chemother.*, **14**, 723–726.

47. Foglesong, M. A., Lamb, J. W., and Dietz, J. V. 1978. *J. Antimicrob. Chemother.*, **13**, 49–52.

48. Fong, I. W., Engelking, E. R., and Kirby, W. M. M. 1976. *Antimicrob. Agents Chemother.*, **9**, 939–944.

49. Foord, R. D. 1976. *Antimicrob. Agents Chemother.*, **9**, 741.

50. Garcia, M. J., Dominguez-Gil, Tabernero, J. M., and Bondia Roman, A. 1979. *Int. J. Clin. Pharmacol. Biopharmacol.*, **17**, 366–370.

51. Geddes, A. M., Schnurr, L. P., Ball, A. P., McGhie, D., Brookes, G. R., Wise, R., and Andrews, J. 1977. *Br. Med. J.*, **1**, 1126–1128.

52. Gillett, A. P. and Wise, R. 1978. *Lancet*, **i**, 962.

53. Ginsburg, C. M. and McCracken, G. H., Jr. 1979. *Antimicrob. Agents Chemother.*, **16**, 74–76.
54. Ginsburg, C. M., McCracken, G. H., Jr., Clackson, J. C., and Thomas, M. 1978. *Antimicrob. Agents Chemother.*, **13**, 845–848.
55. Glynne, A., Goulbourn, R. A., and Ryden, R. 1978. *J. Antimicrob. Chemother.*, **4**, 343–348.
56. Goodwin, C. S., Dash, C. H., Hill, J. P., and Goldberg, A. D. 1977. *J. Antimicrob. Chemother.*, **3**, 253.
57. Goto, S. 1977. *Proc. Roy. Soc. Med.*, **70** (Suppl. 9), 56.
58. Gower, P. E. and Dash, C. H. 1977. *Eur. J. Clin. Pharmacol.*, **12**, 221.
59. Gower, P. E., Kennedy, M. R. K., and Dash, C. H. 1977. *Proc. Roy. Soc. Med.*, **70** (Suppl. 9), 151.
60. Grassi, G. G., Dionigi, R., Ferrara, A., and Pozzi, E. 1980. *Curr. Chemother. Infect. Dis.*, **1**, 120–121.
61. Greene, D. S. Flanagan, D. R., Quintiliani, R., and Nightingale, C. H. 1976. *J. Clin. Pharmacol.*, **16**, 257–264.
62. Greene, D. S., Quintiliani, R., and Nightingale, C. H. 1978. *J. Pharm. Sci.*, **67**, 191.
63. Greene, D. S., Quintiliani, R., and Nightingale, C. H. 1977. *J. Pharm. Sci.*, **66**, 1663.
64. Greene, E., Subramanian, S., Faden, H., Quintiliani, R., and Nightingale, C. H. 1981. *Ann. Thorac. Surg.*, **31**, 155–160.
65. Greene, D. S., Quintiliani, R., Thompson, M. A., and Nightingale, C. H. 1977. *Curr. Ther. Res.*, **22**, 737–740.
66. Griffith, R. S., Black, H. R., Brier, G. L., and Wolny, J. D. 1976. *Antimicrob. Agents Chemother.*, **10**, 814–823.
67. Griffith, R. S., Black, H. R., Brier, G. L., and Wolny, J. D. 1977. *Antimicrob. Agents Chemother.*, **11**, 809–812.
68. Harding, S. M., Eilon, L. A., and Harris, A. M. 1979. *J. Antimicrob. Chemother.*, **5**, 87–93.
69. Hartstein, A. I., Patrick, K. E., Jones, S. R., Miller, M. J., and Bryant, R. E. 1977. *Antimicrob. Agents Chemother.*, **12**, 93–97.
70. Helwig, H. F. 1980. *Curr. Chemother. Infect. Dis.*, **1**, 128–129.
71. Henness, D. M. and Richards, D. 1978. *Curr. Ther. Res.*, **23**, 547–554.
72. Henness, D. M., Richards, D., Santella, P. F., and Rubinfeld, J. 1977. *Clin. Ther.*, **1**, 263–273.
73. Ho, I., Aswapokee, P., Fu, K. W., Matthyssen, C., and Neu, H. C. 1980. *Curr. Chemother. Infect. Dis.*, **1**, 116–118.
74. Hodeges, G. R., Chien, L., Hinthorn, D. R., Harris, J. L., and Dworzack, D. L. 1978. *Antimicrob. Agents Chemother.*, **14**, 454–456.
75. Hoechst-Roussel Pharmaceuticals. Investigational Brochure, 1979.
76. Humbert, G., Leroy, A., Fillastre, J. P., and Godin, M. 1979. *Chemotherapy*, **25**, 189–195.

77. Jalava, S., Saarimoa, H., and Elfoing, R. 1977. *Scand. J. Rheumatol.*, **6** 250–252.
78. Jolly, E. R., Henness, D. M., and Richards, D., Jr. 1977. *Curr. Ther. Res.*, **22** 727–736.
79. Kafetzis, D. A., Kanarios, J., Simamiotis, C. A., and Papadatos, C. J. 1980. *Curr. Chemother. Infect. Dis.*, **1**, 134–136.
80. Kemmerich, B., Lode, H., Gruhlke, G., Dzwillo, G., Koeppe, P., and Wagner, I. 1980. *Curr. Chemother. Infect. Dis.*, **1**, 130–132.
81. Kiss, J. J., Farango, E., and Pinter, J. 1976. *Br. J. Clin. Pharmacol.*, **3**, 891–895.
82. Korzeniowski, O. M., Scheld, W. M., and Sande, M. A. 1977. *Antimicrob. Agents Chemother.*, **12**, 157–160.
83. Kosmidis, J., Stathakis, C., Anyfantis, A., and Daikos, G. K. 1977. *Proc. Roy. Soc. Med.*, **70** (Suppl. 9), 139.
84. Lane, A. Z., Chudzik, G. M., and Siskin, S. B. 1977. *Curr. Ther. Res.*, **21**, 117–127.
85. Levison, M. E., Santoro, J., and Agarwal, B. N. 1979. *Postgrad. Med. J.*, **55**, (Suppl. 4), 12–16.
86. Liu, C., Hinthorn, D. R., Hodges, G. R., Harms, J. L., Conchonnal, G., and Dworzack, D. L. 1979. *Rev. Infect. Dis.*, **1**, 127–131.
87. Lode, H., Stahlmann, R., and Koeppe, P. 1979. *Antimicrob. Agents Chemother.*, **16**, 1–6.
88. McCracken, G. H., Jr., Ginsburg, C. M., Clakson, J. C., and Thomas, M. L. 1978. *J. Antimicrob. Chemother.*, **4**, 515–521.
89. McCracken, G. H., Jr., Ginsburg, C. M., Clakson, J. C., and Thomas, M. L. 1978. *Pediatrics*, **62**, 738–743.
90. McKendrick, M. W., Geddes, A. M., and Wise, R. 1980. *Curr. Chemother. Infect. Dis.*, **1**, 123–125.
91. Meyers, B. R. and Hirschman, S. Z. 1977. *Antimicrob. Agents Chemother.*, **11**, 248–250.
92. Meyers, B. R., Hirschman, S. Z., Wormser, G., Gartenberg, G., and Srulevitch, E. 1978. *J. Clin. Pharmacol.*, **18**, 174–179.
93. Miller, K. W., Chan, K. K. H., McCoy, H. G., Fischer, R. P., Lindsay, W. G., and Zaske, D. E. 1979. *Clin. Pharmacol. Ther.*, **26**, 54–62.
94. Mischler, T. W., Corson, S. L., Larranaga, A., Bolognese, R. J., Neiss, E. S., and Bakovich, R. A. 1978. *J. Reprod. Med.*, **21**, 130–136.
95. Mowton, R. P., Bongaerts, G. P. A., and Van Gestel, M. 1980. *Curr. Chemother. Infect. Dis.*, **1**, 144–146.
96. Neu, H. C. 1978. *J. Infect. Dis.*, **137** (Suppl.), S80–S87.
97. Nightingale, C. H. 1979. *In* "Cephalosporins Today," Biomedical Information Corp., Inc., New York, pp. 33–37.
98. Nightingale, C. H., Bassaris, H., Tilton, R., and Quintiliani, R. 1975. *J. Pharm. Sci.*, **64**, 712.
99. Nightingale, C. H., Greene, D. S., and Quintiliani, R. 1975. *J. Pharm. Sci.*, **64**, 1899–1927.

100. Nightingale, C. H., Klimek, J., and Quintiliani, R. *J. Infect. Dis.*, in press.
101. Nightingale, C. H. and Quintiliani, R. Unpublished data.
102. Nilsson-Ehle, I. and Nilsson-Ehle, P. 1979. *J. Infect. Dis.*, **139**, 712–716.
103. Nishida, M., Murakawa, T., Kamimura, T., and Okada, N. 1978. *Antimicrob. Agents Chemother.*, **14**, 6–12.
104. Norrby, R., Foord, R. D., Price, J. D., and Hedlund, D. 1977. *Proc. Roy. Soc. Med.*, **70** (Suppl. 9), 25.
105. O'Callaghan, C. H. and Harding, S. M. 1977. *Proc. Roy. Soc. Med.*, **70** (Suppl. 9), 4.
106. Oles, K., Quintiliani, R., and Nightingale, C. H. Unpublished data.
107. Olson, N., Nightingale, C. H., and Quintiliani, R. 1980. *Ann. Thorac. Surg.*, **29**, 104.
108. Papathanassion, B., Kosmidis, J., Stathakis, C., Mantopoulos, K., and Daikos, G. K. 1980. *Curr. Chemother. Infect. Dis.*, **1**, 666–667.
109. Paradelis, A. G., Stalhopoulos, G., Trianthoplyllidis, C., and Logaras, G. 1977. *Arzneim-Forsch.*, **27**, 2167–2170.
110. Patel, D., Moellering, R. C., Thrasher, K., Fahmy, N. R., and Harris, W. H. 1979. *J. Bone Joint Surg.*, **61-A**, 531–538.
111. Peterson, L. R., Gerding, D. N., Hall, W. H., and Schierl, E. A. 1978. *Antimicrob. Agents Chemother.*, **13**, 665–668.
112. Pfeffer, M., Jackson, A., Ximens, J., and Perde-DeMenezes, J. 1977. *Antimicrob. Agents Chemother.*, **11**, 331–338.
113. Polk, R. E., Archer, G. L., and Lower, R. 1978. *Clin. Pharmacol. Ther.*, **23**, 473–480.
114. Pursiano, T. A., Misied, M., Leitner, F., and Price, K. E. 1973. *Antimicrob. Agents Chemother.*, **3**, 33–39.
115. Quinn, E. L., Madhaven, T., Wixson, R., Guise, E., Levin, N., Block, M., Burch, K., Fisher, E., Suarez, A., and DelBusto, R. 1978. *Curr. Chemother.*, **2**, 803–804.
116. Quinn, E. L., Phohol, D., Madhavan, T., Burch, K., Fisher, E., and Cox, F. 1973. *J. Infect. Dis.*, **128** (Suppl.), S386–S389.
117. Quintiliani, R. 1979. *In* "Cephalosporins Today," Biomedical Information Corp. Inc., New York, pp. 4–9.
118. Quintiliani, R., Klimek, J., and Nightingale, C. H. 1979. *J. Infect. Dis.*, **139**, 348–352.
119. Quintiliani, R. and Nightingale, C. H. 1978. *Ann. Intern. Med.*, **89**, 650–656.
120. Ram, M. D. and Watanatillan, S. 1974. *Arch. Surg.*, **108**, 540–545.
121. Ram, M. D. and Watanatillan, S. 1974. *Arch. Surg.*, **108**, 187–189.
122. Ratzan, K. R., Baker, H. B., and Lauredo, I. 1978. *Antimicrob. Agents Chemother.*, **13**, 985–987.
123. Ratzan, K. R., Ruiz, C., and Irvin III, G. L. 1974. *Antimicrob. Agents Chemother.*, **6**, 426–431.
124. Regamey, C., Libke, R. D., Engelking, E. R., Clarke, J. T., and Kirby, W. M. M. 1975. *J. Infect. Dis.*, **131**, 291–294.

125. Renlund, M. and Pettay, O. 1977. *Proc. Roy. Soc. Med.*, **70** (Suppl. 9), 179.
126. Richards, A. B., Bron, A. J., McLendan, B., Kennedy, M. R. K., and Walker, S. R. 1979. *Br. J. Ophthal.*, **63**, 687.
127. Rolewicz, T. F., Mirkin, B. L., Cooper, M. J., and Anders, M. W. 1977. *Clin. Pharmacol. Ther.*, **22**, 928–935.
128. Rosin, H. and Uphaus, W. 1980. *Curr. Chemother. Infect. Dis.*, **1**, 148–150.
129. Rubi, R. and Galan, H. M. 1979. *Int. J. Clin. Pharmacol. Biopharmacol.*, **17**, 87–89.
130. Sabath, L. D., Gardner, C., Wilcox, C., and Finland, M. 1975. *Antimicrob. Agents Chemother.*, **8**, 344–349.
131. Sales, J. E. L. and Rimmer, D. M. D. 1977. *Proc. Roy. Soc. Med.*, **70** (Suppl. 9), 95.
132. Santoro, J., Agarwal, B. N., Martinelli, R., Wenger, N., and Levison, M. E. 1978. *Antimicrob. Agents Chemother.*, **13**, 951–954.
133. Schneider, H., Nightingale, C. H., Quintiliani, R., and Flanagan, D. R. 1978. *J. Pharm. Sci.*, **67**, 1620–1622.
134. Scheld, W. M., Korzeiniowski, O. M., and Sande, M. 1977. *Antimicrob. Agents Chemother.*, **12**, 290–297.
135. Schrogie, J. J., Davies, R. O., Yeh, K. C., Rogers, D., Holmes, G. I., Skeggs, H., and Martin, C. M. 1978. *J. Antimicrob. Chemother.*, **4** (Suppl. B), 69–78.
136. Schurman, D. J., Hirshman, H. P., Kajiyama, G., Moser, K., and Burton, D. S. 1978. *J. Bone Joint Surg.*, **60-A**, 359–362.
137. Shuford, G. M. 1979. *J. Am. Dental Assoc.*, **99**, 47–50.
138. Simon, C. and Gutzemeier, U. 1979. *Postgrad. Med. J.*, **55** (Suppl. 4), 30–34.
139. Sinagowitz, E., Pelz, K., Burgert, A., and Kaczkowski, W. 1976. *Infection*, **4**, 192–195.
140. Singhvi, S. M., Heald, A. F., and Schreiber, E. C. 1978. *Chemotherapy*, **24**, 121–133.
141. Sonneville, P. F., Albert, K. S., Skeggs, H., Gentner, H., Kwan, K. C., and Martin, C. M. 1977. *Eur. J. Clin. Pharmacol.*, **12**, 273–279.
142. Spyker, D. A., Thomas, B. L., Sande, M. A., and Bolton, W. K. 1978. *Antimicrob. Agents Chemother.*, **14**, 172–177.
143. Steinberg, E. A., Overturf, G. D., Baraff, L. J., and Wilkins, J. 1977. *Antimicrob. Agents Chemother.*, **11**, 933–935.
144. Tetzloff, T. R., McCracken, G. H., and Nelson, J. D. 1978. *J. Pediatr.*, **91**, 485.
145. Tsuji, A. and Yamana, T. 1979. Abstr. 27th Academy of Pharmaceutical Sciences, National Meeting, Am. Pharm. Assoc., Kansas City, p. 84.
146. Usuda, Y., Sekino, O., Aoki, N., Shimizu, T., Hirasawa, Y., Aoki, T., Omosu, M., and Kasai, K. 1980. *Curr. Chemother. Infect. Dis.*, **1**, 137–140.
147. Walker, S. H. and Gahol, V. P. 1978. *Antimicrob. Agents Chemother.*, **14**, 315–317.
148. Weingarten, C. M. 1979. *J. Lab. Clin. Med.*, **86**, 51–54.
149. Welling, P. G., Dean, S., Selen, A., Kendall, M. J., and Wise, R. 1979. *Int. J. Clin. Pharmacol. Biopharmacol.*, **17**, 397–400.

150. Wiggins, C. E., Nelson, C. L., Clarke, R., and Thompson, C. H. 1978. *J. Bone Joint Surg.*, **60-A**, 93–96.
151. Wilkinson, P. J., Belohradsky, B. H., and Marget, W. 1977. *Proc. Roy. Soc. Med.*, **70**, (Suppl. 9), 183.
152. Wise, R., Andrews, J. M., Hammond, D., Wills, P. J., Geddes, A. M., and McKendrick, M. W. 1980. *Curr. Chemother. Infect. Dis.*, **1**, 118–119.
153. Wittman, D. H., Schassan, H. H., and Freitag, V. 1980. *Curr. Chemother. Infect. Dis.*, **1**, 114–116.
154. Wright, N. and Wise, R. 1980. *Curr. Chemother. Infect. Dis.*, **1**, 133–134.
155. Yoshioka, H., Cho, K., Masatoshi, T., Maruyama, S., and Shimizu, T. 1979. *J. Pediatr.*, **94**, 151–152.

7 ALLERGY

ALLERGY TOWARDS β-LACTAM ANTIBIOTICS

C. H. Schneider and A. L. de Weck

Institute for Clinical Immunology*

Allergic reactions remain one of the major side-effects of β-lactam antibiotics and it is generally estimated that 3 to 5% of the individuals in populations of industrialized nations are allergic to penicillins. Being small molecules of less than 500 daltons, the β-lactam antibiotics are as such neither capable of inducing antibody responses nor delayed cellular reactions. They require, according to accepted immunochemical rules, chemical attachment to larger carriers in order to become sensitizers.

In the early years of penicillin allergy research the β-lactam reactivity was underestimated and the opinion prevailed that penicillins are incapable of directly reacting with nucleophilic carriers. Therefore the emphasis was on a search for reactive metabolites and *in vivo* degradation products which may bind covalently to macromolecular carriers of the body and thus give rise to sensitizing conjugates. For a number of years penicillenic acid and some of its derivatives were thought to be the only intermediates responsible for sensitization (*17, 46*). This notion could not be upheld since a number of semisynthetic penicillins showed sensitizing capacities in animals which did not correlate with their rates of transformation into penicillenic acid *in vitro* (*47*). Furthermore it was realized that penicillenic acid formation at blood pH is insignificant and amounts formed are rapidly hydrolyzed to penicilloate (*17*). Penicillenic acid derivatives preformed *in vitro* and measurable in penicillin solutions *e.g.*, by a strong band at 320 nm, may on the other hand be important sensitizing components and the sensitizing pathways they imply could be effective in those instances where unbuffered penicillin solutions are kept for some time before injection. By the same token, insufficiently purified penicillins as well as inadequately stored solid preparations could become particularly effective sensitizers.

In 1965 the capacity of the β-lactam ring of penicillin to directly react with nucleophiles at neutral pH was finally established (*17, 37*) and it was shown that dinitrophenylated 6-aminopenicillanic acid (6-APA), a pseudo-penicillin which cannot

* Inselspital, 3010 Bern, Switzerland.

form penicillenic acid acylates amines about as fast as benzylpenicillin and induces antibody formation in rabbits (36, 37). The significance of these results was questioned by some workers since the reaction rates reported for neutral penicilloylations of amines or protein carriers are considered to be quite low (second order rate constant for the reaction of benzylpenicillin with 6-aminocaproate: 2.6×10^{-2} M^{-1} hr^{-1} (34)). However it should be kept in mind that at neutral pH many conjugations to primary amino functions are quite slow, including those of chlorodinitrobenzenes well known as "reactive reagents" in organic chemistry and as "classical sensitizers" in allergy. This point has recently been discussed in some detail by Bundgaard (5). It should also be noted that faster penicilloylations, e.g., of 1,2-aminothiols or oligoglycine chains, are known (34) and that the nature of the constituents eventually becoming involved in sensitization after penicilloylation has not been established. As we shall show in the following paragraph, cellular conjugates, in particular penicilloylated lymphocytes, may be implicated as sensitizing agents and in this case molecular kinetic data might be of little predictive value in the first place.

In 1967 British workers drew attention to the possibility that the sensitizing behavior of penicillins may be due predominantly if not exclusively to contaminants arising during the manufacturing process (3, 13, 44). Indeed it was found that the strong and hitherto unexplained immunogenicity of 6-APA was due to penicilloylated protein impurities (2, 3). Later it was also shown that treatment of 6-APA with the proteolytic enzyme pronase abolished the immunogenicity in rabbits as well as its ability to elicit passive cutaneous anaphylaxis (PCA) in guinea pigs (40). On the other hand the more important question of which role protein impurities play as allergens in clinically used benzylpenicillin and in semisynthetic penicillins was not definitely resolved. Theoretically, penicilloylated foreign proteins are to be regarded as potent immunogens but the question remained of what amounts are present in the various clinically-used penicillin preparations. It seems that the levels actually observed by different workers were quite variable (10–300 ppm) and that technical difficulties in isolating and separating the very small amounts of contaminants in many penicillins as well as the eventual presence of polymers, obscured the picture (8).

Recently Swedish workers have reemphasized the importance of penicilloylated protein contaminants in penicillin allergy. They have set up a sensitive radioimmunoassay specially adapted for the determination of penicilloylated protein contaminants in penicillins of the order of 1 ppm (15). The method, when applied to sixty commercial ampicillin preparations, revealed markedly different levels of contaminants but seemed to indicate in most of the contaminated preparations impurity levels equivalent to 1 to 3 ppm (1). That such low levels may be significant in sensitization was shown experimentally by sensitizing mice with pure benzylpenicillin to which 3 to 15 ppm of penicilloyl-bovine γ-globulin (BGG) was added. With the schedule used the contaminated but not the pure penicillin induced penicilloyl-specific IgE, IgG, and IgM antibody production (14). These data are discussed further in the following paragraph.

With regard to the immunological specificities involved in penicillin allergy, the notion established in the 1960's that the penicilloyl group attached predominantly

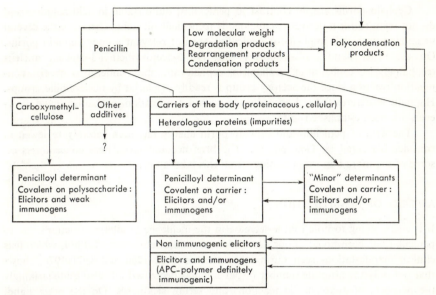

FiG. 1.   Immunogens and elicitors in penicillin allergy.
The low molecular weight penicillin derivatives include penicilloate, penamaldate, penaldate, penilloaldehyde, penicillenate, penillate, and oligomers.

to ε-lysine functions constitutes a major antigenic determinant remains valid. However a variety of other determinants sometimes classified as "minor determinants" may also be involved. A diagram first used in 1970 (23) to summarize the various pathways which afford sensitizing and/or eliciting antigens is still applicable with some modification (Fig. 1).

Cephalosporins are immunochemically about as complex as penicillins but possess a β-lactam ring which proves generally somewhat less reactive than that of most penicillins. Detailed studies on the reactivity with amines have suggested that cephalosporoyl amide, the equivalent of the penicilloyl antigenic determinant, is of low stability and may decompose to a penaldate derivative. Cephalosporin-based determinants that have undergone such degradation retain the R_1-side chain but lack the dihydrothiazine moiety (11, 10, 43). Accordingly, cephalosporin- and penicillin-based haptenic structures are not expected to share structural elements of sufficient immunochemical importance to form a basis for antibody crossreactivity provided the respective side chains are distinct. Indeed, reports of immediate reactions to cephalosporins in penicillin-allergic patients are infrequent and involve mostly cephalosporins with a thiophene side chain such as cephalothin (39). Since the thiophene ring (22) is immunochemically similar to the benzene side chain of penicillin G (PCG), penicillin V (PCV), and others, the observed crossreactions may be due to side chain similarity in most instances.

Cephalosporins are, in contrast to penicillins, quite stable in acid solution and do not seem to form derivatives analogous to penicillenic acid. Therefore the several sensitizing pathways implied for penicillins are not relevant among cephalosporins. On the other hand cephalosporins with the 3-acetoxymethyl-3-cephem nucleus (cephaloglycin, cephalothin, cephapirin, cephaloram) may undergo a special conjugation reaction since the acetoxy group is readily displaced by nucleophilic groups. Haptenic structures formed according to such a conjugation mechanism have, however, not been established so far.

The field of penicillin and cephalosporin allergy has been recently reviewed in considerable detail by Dewdney (8). The brief account given here concentrates on some of the more important findings from this laboratory.

ASPECTS OF SENSITIZATION

It is encouraging to note that a decrease in the incidence of allergic reactions due to penicillin has been noted in our department as well as elsewhere. Table I, which lists clinical manifestations seen during the intervals 1962–1966 and 1971–1976, shows that not only the absolute number of patients has decreased but also quite strikingly the numbers of anaphylactic reactions and serum sicknesses. On the other hand, generalized exanthemas have become more numerous.

Obviously it is not possible to correlate these observations with a single measure. We are inclined to think that the following features may have been contributing to

TABLE I. Clinical Symptoms of Penicillin Allergy at the "Inselspital"

	1962–1966		1971–1976	
	311	cases (%)	236	cases (%)
Generalized urticaria	102	(33)	90	(38)
Anaphylactic shock	59	(19)	8	(3.5)
Anaphylactic symptoms			7	(3)
Serum-like disease	43	(14)	11	(4.5)
Angioneurotic edema	28	(9)	31	(13)
Generalized exanthema	25	(8)	65	(27.5)
Contact eczema	15	(5)	3	(1.5)
Blood dyscrasias	13	(4)	4	(2)
Pruritus	6	(2)	7	(3)
Local reactions	7	(2)	4	(1.5)
Asthma	4	(1)	0	(—)
Varia	9	(3)	6	(2.5)

(6.5)

incidence lowering: 1) a better awareness of clinicians that penicillin therapy may lead to untoward reactions in sensitized and in easily sensitizable patients, producing a reluctance to use penicillins in these cases; 2) the banning (at least in Switzerland) of penicillins and other antibiotics used in human medicine from application in cattle raising; 3) the increasing awareness that storing of penicillin solutions may develop complex mixtures of degradation products of potential allergological significance; and 4) the better quality of penicillins on the market, *i.e.*, with regard to the relative absence of contaminants and degradation products and the absence of additives of potential allergological significance.

Storage of penicillin no doubt gives rise to degradation products of allergological importance. In early studies we found that PCG kept in phosphate buffer between pH 6.9 and 7.5 at room temperature for one week gave several fractions upon gel chromatography which were all able to elicit skin reactions in penicillin-sensitive patients. It was concluded that compounds of comparatively low molecular weight, such as small polymers, and reactive derivatives conjugating *in vivo* were mainly responsible for the allergic reactions observed (*53*). More recently we studied the degradation of PCG in concentrated unbuffered solution and found that within 2 days at room temperature upto about 10% of the initial penicillin was transformed into a heterogeneous fraction moving ahead of penicillin on a Sephadex G-25 column (*29*). Therefore the possible formation of multivalent elicitors and reactive allergens during storage of penicillins already in the dry state but certainly after dissolution should not be underestimated as a cause for allergy.

In our 1968 paper we had concluded that the presence of minute amounts of protein impurities in commercial PCG (at least in preparations of good quality) played but a very minor role in elicitation of allergic reactions in sensitized patients (*53*). The possibility remained, however, that very lightly substituted benzyl-penicilloyl-(BPO)-proteins of weak capacity to elicit skin reactions, but nevertheless potentially good immunogens, might have gone undetected. It was subsequently found that in a group of 22 penicillin-allergic patients about half of them did not react at all to fractions of broth and mycelium from penicillin fermentation media. In the other cases it was considered that the observed sensitization towards penicillium residues may have originated from contact with penicillium organisms (*20*).

Yet another approach was employed to differentiate between intrinsic immunogenicity based on the *in vivo* reactivity of the intact penicillin molecule and extrinsic immunogenicity which may be due to contaminants and *in vitro* degradation products (*32*). By treating penicillins with 3,6-bis-(dimethylaminomethyl)-catechol at pH 7.4 the β-lactam is rapidly hydrolyzed. Thus the ability of penicilloylating carriers *in vivo* is lost whereas the contaminants remain unchanged. Measuring the immunogenicity of the samples before and after such treatment should give an estimate of the overall immunogenicity *versus* that of the contaminants. When the method was applied to a commercial PCG and a PCV using rabbits and a schedule with complete Freund's adjuvant for immunization it was found that the penicilloyl-specific immunogenicities of both preparations were mainly due to the intact penicillin molecules, since the catalytic hydrolysis with the catechol considerably reduced the immunogenicity of the preparations and left but a marginally detectable immunogenic effect.

Catechol-hydrolyzed penicillin was also used in the study by Kristofferson mentioned in the introduction (14). Pure penicillin as well as hydrolyzed penicillin induced apparently similar levels of penicilloyl-specific IgM antibody in mice with B. pertussis as adjuvant. This result is not easily explained since penicilloic acid has thus far only been invoked as a potential source for minor determinants (28). More important seems the observation that pure penicillin does not induce penicilloyl-specific antibody formation when given to mice without adjuvant but becomes effective in combination with 15 ppm of a good BPO-immunogen (BPO$_{26}$-BGG). If residual BPO-proteins in commercial benzylpenicillins are of comparable immunogenicity, this result should certainly encourage penicillin manufacturers to further refine their preparations, since it implies that not only gross contamination but trace amounts of penicilloylated proteins could be significant. Although a further reduction of patient sensitization thus becomes conceivable, the goal of virtual abolishment of such sensitization remains elusive. Penicillin is a fragile molecule which is reactive in various ways and to

TABLE II. Development of Anaphylactic Antibody in Outbred Guinea Pigs Treated with "Pure Benzylpenicillin"[a]

Animal No.	PCA reactions in mm² in guinea pigs sensitized by antisera taken after[b]							
	91 days			171 days		192 days		
	1/10 BPO-PLL	1/100 BPO-PLL	1/10 PCG	1/10 BPO-PLL	1/10 PCG	1/10 BPO-PLL	1/100 BPO-PLL	1/10 PCG (serum dilution) (elicitor)
2316	—	—	—	—	—	37	—	—
2317	—	—	—	—	—	—	—	—
2318	—	—	—	639	—	1.044	402	47
2320	—	—	—	107	—	306	—	—
2321	639	189	—	490	—	598	204	—
2322	66	—	—	—	—	177	—	—
2323	—	—	—	—	—	—	—	—
2324	—	—	—	—	—	—	—	—
2325	—	—	—	—	—	—	—	—
2326	—	—	—	—	—	—	—	—

[a] Pure PCG (courtesy Dr. Ahlstedt) in PBS (40 mg/3.8 ml) was mixed with 2 mg Al(OH)$_3$ in 0.2 ml, 0.1 M, NaOH. Animals received intradermally into the back 0.1 ml freshly prepared mixture at days 0, 21, 42, 63, 84, 164, 185. [b] PCA evaluation was in guinea pigs after intradermal injection of 0.1 ml antiserum dilution. Elicitation was performed 24 hr later by giving the elicitor (BPO-PLL, 0.1 μmol BPO; PCG as used for sensitization, 25 mg) i.v. (19). The area of the blue spots is expressed as the product of two perpendicular diameters.

conclude from mice experiments that these reactivities are of no allergological significance would certainly seem premature.

No doubt the Swedish observation that PCG when administered to mice in a schedule simulating clinical use of penicillins does not evoke any anti-penicilloyl antibody in contrast to results with contaminated penicillin is impressive. On the other hand, by slightly changing the schedule and by using $Al(OH)_3$ as an adjuvant, guinea pigs can be made to produce BPO-specific antibody (Table II). Furthermore the notion that only heavily penicilloylated conjugates can induce IgE antibody (which would weaken the argument for *in vivo* conjugation) is not generally valid and depends on the carriers involved. In fact we recently found that BPO-ovalbumin with a haptenic density of 2 to 7 BPO-groups per molecule elicited a persistent BPO-specific IgE response in mice while heavily substituted conjugates (BPO_{38}-BGG) induced only a transient response (*21*). Since it is well established that hapten-specific IgE antibody production is completely T-cell dependent (*12*), it follows that both haptenic as well as T-cell determinants must be available on an antigen inducing such responses. There is at present no reason to believe that this requirement cannot be met by certain (although not by all) haptenated and slightly altered autologous carriers.

Unfortunately, the question of which carriers of the body become actually penicilloylated as well as involved in sensitization remains open and difficult to answer by direct experiment. Obviously, upon ingestion or injection of a reactive chemical a variety of carriers becomes available within the organism for conjugation. These include soluble proteins, carbohydrates, and more complex high molecular weight materials or structural elements such as collagen fibers and also cellular membranes. One may follow the drug in its radiolabeled form after injection into animals and establish the distribution and amounts of conjugates formed. However this does not reveal whether the radioactive components identifiable at various locations represent immunologically active conjugates. This approach has therefore been used on a very limited scale thus far. A different method, namely the *in vitro* evaluation of the effect of various types of penicillin conjugates on lymphocytes from sensitized patients, has been used in this laboratory for some time. It showed that penicilloylated lymphocytes as well as other cells may be immunologically effective conjugates.*

The studies (*42, 54*) involved peripheral blood lymphocytes from patients allergic to penicillin. Intact penicillin added to such cultures regularly induces within 3 to 5 days a marked lymphocyte proliferation as detected by thymidine-H^3 incorporation. It seems certain that this effect depends on the formation and efficiency of penicilloyl conjugates in the cell culture since prehydrolyzed penicillin does not show any stimulating effect. On the other hand, maximally penicilloylated poly-L-lysine (PLL) or penicilloylated proteins such as BPO_{17}-HSA possess a definite although usually limited stimulating capacity. Some stimulation may eventually also be seen with BPO-groups on inert particles or on autologous or homologous erythrocytes, whereas small biva-

* The following two paragraphs have in essence been presented previously in Spanish (*31*) and in Italian (*30*).

lent BPO-haptens are nonstimulating. A striking stimulation is, however, observed with BPO-coated lymphocytes prepared by incubating mitomycin-treated autologous cells obtained from a Ficoll-Isopaque gradient with PCG at 37°C for 3 hr. Their stimulation index varies between 15 and 50 and may thus be as high as or higher than culture stimulation obtained with 500 μg/ml PCG. It thus appears possible that BPO-coated lymphocytes provide a particularly effective means of specific sensitization.

With regard to the specificity of the effect, it may be noted that lymphocytes from normal persons or from patients allergic to nonpenicillin antigens do not show stimulation with BPO-lymphocytes. The presence of BPO groups on penicillin-treated lymphocytes, although quite minimal, could be established by immunofluorescence with fluorescein-labeled anti-BPO antibody. BPO-lymphocytes, on the other hand, do not provide the only efficient stimulation thus far observed. When peripheral blood lymphocytes which usually contain about 10% monocytes are depleted of monocytes by passage through a nylon fiber column, stimulation of the cultured cells by penicillin becomes almost insignificant whereas the high stimulation by BPO-lymphocytes is not affected. Progressive addition of monocytes in reconstitution experiments restores stimulation by penicillin to normal indices.

With regard to cephalosporin sensitization, our limited experience, in particular with cefuroxim and cefotaxim, shows that they are less immunogenic experimentally than PCG or semi-synthetic penicillins (50). In guinea pigs with high titers of antibodies raised by cefuroxim-BGG conjugates there was practically no PCA-reaction with PCG or BPO-polylysine. Even with other cephalosporins such as cephalexin (CEX), cephaloridine (CER), or cephalotin (CET) only a low grade of crossreactivity was found which suggests that the bulk of the antibodies raised by cefuroxim-protein conjugates is directed against the R_1 side chain and not against the entire cephalosporoyl moiety. Among 22 patients allergic to penicillin who showed high levels of BPO-specific IgE antibodies in the radioallergosorbent test (RAST), no IgE antibodies against cefuroxim could be detected by the RAST. Similarly, RAST inhibition experiments showed that BPO-specific RAST binding can hardly be inhibited by cefuroxim or cefotaxim. These studies on the specificity of antibodies induced in humans or in animals suggest that no crossreactivity is to be expected between penicillins and cephalosporins provided the side chains are sufficiently different. On the other hand, lymphocytes from penicillin-sensitized patients can be stimulated to proliferate in culture not only by penicillins but also by most of the cephalosporins including cefuroxim and cefotaxim. It thus appears that cross allergic manifestations based on cellular reactivity may be expected to be quite common in penicillin-sensitized patients treated with cephalosporins (50).

As indicated by our lymphocyte cultures, some cephalosporins appear to be rather toxic for lymphocytes. This seems by now to be a well-known phenomenon (7). Whereas little difference in toxicity for lymphoid cells is found among penicillins this is not the case for cephalosporins. Indeed, some cephalosporins appear to impair markedly both lymphocyte and macrophage functions whereas others such as cefotaxim and cefuroxim are rather well tolerated by lymphoid cells (Fig. 2) and also

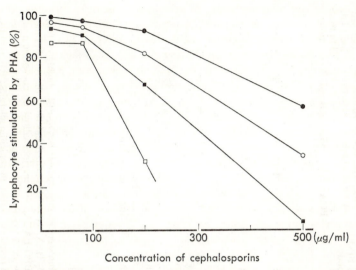

FIG. 2. Inhibition of phytohemagglutinin-induced lymphocyte stimulation by some cephalosporins.
The peripheral blood lymphocytes were from normal human donors. □ CER; ■ CET; ○ CXM; ● CTX.

by macrophages. While the usual therapeutic levels of cephalosporins of the order of 1 to 2 g per day appear to be below the levels required for detectable toxicity on lymphoid cell functions *in vitro*, this is not the case for the higher doses which are sometimes used. Obviously, it should not be unimportant to the infected patient receiving such drugs to see his own defence mechanisms impaired by the toxic effect of the antibiotic on lymphoid cells or macrophages.

ASPECTS OF ELICITATION AND INHIBITION OF IMMEDIATE REACTIONS

It is important to realize within the field of drug allergy that eliciting antigens need not necessarily be immunogenic (sensitizing) at the same time. This is no new insight and in fact the term "hapten" in its classical meaning defined a substance with the capacity to react with antibody but not to immunize and was first used by Landsteiner (*16*) to describe the immunogenicity of tissue extracts containing the Forssmann antigen. In this particular instance the hapten was a relatively large polysaccharide representing a segment of an immunogenic molecule. When a spectrum of haptenic conjugates became accessible by synthesis, other examples of antigens with a restricted number of functions became known. By using penicillin allergy as a model and BPO-antigens as examples, an antigen classification based on the number of haptenic groups per molecule was proposed in order to help clarify the relationship between molecular organization and antigenic function (*33, 45, 52*). This is recapitu-

TABLE III. Some Antigenic Functions of BPO-conjugates

Antigens[a]	Immunogenicity			Elicitation of hypersensitivity[b]					
	Induction of anti-BPO antibody	Induction of delayed hypersensitivity	Precipitation of anti-BPO antibody	Anaphylactic-type reactions			Arthus reactions in		Delayed local i.d. skin reactions
				PCA	SA	WE	RB	GP	
Multivalent									
BPO-protein (BPO-BPO-BPO-BPO-BPO-BPO)	+	+	+	+	+	+	+	+	+
BPOH-PLL (BPO BPO BPO / BPO BPO BPO)	−	−	+	+	+	+	+	+	−
Bivalent									
BPO2-HEX (BPO——BPO)	−	−	−	+	+	+	−	−	−
Monovalent									
BPO-BAC (BPO-)	+	+	− inh	−	−	−	−	−	−
BPO-EACA (BPO——)	− inh	−	− inh	− inh	− inh	inh	−	−	−
Pseudo-monovalent									
BPO1-PLL (BPO +−+)	+	+	− inh	+	+	+	+[c]	+[c]	+

[a] BPO-protein, highly penicilloylated bovine γ-globulin and human serum albumin were mainly studied; BPOH-PLL, highly or fully penicilloylated poly-L-lysine (chain length 12 or 20 lysines) were studied; BPO2-HEX, N1-N6-bis-benzylpenicilloyl diaminohexane; BPO-BAC, bacitracin F, monopenicilloylated at the ε-amino function of lysine; BPO-EACA, Nε-benzylpenicilloyl aminocaproic acid; BPO1-PLL, poly-L-lysine (12 lysines) carrying on the average one BPO-group. [b] PCA, passive cutaneous anaphylaxis in the guinea pig; SA, systemic anaphylactic shock in the guinea pig; WE, wheal and erythema reactions in human penicillin allergics; RB, rabbits; GP, guinea pigs; inh, specific inhibition. [c] In part nonspecific reactions: reaction elicitable at higher dosage also in nonsensitized animals.

lated in part in Table III. It is obvious that the highly or fully penicilloylated PLL is an "incomplete antigen" since it is not immunogenic under the experimental conditions thus far studied. However, it elicits the various types of allergic responses and thus represents a competent multivalent hapten in the classical sense. Its counterpart is BPO-bacitracin, a "pure immunogen," which induces antibody formation or delayed-type hypersensitivity yet does not elicit the manifestations of allergy and may even inhibit, e.g., BPO-specific antibody precipitation in sufficient excess. A simple monovalent inhibitor is BPO-ε-aminocaproic acid (BPO-EACA) which is neither immunogenic nor usually eliciting and which can be used, e.g., as an inhibitor of anaphylactic reactions. In contrast to BPO-EACA the peptidic BPO-bacitracin presumably contains either a T-cell stimulating determinant or else may be able to associate firmly with carriers exhibiting such determinants.

The so-called pseudomonovalent BPO_1-polylysine in Table III is immunogenic and elicits most hypersensitivity responses. It constitutes an exception since it is otherwise well established that elicitation of hapten-specific antibody-mediated hypersensitivity is most efficiently accomplished by multivalent molecules. Furthermore trivalent antigens for immune complex mediated reactions and divalent antigens for anaphylactic-type reactions are minimally required as a rule. However there is evidence that a series of discrete monovalent conjugates in addition to BPO_1-polylysine may be elicitors of anaphylaxis. For instance, monohaptenic carbohydrates such as slightly substituted BPO-carboxymethyl cellulose (38) and slightly penicilloylated dextran, inulin, or raffinose (19) are elicitors of BPO-specific PCA. It was also found that 1,6-diaminohexan carrying a dinitrocarboxyphenyl (DNCP) haptenic group on one amino terminus and a BPO on the other one was an elicitor of PCA in guinea pigs sensitized by anti-DNCP antiserum but not in anti-BPO sensitized animals. This monovalent elicitation required intravenous administration of the elicitor whereas intradermal injection was always ineffective. Intradermal elicitation was possible, however, in animals doubly-sensitized by anti-DNCP and anti-BPO antisera at the same time (24). The data on DNCP-haptenic elicitation are thus far interpreted on the basis of hydrocarbon residues present on the molecule at some distance from the haptenic part and which may act as helper groups enabling a monovalent hapten to become an elicitor of anaphylaxis under certain conditions. The benzyl side chain of PCG represents such a helper group but recent unpublished evidence shows that the thiazolidine moiety is probably an even more capable auxiliary group.

Our observations are at present restricted to guinea pig anaphylaxis; they also require relatively large doses of the monovalent DNCP-BPO elicitor (24). Nevertheless it must seem somewhat disturbing to the allergist to note that monovalent compounds exist which may not evoke reactions in a skin test but could, on the other hand, elicit anaphylaxis when given intravenously.

Monovalent elicitation may also be a mechanism by which large molecules i.e. proteins are able to evoke anaphylaxis. Thus PCA-elicitation with monohaptenic model peptides has shown that fairly large distances between the hapten and the helper hydrocarbon moiety do not hamper anaphylactogenicity. It is therefore conceivable that covalent reaction *in vivo* of a drug with a protein or peptide producing a single haptenic group in some distance, *e.g.*, to a phenylalanine as auxiliary moiety, may establish an anaphylactogen (*26*). By the same token glycoproteins with a single haptenic group may act as anaphylactogens as well (*25*).

The anaphylactogenic penicilloylated carbohydrates mentioned above are quite directly related to practical issues of penicillin allergy, since carboxymethyl cellulose is used in some penicillin preparations as an additive. As described in detail, 2 to 3 BPO groups per 100 glucose units are bound to the cellulose over a 20-hr period at 4°C in neutral penicillin solution but conjugates with an average of 0.2 BPO per 100 glucose units which may form in less than 1 hr are still anaphylactogenic (*38*). Penicilloyl carbohydrate formation has been studied in some detail (*35*) and provides a basis for the early observation of Siegel that PCG incubated with carboxymethyl cellulose produces wheal and flare reactions in sensitive patients (*41*). It may be noted that penicilloyl polysaccharides are also immunogenic. They regularly induced hapten-specific and carrier-specific delayed-type hypersensitivity and occasionally anaphylactic antibody in the guinea pig (*27*).

The inhibiting function of monovalent haptens was used a number of years ago for abolishing penicillin-induced allergic reactions in patients (*48, 51*). The inhibitor used in particular, N$^\epsilon$-benzylpenicilloyl-N$^\alpha$-formyl-L-lysine (BPO-FLYS), has been evaluated in a more recent clinical trial which involved investigators from 9 different European groups and 90 patients hypersensitive to penicillin (*49*). The results show that the effect of BPO-FLYS in combination with penicillin therapy was clinically successful in 42 out of 46 cases (91%) since treatment of penicillin could be pursued or resumed without adverse reactions. The effect of the inhibitor alone on acute allergic symptoms was also evaluated and was considered satisfactory in 17 of 26 patients. Definite failures to inhibit allergic manifestations were reported in 11 cases. They were due in some instances to insufficient inhibitor doses employed and in others to probably insufficient crossreactivity between the BPO hapten and anti-minor determinant antibodies involved. It also appeared that in a few cases the allergic symptoms were due to chronic urticaria or asthma of unrelated etiology but prevalent in the presence of an established penicillin hypersensitivity. The major obstacle to a more general use of BPO-FLYS at the time being is the occurrence of positive skin reactions to the inhibitor in up to 15% of patients allergic to penicillin.

DIAGNOSTIC TESTS

Among diagnostic *in vivo* methods only skin testing is in frequent use. In penicillin allergy a number of test reagents have been developed and evaluated over the years, whereas the arsenal in cephalosporin allergy is more restricted. In most cases skin testing allows us to assess with confidence whether a patient is allergic to penicillin or not.

Skin tests by the scratch, prick, or intradermal technique with penicillin may give positive results when anaphylactic reactivity is involved. On the other hand, epicutaneous tests are frequently positive in cases of exanthema, which are manifestations of delayed-type hypersensitivity. In a number of cases BPO-polylysine is the reagent of choice for detecting anaphylactic sensitization. It is expected to react with BPO-specific antibodies and also with antibody directed against the penicillin side chain only. Further skin test reagents include penicillamine-PLL (PENAM-PLL), which should reveal penicillamine-specific sensitization (23, 28), and the monovalent compounds benzylpenicilloic acid (BPOH), BPO-FLYS, and N^ϵ (N-formyl-benzylpenicilloyl)-aminocaproic acid (FORM-BPO-EACA). These derivatives do normally inhibit BPO-specific reactions; they act however as elicitors of skin reactions in some cases. The reactions may involve multivalent conjugate formation *via* opening of the thiazolidine ring of BPOH and BPO-FLYS and reaction of the newly generated thiol group with disulfides of skin proteins in some instances. On the other hand, with FORM-BPO-EACA, which contains a formylated thiazolidine nitrogen, this reaction path is blocked on chemical grounds (28).

The frequency of positive skin tests with the above reagents is shown in Table IV. The tests involved 206 patients with symptoms of penicillin allergy and 43 patients

TABLE IV. Frequency of Positive Skin Tests in Penicillin Allergy during 1971–1976

	High reactor[a] (%)		Low reactor[a] (%)		Negative (%)	
BPO_{max}-PLL	97	(39)	68	(27.5)	83	(33.5)
PCG	68	(27.5)	42	(17)	137	(55.5)
BPOH	39	(15.1)	37	(14.9)	172	(69.3)
BPO-FLYS	15	(6)	21	(8.5)	212	(85.5)
FORM-BPO-EACA	24	(11.8)	33	(16.3)	145	(71.8)
PENAM-PLL	34	(35)	16	(16.5)	47	(48.5)

[a] High reactor:

BPO-PLL:	scratch 500 nmol/ml	╫/╫/+	and/or
	i.d. 25	╫/╫/+	
PCG:	scratch 200,000 U/ml	╫/╫/+	and/or
	i.d. 10	╫/╫/+	and/or
	i.d. 100	╫/╫	and/or
	i.d. 1,000	╫/╫	

Low reactor:

BPO-PLL:	scratch 500 nmol/ml	(+)/−	and/or
	i.d. 25	(+)/−	and/or
	i.d. 250	╫/╫/+	
PCG:	scratch 200,000 U/ml	(+)/−	and/or
	i.d. 10	(+)/−	and/or
	i.d. 100	+/(+)	and/or
	i.d. 1,000	+/(+)	

Classification with the other reagents is accordingly.

without history but positive skin reactions examined at the Inselspital during 1971–1976. It is obvious that all skin reagents are efficient elicitors in a number of cases. If one disregards the distinction between high and low reactors, the percentage of positive reactions elicited by the various reagents shows the following order: BPO-PLL, 66.5%; PENAM-PLL, 51.5%; PCG, 45.5%; BPOH, 30.7% BPO-FLYS, 30.7%; FORM-BPO-EACA, 28.2%. A more detailed analysis of the importance of skin test reagents is possible by listing the percentage of patients which reacts positively to both of two major reagents, e.g., BPO-PLL and PCG. It is then established whether the inclusion of positive reactions of a third reagent increases the combined percentage of positive tests. The gain in positive percentage is a measure of the importance of the third reagent (cf. also refs. 31, 30). One such analysis of our data is shown in Table V where PENAM-PLL appears as an important reagent since it gains an additional 10.5% of positive reactions bringing the combined percentage of positive responses to almost 90%. Also important are ampicillin and ampicilloyl-polylysine, two reagents not included in Table IV. These data show that in addition to reactions detectable by BPO-PLL and PCG other specificities play a role, and imply that a skin test for diagnosis of penicillin allergy should include more reagents than penicilloyl-polylysine and penicillin.

Some of the *in vitro* cellular methods seem closely related to *in vivo* testing but at present only lymphocyte transformation test (LTT) data are available to us on a larger scale. There is quite a good correlation between skin tests and LTT. About 65% of positive skin reactors also show significant lymphocyte stimulation by PCG. This figure is around 50% when BPO-polylysine stimulation is considered. On the other hand, a high percentage (44.4–64.7%) of skin test-negative patients show positive LTT. This is not unexpected since only immediate skin reactions are considered   in the comparison whereas in lymphocyte culture delayed-type reactions may also become apparent, e.g., from patients with generalized exanthemas. The results discussed here are all taken from cultures with AB sera. In cultures with autologous sera lower stimulations are often found and concomitantly also somewhat

TABLE V. Percentage of Positive Skin Tests Elicited by BPO-PLL and PCG Alone and in Combination with a Third Reagent

Number of patients tested	BPO-PLL- and PCG-positives (%)	Third test reagent	Combination positives (%)	Gain (%)
244	79.9	BPOH	82.4	2.5
95	77.9	PENAM-PLL	88.4	10.5
200	78.0	FORM-BPO-EACA	81.0	3.0
244	79.9	BPO-FLYS	80.7	0.8
66	69.7	Ampicillin	81.8	12.1
59	67.7	Ampic.-PLL	91.4	23.7

TABLE VI. Comparison of Skin Tests and *In Vitro* Tests of Penicillin-allergic Patients 1971–1976

Test antigens		% of all skin test-positives being *in vitro*		% of all skin test-negatives being *in vitro*	
In skin	*In vitro*[a]	Positive + +	Negative + −	Negative − −	Positive − +
BPO-PLL	BPO-PLL culture	47.3	52.7	35.3	64.7
BPO-PLL	PCG culture	65.0	35.0	55.5	44.4
PCG	BPO-PLL culture	51.3	48.6	50.0	50.0
PCG	PCG culture	64.3	35.7	42.9	57.1
BPO-PLL	BPO-phages	46.3	53.6	67.6	32.4
PCG	BPO-phages	49.0	51.0	63.1	36.9
Ampic.-PLL	BPO-phages	52.8	47.2	57.9	42.1
BPOH	BPO-phages	43.7	56.3	59.5	40.5
BPO-PLL	BPO-RAST	32.5	67.5	96.0	4.0
PCG	BPO-RAST	29.9	70.1	81.0	19.0
Ampic.-PLL	BPO-RAST	6.4	93.6	94.4	5.6
BPOH	BPO-RAST	28.6	71.4	78.7	21.3
BPO-PLL	RIST (IgE)	27.5	72.5	79.3	20.3
PCG	RIST (IgE)	18.2	81.8	68.5	31.5
Ampic.-PLL	RIST (IgE)	15.4	84.6	60.0	40.0
BPOH	RIST (IgE)	29.0	71.0	75.8	24.2

[a] Culture: lymphocyte transformation test with peripheral blood lymphocytes (*6*, *18*) with BPO-PLL or PCG as stimulators; BPO-phages, bacteriophage assay (*9*); BPO-RAST (*55*, *56*); RIST (*55*, *56*).

lower correlations with skin tests. It could be that in the presence of specific antibodies the stimulation of lymphocytes by penicillin conjugates is hampered. In general the presence of penicillin-specific lymphocytes in peripheral blood is the most stable parameter of the immune response, since positive results may frequently be observed for many years (more than 10 years in some instances) after the first sensitization.

The correlation between skin testing and *in vitro* tests measuring specific antibody was lower than with LTT. Table VI lists the percentage of all skin test-positive patients showing positive (+ +) and negative (+ −) *in vitro* tests. Similarly the percentage of all skin test negatives showing negative (− −) or positive (− +) *in vitro* tests is shown. The bacteriophage test, the most sensitive method for detecting circulating antibody, correlates well in about half the cases with positive skin tests. On the other hand, it detects antibody in 30 to 40% of patients with negative skin tests. The RAST detecting anti-BPO IgE in about 30% of skin test positives correlates better when only high skin reactors towards BPO-polylysine are considered. In this case 50% of the skin reactors show also a positive RAST. The proportion of patients with a positive skin test and elevated IgE as measured by radioimmunosorbent test (RIST) varies between 15.4% (ampicilloyl-polylysine) and 29.0% (BPOH). On the other hand between 20.7% (BPO-polylysine) and 40.0% (ampicilloyl-polylysine) of the skin test negatives show positive RIST. Elevated IgE thus does not discriminate well between skin test positive and skin test negative patients.

Acknowledgments

This work was supported in part by grants (3.468.75, 3.944.78) from the Swiss National Science Foundation.

REFERENCES

1. Ahlstedt, S., Kristofferson, A., and Petterson, E. 1979. *Int. Arch. Allerg. Appl. Immun.*, **58**, 20–29.
2. Batchelor, F. R. and Dewdney, J. 1968. *Proc. Roy. Soc. Med.*, **61**, 897–899.
3. Batchelor, F. R., Dewdney, J., Feinberg, J. G., and Weston, R. D. 1967. *Lancet*, i, 1175–1177.
4. Batchelor, F. R., Dewdney, J. M., and Gazzard, D. 1965. *Nature*, **206**, 362–364.
5. Bundgaard, H. 1976. *Arch. Pharm. Chem. Sci. Ed.*, **4**, 91–102.
6. Chalmers, D. G., Cooper, E. H., Coulson, A. S., Evans, C., and Topping, N. E. 1967. *Int. Arch. Allerg.*, **32**, 117–130.
7. Chaperon, E. A. and Sanders, W. E. 1978. *Infect. Immun.*, **19**, 378–384.
8. Dewdney, J. 1977. *In* "The Antigens," ed. by M. Sela, Academic Press, New York, Vol. IV, pp. 73–245.
9. Haimovich, J., Sela, M., Dewdney, J. M., and Batchelor, F. R. 1967. *Nature*, **214**, 1369–1370.
10. Hamilton-Miller, J. M. T. and Abraham, E. P. 1971. *Biochem. J.*, **123**, 183–190.
11. Hamilton-Miller, J. M. T., Newton, G. G. F., and Abraham, E. P. 1970. *Biochem. J.*, **116**, 371–384.
12. Ishizaka, K. 1976. *Adv. Immunol.*, **23**, 1–75.
13. Knudsen, E. T., Robinson, O. P. W., Croydon, E. A. P., and Tees, E. C. 1967. *Lancet*, i, 1184–1188.
14. Kristofferson, A., Ahlstedt, S., and Hall, E. 1979. *Int. Arch. Allerg. Appl. Immun.*, **60**, 295–301.
15. Kristofferson, A., Ahlstedt, S., Petterson, E., and Swärd, P. O. 1977. *Int. Arch. Allerg. Appl. Immun.*, **55**, 13–22.
16. Landsteiner, K. 1921. *Biochem. Z.*, **119**, 294–306.
17. Levine, B. B. 1961. *Arch. Biochem. Biophys.*, **93**, 50–55.
18. Ling, N. R. and Kay, J. E. 1975. "Lymphocyte Stimulation," North-Holland, Amsterdam, pp. 25–67.

19. Molinari, M., Schneider, C. H., de Weck, A. L., Gruden, E., and Pfeuti, Ch. 1973. *Z. Immun.-Forsch.*, **146**, 225–238.
20. Müller, E., Schneider, C. H., and de Weck, A. L. 1970. *Z. Immun.-Forsch.*, **140**, 18–42.
21. Nakagawa, T., Blaser, K., and de Weck, A. L. 1980. *Int. Arch. Allerg. Appl. Immun.*, in press.
22. Pressman, D. and Grossberg, A. L. 1968. "The Structural Basis of Antibody Specificity," Benjamin, New York, pp. 50–52.
23. Schneider, C. H. 1970. *In* "Penicillin Allergy, Clinical and Immunologic Aspects," ed. by G. T. Stewart and J. P. McGovern, Thomas, Springfield, pp. 23–58.
24. Schneider, C. H., Gruden, E., Wälti, M., Toffler, O., de Weck, A. L., and Jost, R. 1979. *Mol. Immunol.* **16**, 269–279.
25. Schneider, C. H. and Guenin, R. 1980. Preliminary observations.
26. Schneider, C. H., Guenin, R., and Toffler, O. 1979. *In* "Peptides, Procceedings of the 6th American Peptide Symposium," ed. by E. Gross and J. Meienhofer, Pierce, Rockford, Ill., pp. 941–944.
27. Schneider, C. H., Michl, J., and de Weck, A. L. 1971. *Eur. J. Immunol.*, **1**, 98–106.
28. Schneider, C. H., Pfeuti, Ch., and de Weck, A. L. 1973. *Helv. Chim. Acta*, **56**, 1235–1243.
29. Schneider, C. H., Rolli, H. P., and de Weck, A. L. 1980. Unpublished observations.
30. Schneider, C. H. and de Weck, A. L. 1978. *In* "Atti Del 7. Corso Nazionale di Aggiornamento in Rianimazione," ed. by A. Fantoni, Ghia'Ghedini, Milano, pp. 211–225.
31. Schneider, C. H. and de Weck, A. L. 1977. *In* "Alergia a Medicamentos. II Simposium Nacional," ed. by E. Lopez Botet, Liade, Madrid, pp. 369–383.
32. Schneider, C. H. and de Weck, A. L. 1970. *Immunochemistry*, **7**, 157–166.
33. Schneider, C. H. and de Weck, A. L. 1970. *Chimia*, **24**, 10–12.
34. Schneider, C. H. and de Weck, A. L. 1968. *Biochim. Biophys. Acta*, **168**, 27–35.
35. Schneider, C. H. and de Weck, A. L. 1967. *Immunochemistry*, **4**, 331–343.
36. Schneider, C. H. and de Weck, A. L. 1966. *Helv. Chim. Acta*, **49**, 1707–1714.
37. Schneider, C. H. and de Weck, A. L. 1965. *Nature*, **208**, 57–59.
38. Schneider, C. H., de Weck, A. L., and Stäuble, E. 1971. *Experientia*, **27**, 167–168.
39. Scholand, J. F., Tennenbaum, J. I., and Cerilli, G. J. 1968. *J. Am. Med. Assoc.*, **206**, 130–133.
40. Shaltiel, S., Mizrahi, R., Stupp, Y., and Sela, M. 1970. *Eur. J. Biochem.*, **14**, 509–515.
41. Siegel, B. B. 1962. *J. Allerg.*, **33**, 349–355.
42. Spengler, H., de Weck, A. L., and Geczy, A. 1974. *In* "Lymphocyte Recognition and Effector Mechanisms. Proceedings of the 8th Leucocyte Conference," ed. by K. Lindahl-Kiessling and D. Osoba, Academic Press, New York, pp. 501–507.
43. Stemberger, H. and Wiedermann, G. 1970. *Z. Immun.-Forsch.*, **140**, 43–49.
44. Stewart, G. T. 1967. *Lancet*, **i**, 1177–1183.

45. de Weck, A. L. 1974. *In* "The Antigens," ed. by M. Sela, Academic Press, New York, Vol. II, pp. 141–248.
46. de Weck, A. L. 1962. *Int. Arch. Allerg.*, **21**, 20–37.
47. de Weck, A. L. 1962. *Int. Arch. Allerg.*, **21**, 38–50.
48. de Weck, A. L. and Girard, J. P. 1972. *Int. Arch. Allerg.*, **42**, 798–815.
49. de Weck, A. L. and Jeunet, F. 1975. *Z. Immun.-Forsch.*, **150**, 138–160.
50. de Weck, A. L. and Schneider, C. H. 1980. *Antimicrob. Chemother.* (Suppl.), in press.
51. de Weck, A. L. and Schneider, C. H. 1972. *Int. Arch. Allerg.*, **42**, 782–797.
52. de Weck, A. L. and Schneider, C. H. 1969. *In* "Current Problems in Immunology," ed. by O. Westphal, H. E. Bock, and E. Grundmann, Springer-Verlag, Berlin, pp. 32–46.
53. de Weck, A. L., Schneider, C. H., and Gutersohn, J. 1968. *Int. Arch. Allerg.*, **33**, 535–567.
54. de Weck, A. L., Spengler, H., and Geczy, A. F. 1974. *Monogr. Allerg.*, **8**, 120–124.
55. Wide, L., Benich, H., and Johansson, S. G. O. 1967. *Lancet*, **ii**, 1105–1107.
56. Wide, L. and Juhlin, L. 1971. *Clin. Allerg.*, **1**, 171–177.

NAME INDEX

318

SUBJECT INDEX

319

MATERIAL INDEX